Pharmacovigilance Essentials

Mukesh Nandave • Anoop Kumar
Editors

Pharmacovigilance Essentials

Advances, Challenges and Global Perspectives

Springer

Editors
Mukesh Nandave
Department of Pharmacology
Delhi Pharmaceutical Sciences and
Research University
New Delhi, India

Anoop Kumar
Department of Pharmacology
Delhi Pharmaceutical Sciences and
Research University
New Delhi, India

ISBN 978-981-99-8948-5 ISBN 978-981-99-8949-2 (eBook)
https://doi.org/10.1007/978-981-99-8949-2

This Springer imprint is published by the registered company Springer Nature Singapore Pte Ltd.
The registered company address is: 152 Beach Road, #21-01/04 Gateway East, Singapore 189721, Singapore

Paper in this product is recyclable.

Foreword

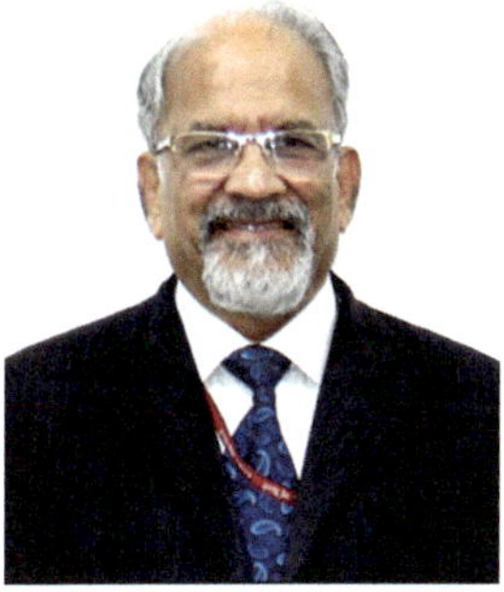

Pharmacovigilance is increasingly important in improving drug safety for patients and reducing risk within the practice of pharmaceutical medicine. It has changed over time, moving from its original emphasis on the safety of medicines to the integration of benefit analysis as well as artificial intelligence technologies, which offer significant advantages, including early detection of ADRs, improved data quality, and faster response times.

The book entitled *Pharmacovigilance Essentials: Advances, Challenges and Global Perspectives* by *Dr. Mukesh Nandave and Dr. Anoop Kumar* has not only given a simple yet complete view of pharmacovigilance with the methodological approach across the globe. This book has also described vaccine safety surveillance, herbovigilance, materiovigilance, and hemovigilance, along with the role of pharmacogenetics and artificial intelligence in the field of pharmacovigilance. Several individuals with diverse expertise in drug safety have written all chapters. Dr. Mukesh Nandave and Dr. Anoop Kumar have rich experience in the field of pharmacovigilance, as evidenced by their publications in international journals of repute and comprehensive view in this must-read and essential book. I must appreciate both of them in the way they have edited this book. That is very special indeed!

This book will serve as a guide for everyone working within pharmaceutical companies, contract research organizations, and medicine regulatory agencies, and for all researchers and students of medical as well as pharmaceutical sciences. The editors and the publisher, Springer Nature, need to be commended and congratulated for providing useful information.

Pharmacovigilance Program of India (PVPI) Y. K. Gupta
Ghaziabad, India
Global Antibiotics Research and Development
Partnership (GARDP), Geneva, Switzerland
AIIMS-Vijaynagar, Jammu, Jammu and Kashmir, India

Preface

Pharmacovigilance is a discipline involved in identifying, assessing, understanding, monitoring, and preventing adverse effects or any other intervention-related problems. The pharmacovigilance process involves multiple steps, starting from ADR reporting to aggregate reporting, to keep regular check on the safety of interventions (drugs, herbals, medical devices, and blood products) in the market. The process of pharmacovigilance may look simple, but it is complex. This book entitled *Pharmacovigilance Essentials: Advances, Challenges and Global Perspectives* intends to provide more rigorous knowledge on pharmacovigilance. This book is divided into four sections and presented in a logical sequence. The first section introduces pharmacovigilance, historical aspects, and commonly used databases across the globe. The second section contains chapters on processing and reporting individual case safety reports across the globe. The third section of book explains pharmacovigilance systems in India, the USA, EU, and non-EU countries. The last section of the book describes specialized pharmacovigilance areas like vaccine safety surveillance, herbovigilance, materiovigilance, and hemovigilance. The role of pharmacogenetics in pharmacovigilance, signal detection and assessment, and the role of artificial intelligence in pharmacovigilance are also described in detail. The book not only covers global processes but is also packed with examples and annexures for better understanding of readers.

The editors wish to express their considerable appreciation to Dr. Naren Aggarwal, Swati Sharma, Yogitha Subramani, and Saraniya Vairamuthu from Springer Nature who managed the production of this book in difficult circumstances, and their contribution is much appreciated. I trust this book will be useful to researchers, faculty members, and medical and pharmacy students who want to learn about pharmacovigilance.

New Delhi, India — Mukesh Nandave
New Delhi, India — Anoop Kumar

Contents

Editors and Contributors

About the Editors

Mukesh Nandave is an associate dean (research & development) and head of the Department of Pharmacology and Pharmaceutical Biotechnology at Delhi Pharmaceutical Sciences and Research University, Govt. of NCT of Delhi, New Delhi, India. He has earlier served as associate professor and head of the Department of Pharmacology at NMIMS University, Mumbai (2010–2017). He has also worked as a research scientist in the medical affairs and clinical research department of Ranbaxy Research Laboratories (currently known as Sun Pharmaceutical Industries Limited, Gurugram). Dr. Nandave earned his Ph.D. in pharmacology from AIIMS, Delhi, and received his postdoctoral training from the Ohio State University Medical Center, Ohio, Columbus, USA.

For more than 20 years, Dr. Nandave has investigated the role of nutraceuticals, herbomineral formulations, and phytoconstituents for myocardial ischemia and reperfusion injury, diabetes, obesity, and pain management. He has published numerous papers in peer-reviewed national and international journals and various book chapters. His lab received more than 3.5 crore total funding from Govt. (DBT, DST, ICMR, and AYUSH) as well as industry (Pharmazz, Dabur, Charak, Madhavbaug, Sandu).

Dr. Nandave has received numerous awards. He is secretary-general of the International Academy of Cardiovascular Sciences (IACS)-India section and treasurer of the Society for Promotion and Research of Cardiovascular Sciences (SPARCS). He is a life member of various professional bodies, including the International Society for Heart Research (ISHR), the International Academy of Cardiovascular Sciences (IACS), the Indian Pharmacological Society (IPS), the Indian Pharmaceutical Association (IPA), the Association of Physiologists and Pharmacologists of India (APPI), Association of Pharmaceutical Teachers of India (APTI), and Society for Ethnopharmacology.

Anoop Kumar currently working as an Assistant Professor in the Department of Pharmacology, Delhi Pharmaceutical Sciences & Research University (DPSRU), Govt. of NCT of Delhi, New Delhi, India. Earlier, he worked as an Assistant Professor and Head in the Department of Pharmacology and Toxicology, National

Institute of Pharmaceutical Education and Research (NIPER), Raebareli, and as an officiating Head and Associate Professor in the Department of Pharmacology, ISF College of Pharmacy, Moga, Punjab. He has also worked as a research scientist in the medical affairs and clinical research department of Sun Pharmaceutical Industries Limited, Gurugram, and Translational Health Science Institute (THSTI), Faridabad. He has completed his Ph.D. from Birla Institute of Technology, Mesra, Ranchi, as a DST INSPIRE Fellow. He has also served as an expert member of the Board of Studies (BOS) of the Clinical Research Programme of IKGPTU, Jalandhar, Punjab (2019–2021), and Drug Discovery Hackathon 2020 joint initiative of AICTE, CSIR, and Govt. of India.

He has authored many research and review articles and a few book chapters in reputable international journals and publishers. He has also worked as the member secretary of the Institutional Animal Ethics Committee (IAEC) and Animal House In-charge. Recently, he has also been included in the top 2% list of scientists released by Stanford. His lab also gets funding from DST SERB SRG (30 lakhs), ICMR Mission Project (1.3 crores), and IIT-Delhi (10 lakhs). Dr. Anoop Kumar is Member Secretary of Institutional Ethics Committee for Clinical Trials and BA/BE studies at DPSRU and Treasurer of ISPOR India Chapter.

Contributors

Mohd Amir Department of Pharmacology, Delhi Pharmaceutical Sciences and Research University, New Delhi, India

Vipin Bhati Department of Pharmacology, Delhi Pharmaceutical Sciences and Research University, New Delhi, India

Mohammad Hamid Department of Pharmacology, Delhi Pharmaceutical Sciences and Research University, New Delhi, India

Muntaha Javid Department of Pharmacology, Delhi Pharmaceutical Sciences and Research University, New Delhi, India

Anoop Kumar Department of Pharmacology, Delhi Pharmaceutical Sciences and Research University, New Delhi, India

Prabhakar Kumar Department of Pharmacology, Delhi Pharmaceutical Sciences and Research University, New Delhi, India

Dipali Nandave Department of Dravyaguna Vigyan, All India Institute of Ayurveda, New Delhi, India

Mukesh Nandave Department of Pharmacology, Delhi Pharmaceutical Sciences and Research University, New Delhi, India

Deepika Pandey Department of Pharmacology, Delhi Pharmaceutical Sciences and Research University, New Delhi, India

Deepti Pandita Department of Pharmaceutics, Delhi Pharmaceutical Sciences and Research University, New Delhi, India

Sweta Roy Department of Pharmacology, Delhi Pharmaceutical Sciences and Research University, New Delhi, India

Megha Sahu Department of Pharmacology, Delhi Pharmaceutical Sciences and Research University, New Delhi, India

Priyanka Sharma Department of Pharmacology, Delhi Pharmaceutical Sciences and Research University, New Delhi, India

Ruchika Sharma Centre for Precision Medicine and Pharmacy, Delhi Pharmaceutical Sciences and Research University DPSRU, New Delhi, India

Divya Shukla Department of Pharmacology, Delhi Pharmaceutical Sciences and Research University, New Delhi, India

Rima Singh Department of Pharmacology, Delhi Pharmaceutical Sciences and Research University, New Delhi, India

Deepali Siwan Department of Pharmacology, Delhi Pharmaceutical Sciences and Research University, New Delhi, India

Maneesh Soni Department of Pharmacology, Delhi Pharmaceutical Sciences and Research University, New Delhi, India

Surbhi Soni Department of Pharmacology, Delhi Pharmaceutical Sciences and Research University, New Delhi, India

Jyoti Upadhyay Department of Pharmaceutical Sciences, School of Health Sciences and Technology, UPES University, Dehradun, Uttarakhand, India

Alishan Zia Department of Pharmacology, Delhi Pharmaceutical Sciences and Research University, New Delhi, India

HMO	Health Maintenance Organisation
HvPI	Hemovigilance Programme of India
IBD	International Birth Date
ICH	International Conference on Harmonisation of Technical Requirements
ICSR	Individual Case Safety Report
IHI	Institute of Healthcare Improvement
IMDRF	International Medical Device Regulators Forum
IND	Investigational New Drug
IPAT	Indicator-Based Pharmacovigilance Assessment Tool
IPC	Indian Pharmacopoeia Commission
ISDS	International Society for Disease Surveillance
JMO	Japanese Maintenance Organization
KAERS	Korea Adverse Event Reporting System
KIDS	Korea Institute of Drug Safety and Risk Management
LINCS	Library of Integrated Network-Based Cellular Signatures
MAGs	MedDRA Analytical Groupings
MAH	Marketing Authorization Holders
MAUDE	Manufacturer and User Facility Device Experience
MDAE	Medical Device Adverse Events
MDMC	Medical Device Adverse Event Monitoring Center
MDR-2017	Medical Device Rule-2017
MedDRA	Medical Terminology for Drug Regulatory Authorities
MEDLEE	Medical Language Extraction and Encoding System
MHRA	Medicines and Healthcare Products Regulatory Agency
MMR	Measles, Mumps and Rubella
MoHFW	Ministry of Health and Family Welfare
MS	Mass Spectroscopy
MSs	Member States
MSSO	Maintenance and Support Services Organization
MV	Materiovigilance
MvPI	Materiovigilance Programme of India
NACO	National AIDS Control Organization
NAPs	National Authorised Products
NCA	National Competent Authorities
NCBI	National Center for Biotechnology Information
NCC	National Coordinating Centre
NDA	New Drug Application
NDCT	New Drugs and Clinical Trials Rule
NHSRC	National Health System Resource Centre
NIB	National Institute of Biologicals
NIH	National Institute of Health
NLP	Natural Learning Processing
NOAEL	No Observable Adverse Effect Level
NPVP	National Pharmacovigilance Program

NRA	National Regulatory Authority
NSAIDS	Nonsteroidal Anti-inflammatory Drugs
OMOP	Observational Medical Outcomes Partnership
OMSM	Office of Medicines Safety Monitoring
OPD	Outpatient Department
OTC	Over-the-Counter
PADER	Periodic Adverse Drug Experience Report
PAL	Pharmaceutical Affairs Law
PBRER	Periodic Benefit Risk Evaluation Report
PDUFA	Prescription Drug User Fee Act
PET	Positron Emission Tomography
PIDM	Program for International Drug Monitoring
PMDA	Pharmaceuticals and Medical Devices Agency
PMS	Post-marketing Surveillance
PRAC	Pharmacovigilance and Risk Assessment Committee
PRAC	Pharmacovigilance Risk Assessment Committee
PRISM	Post-licensure Rapid Immunisation Safety Monitoring System
PSUR	Periodic Safety Update Reports
PV	Pharmacovigilance
PvPI	Pharmacovigilance Programme of India
RA	Regulatory Authorities
RCA	Rapid Cycle Analysis
RCT	Randomized Clinical Trials
REMS	Risk Evaluation and Mitigation Strategy
RMM	Risk Minimization Measure
RMP	Risk Management Plan
RNTCP	Revised National Tuberculosis Control Program
RWD	Real World Data
SAE	Serious Adverse Event
SANTE	DG Health and Food Safety (parent DG)
SCTIMST	Sree Chitra Tirunal Institute for Medical Sciences & Technology
SDG	Sustainable Development Goal
SHOT	Serious Hazards of Transfusion
SLA	State Licencing Authority
SMQ	Standardised MedDRA Queries
SoPI	Society of Pharmacovigilance, India
SRS	Spontaneous Reporting System
SSQ	Standardised Search Queries
STEPS	System for Thalidomide Education and Prescribing Safety
SUSAR	Suspected and Unexpected Serious Adverse Reactions
TG	Toxicogenomic
TGA	Therapeutic Goods Administration
UMC	Uppsala Monitoring Centre
UN	United Nations
US	United States

USA	United States of America
VAERS	Vaccine Adverse Event Reporting System
VSD	Vaccine Safety Datalink
WHO PIDM	WHO Programme for International Drug Monitoring
WHO	World Health Organization
WHO-ART	WHO Adverse Reaction Terminology
WHO-DDE	World Health Organization Drug Dictionary Enhanced
WHO-HD	World Health Organization Herbal Dictionary
WHO-UMC	World Health Organization Uppsala Monitoring Centre
YC	Yellow Card

Introduction to Pharmacovigilance

1

Surbhi Soni, Mukesh Nandave, and Anoop Kumar

1.1 Introduction

Pharmacovigilance (PV) deals with the segment of safety of medicines and other treatment options available (World Health Organization 2004a). Adverse drug reactions (ADRs) are defined as "an appreciably harmful or unpleasant reaction resulting from an intervention related to the use of a medicinal product; adverse effects usually predict hazard from future administration and warrant prevention, or specific treatment, or alteration of the dosage regimen, or withdrawal of the product" (Coleman and Pontefract 2016). They are a common clinical manifestation in both in-patients and out-patients. Some of the most routinely used drugs involved in high ADR rates include antiplatelets, anticoagulants combined with non-steroidal anti-inflammatory drugs (NSAIDs), antidiabetics, cytotoxic, immunosuppressants, and diuretics. Self-medication also contributes to ADR, which seems prevalent in public due to easy drug access, expensive doctor visits, and self-diagnosis. Among the common over-the-counter (OTC) medications, NSAIDs account for a considerable proportion of the drugs consumed by people. Risks involved include overdose, wrong medicines, harmful interactions, abuse, and of prime importance is a manifestation of serious ADR (Montastruc et al. 2016).

Before the clinical trial, all medicines and vaccines undergo rigorous screening and testing before being made available to the public. Nevertheless, clinical trials involve a limited number of subjects selected according to the established parameters and for a fixed duration. Long-term and unexpected side effects are only visible once the drug enters the market and is used by a considerable heterogeneous

S. Soni (✉) · M. Nandave · A. Kumar
Department of Pharmacology, Delhi Pharmaceutical Sciences and Research University, New Delhi, India
e-mail: mukeshnandave@gmail.com; anoopdpsru@dpsru.edu.in

M. Nandave, A. Kumar (eds.), *Pharmacovigilance Essentials*,
https://doi.org/10.1007/978-981-99-8949-2_1

population. In scientific terms, pharmacovigilance is defined as "the science and activities relating to the detection, assessment, understanding, and prevention of adverse effects or any other medicine-related problems" (World Health Organization 2004a). The word pharmacovigilance is a combination of two terms. It has roots in the Greek and Latin languages. The Pharmakon is a Greek terminology meaning "medical substances," and Vigilia is a Latin term meaning "keep a watch."

The history of pharmacovigilance is nearly 170 years old. The first incident that led to the need for PV was a chloroform anesthesia tragedy leading to the death of a young girl in Britain, followed by multiple cases. The significant events in the PV timeline from 1893 till 2017 are depicted in Fig. 1.1. The Lancet Journal established its first-ever commission; results were published in 1893. On June 30, 1906, the US Federal Food and Drug Act was formed, which mandated drugs to be pure and free from contamination. In 1937, the sulphanilamide elixir tragedy highlighted the toxicity of diethyl glycol as a solvent; thus, in 1938, the Federal Food, Drug, and Cosmetic Act (FD&C) was enacted to redesign the public healthcare structure. A significant change in EU Pharmacovigilance occurred in 1961 when Dr. McBride wrote a letter to the Lancet editor on the thalidomide tragedy. This measure revolutionized the PV system, making spontaneous reporting more organized. In 1965, the development of European legislation was followed by the World Health Organization (WHO) Programme for International Drug Monitoring. The establishment of the European Medical Agency (EMA) was seen in 1995. Eudravigilance, a European database for official documentation of ADRs, was founded in 2001 and was reintroduced with a modified format in 2017. In 2010, Pharmacovigilance Programme of India (PvPI) was launched (Fornasier et al. 2018).

Pharmacovigilance is a discipline in the healthcare industry established to overcome the shortcomings of the existing healthcare system and is relevant to everyone who have had medical interventions (World Health Organization 2002). Many new ADRs from a new treatment appear in phase 4 after the medicine reaches the market and show an S-shaped curve with three main stages. Namely, they are latent, signal detection, and lengthy phase.

Functions like protecting human subjects during clinical trials by providing review expertise on the protocol involved, selecting the first safe dose (in humans), establishing the safety profile of the drug by maintaining a risk awareness of the drug involved, monitoring safety-related problems of products manufactured by addressing issues arising at any segment of the manufacturing process, inspection readiness, all are looked after by PV personnel and artificial intelligence is making its way into pharmacovigilance. The surge in the availability of healthcare data due to the adaptation of digital tools is helping PV. Thus, several associated disciplines are finding their way into mainstream PV, indicating a bright future for PV (Beninger 2018).

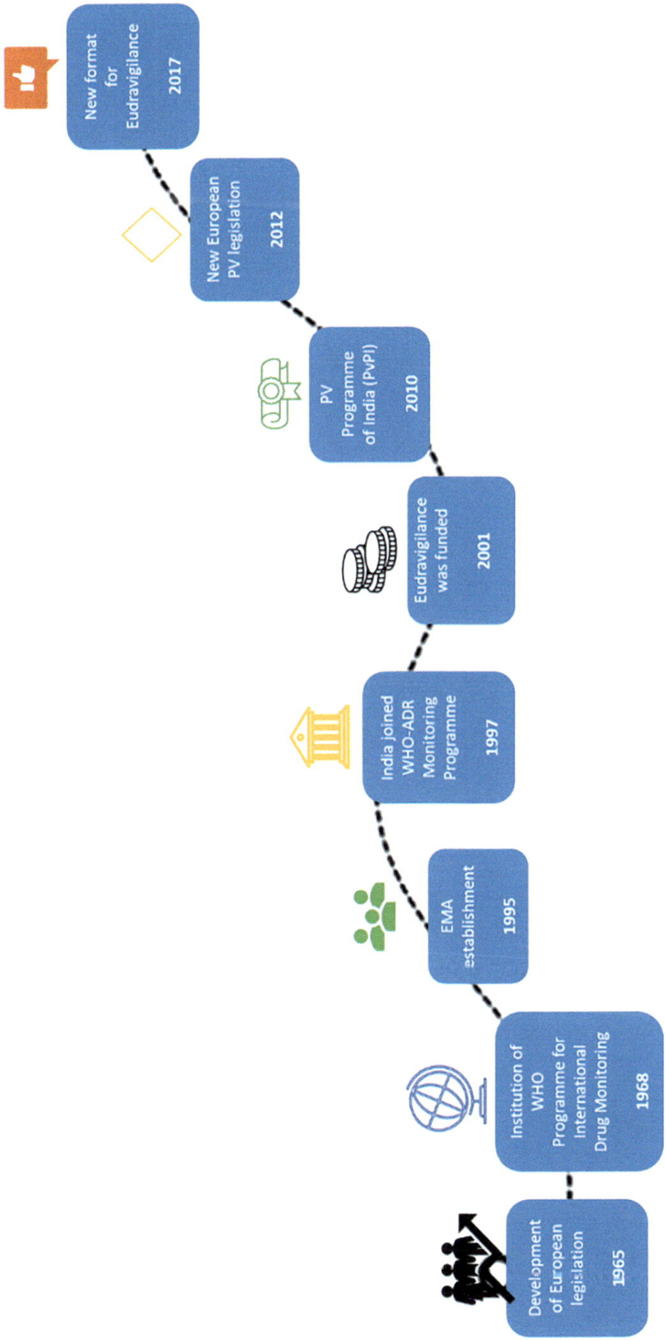

Fig. 1.1 Evolution and establishment of PV

1.2 Needs and Objectives of Pharmacovigilance

Regarding commercial trends in the pharmaceutical industry, the product lifecycle to reach the market is shortened, affecting both the regulatory system and the industrial economies. Conventionally, for a drug to enter the market, it takes 10–15 years, and a high sales rate is required to compensate for the cost involved in the development. With the shortening cycle of drug development, regulatory authorities are reducing evaluation time, thus generating the risk profile of a drug/treatments. Many companies are resorting to mergers/takeovers and outsourcing. However, these actions affect the management cycle of the product. For example, whom to report adverse effects, who are the priority profiles, who is responsible for data collection and analysis, and how will the safety actions be undertaken? (Edwards 2000). Before coming to the market, every new molecule must undergo a rigorous monitoring and trial process. Qualification at each level is needed for the drug to be approved.

1.2.1 Needs

- During clinical trials the safety of the drug is tested in a limited number of subjects/patients.
- The clinical trials have strict inclusion and exclusion criteria for subjects under trial thus limiting the testing of the new medical intervention.
- The duration period for the trials is limited.
- Various drug–drug interactions are involved in ADR reports and screening of them during trials is not possible thus PV is needed to look after it.

A vigilant pharmacovigilance system is required to avoid the possibility of any mishap occurring (Amery and ISPE 1999). Although PV is essential for ensuring the safety of patients and clinical results, certain health conditions require more attention and prompt action, e.g., oncology treatment. Drugs in this category have a narrow safety index, making it of higher priority for the PV. The aim of PV lies in patient care and safety and communicating reliable information for assessing the risk-benefit profile of drug/treatment (Pitts et al. 2016).

1.2.2 Objectives

- To ensure safe and effective medications are provided to the patients.
- To prevent any tragedies associated with the drugs and continuous monitoring of drugs/treatment even after they have entered the market is a prime objective of PV.
- To ensure patient safety. Continuous monitoring and identification of any ADR that concerns the security of a patient about any pharmaceutical product.
- To collect and oversee information on the safety of medicines. It includes assessing the risk–benefit profile, ensuring the collection and analysis of the

safety and ADR profile, and influencing regulatory policies and medical practices directly.
- To obtain "signals" by studying individual case reports of market-approved drugs. PV detects strong signals of a pre-existing yet unrecognized adverse effect, thus helping to understand drug safety better and allowing necessary investigations if required.
- To identify the alternate use of available drugs by repurposing them.
- They are proactively managing the risk associated with the drugs and decreasing the potential side effect frequency. Measures to control include changing the labels, dose, restricted use, and post-marketing surveillance.
- Ensuring transparency in communication between the patients and the shareholders, including the healthcare personnel, is essential. This could be achieved by accurately sharing pharmacovigilance data. It is done to avoid losing trust among the public stakeholders and loss of lives.
- To use PV in the optimization process by early identifications of safety concerns during the clinical trials.
- To assist drug regulation protocols.

1.3 Pharmacovigilance in Drug Development

Drug discovery and development is time-consuming, competitive, expensive, and complicated. Various stages of the process are depicted in Fig. 1.2, starting from target identification to drug approval. Developing a drug from the idea of it to making it available on store shelves takes sustained and substantial investment (Dimasi 2001). Collaborative work is seen between investors, industry people, academia, patent lawyers, regulatory authorities, and marketing personnel. Safety monitoring of medicines is an ongoing, dynamic, and multi-step process. Each step has a valid, predetermined, and reasonable reason. Testing and optimization of the selected compound is done under stringent conditions to identify the "drug candidate" with acceptable safety, dosage, efficacy, and toxicity profile. In vitro and In vivo (preclinical) studies are conducted, which aim to generate human-safe doses and parameters that include pharmacokinetics and dynamics data (Agrawal 2014). The role of PV in preclinical studies is to analyze and assess the drug candidate's toxicity, safety, and ADR profile.

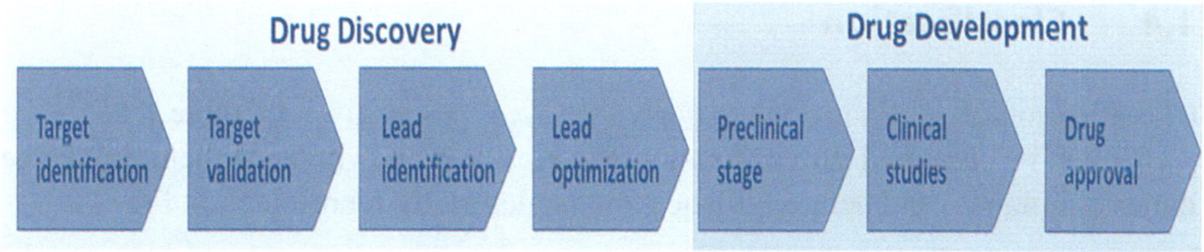

Fig. 1.2 Drug discovery and development

A new drug application (NDA) that includes all the relevant data on the drug development process, including the quality of the drug and preclinical and clinical information, is submitted to the appropriate regulatory authority, for example, the US FDA, which oversees the drug approval, development, and marketing process. After the regulation, the drug is commercialized. Once the drug reaches the store shelves, post-marketing surveillance (PMS) checks the drug's safety and efficacy profile. Vigilant monitoring and reporting of any adverse event to the FDA is encouraged in this phase. The report contains information on the failure of treatment, ADR, off-label use, poor quality of drugs, and drug interactions (Saha 2014).

The clinical phase of drug development is divided into four stages: phase I, II, III, and IV. During the first three phases, PV is accountable for drug safety in human subjects and closely monitor the ADRs, if any are present. The PV team evaluates the risk–benefit profile to ensure patient safety. However, phase I, II, and III are bound by limitations of fewer subjects and shorter duration, thus restricting the exhaustive evaluation of the drug's safety profile. The inclusion and exclusion criteria for subject selection are limited. Therefore, phase IV of the clinical trial is critical, since it involves post-marketing surveillance (PMS) (Trifirò and Crisafulli 2022). During PMS, PV personnel collect and analyze the ADRs reported by healthcare professionals or patients. If supporting data is collected, an update of label information also follows. With efficient methods and protocols, risk minimization can be done for the ADR detected during the PMS. During the clinical phase, PV personnel have reported new ADRs to regulatory bodies, investigators, and ethics committees. However, if the drug does not meet the safety criteria, it is withdrawn from the market (Saha 2014). The entire drug development process is very costly. For a new drug entity to come into the market, around \$0.8–1.0 billion are incurred and roughly 10–15 years of timeline. PV plays a vital role at various stages of the drug development process. Another concept, "drug repurposing," is of great value in drug development. The signals generated from medication during the PMS are collected and analyzed to find a possibility of positive or novel indications. Furthermore, early signal alerts also indicate potential alternate use of drugs for a different medical condition. Thus, drug repurposing can assist in drug development and can be of economic aid.

Additionally, annual report submissions are a part of the routine. During PMS, safety review reporting is mandatory for companies (Agrawal 2014). PV is focused on recognizing safety concerns and identifying and minimizing risk factors, thus emphasizing their importance.

1.4 Classification

Classification of ADRs is done majorly into six types as given in Table 1.1.

PV can be classified into different categories: vaccine vigilance, hemovigilance, materiovigilance, and hemovigillance and is pictorially represented in Fig. 1.3.

Table 1.1 Types of ADRs

Type A	Augmented reaction, due to the kinetic and dynamic profile of the drug
Type B	Bizarre reaction that arises due to immunological response
Type C	Occur due to chronic use of the drug
Type D	Regular drug usage accompanied by organ damage
Type E	Drug treatment withdrawal effects
Type F	Failure of treatment due to multiple ongoing treatment

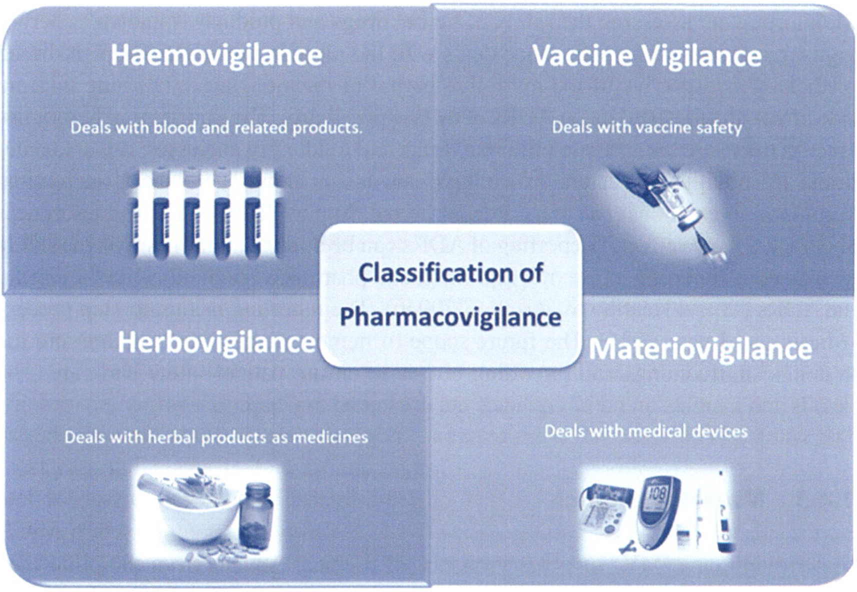

Fig. 1.3 Classification of Pharmacovigilance

1.4.1 Vaccine Vigilance

Immunization is the most prosperous and cost-effective healthcare measure (From the Centers for Disease Control and Prevention 1999). It has effectively prevented mortality from diphtheria, tetanus, whooping cough, and several life-threatening diseases (World Health Organization 2017). Vaccine vigilance involves detecting, identifying, assessing, and communicating Adverse Events Following the Immunization (AEFI) (Heininger et al. 2017). AEFI is an unfavorable event after immunization with no causal relationship with the vaccine. An efficient vaccine monitoring system is required to deal with the safety concerns of immunization and the after-effects. The ADRs of immunization fall into either potential side effects or vaccine-related problems (Nuwarda et al. 2022). Multiple vaccine vigilance systems and databases are available, and are discussed in a different chapter. The causality assessment of vaccines is a four-step process, including an eligibility check, checklist, algorithm, and classification of the AEFIs (World Health Organization 2016a). Vaccine surveillance protects and safeguards the public from preventable adverse reactions. Further details on vaccine vigilance can be found in Chap. 11.

1.4.2 Herbovigilance

Monitoring and assessing the safety of herbal drugs and products is known as herbovigilance. This branch of vigilance deals with the reporting of ADRs for plant-based medicines. Irrespective of the myth that herbal medications are 100% safe with no side effect profile, the data on ADRs deny this possibility. The objective of herbovigilance is to ensure the safe use of herbal drugs and to identify and assess adverse reactions. Herbovigilance caters to multiple needs, including herb–drug interaction, herb–food interactions, and standardized herbal drug availability, to raise awareness and track adverse effects. Reporting of ADRs can be done in multiple ways, including spontaneous reporting, consumer reporting, and pharmacists/manufacturers reporting the ADRs (World Health Organization 2004b). The reporting is a multi-step process (Martin and Lucas 2021). The future scope of hemovigilance lies in addressing the system's shortcomings and providing efforts to ensure patient safety and care. The details and insights on herbovigilance are explained in Chap. 12.

1.4.3 Materiovigilance

Materiovigilance (MV) involves vigilance of medical devices from the point they are manufactured until the patient receives the benefit. Every device must be assessed for its safety during and after the use by the patient. Many medical devices in the global market are reported to cause injuries and cause death. For example, breast implants, pacemakers, contraceptives, and incubators are high-risk devices and require a robust surveillance system. If a complaint about medical devices remains unresolved, the product is recalled as a part of safety measures. National and international regulatory guidelines are in place, and harmonization is needed. PMS is one of the essential ways the adverse events associated with medical devices are studied and reported, thus ensuring continuous improvement in them for a better patient experience. Different countries have different systems established for the MV. Medical devices are subjected to harsh legislation to ensure patient safety. As with the coming years, medical device usage is expected to rise; thus, a stringent MV system is needed (Joshi et al. 2021). Furthermore, materiovigilance are discussed in detail in Chap. 13.

1.4.4 Hemovigilance

Hemovigilance involves monitoring and surveillance of blood transfusion and products to ensure patient safety. Both the donor and patient safety are taken into consideration (World Health Organization 2016b). The practice was started in France in 1994, later followed by multiple countries. The need arises from the history of infection transmissions occurring via blood products, thus prioritizing blood transfusion safety. The scope of hemovigilance includes identifying and issuing safety alerts, trends in ADRs, and implementing improved practices for transfusion processes. The ADR can range from a local hematoma, thrombophlebitis, delayed bleeding, and nerve irritation to something serious like hemolysis, cardiac problems, cerebrovascular damage, or death (Mukherjee and Maiti 2016; Khobragade et al. 2022). Various recommendations are being implemented at national and global levels. The principal aim of hemovigilance is to identify the trends in adverse reactions and improve the entire process, stimulate research, raise awareness, and improve the safety of blood and blood products. For more detailed information on hemovigilance, refer to Chap. 14.

1.5 Case Reporting

Collecting information on drug-related events, assessing and documenting, and finally submitting it comes under case reporting and is an integral part of ADR management. Different organizations in different countries overlook the reporting. For India, the Pharmacovigilance Programme of India (PvPI) oversees case reporting. For the US, the FDA has a robust system of case reporting under the FDA Adverse Event Reporting System (FAERS); and in Europe, it is done through Eudravigilance. ADRs are unwanted effects caused to the patient by medical intervention and can even be dangerous if not taken care of and managed in time. There are various occasions where the reporting of ADRs proves to be a valuable aid. Ensuring patient safety and care is one significant aspect of it. PMS, signal generation of unusually identified adverse events, and regulatory decisions are influenced based on the case reports. The merits of case reporting are multiple. Potential medication responsible for the ADR is identified, assists in signal detection and generation, and improvised risk management. Patient confidence and participation are boosted, ultimately leading to a better impact on patient safety and care (Singh et al. 2020). Countries have different reporting protocols, which are discussed in detail in Chap. 6. The various components of case reporting include a national coordination center for PV, a reporting organization responsible for ADR reporting, a robust database, healthcare professionals, patients, pharmaceutical industries, an ADR monitoring center, and analyzing and regulatory authorities (Joshi et al. 2022).

The reporting of ADRs was initially started as spontaneous reporting. Spontaneous Reporting System (SRS) involves reporting by healthcare professionals. It was the primary source of information for PV and drug regulations. National vigilance centers were established. Spontaneous reporting aids in yielding continuous helpful information, thus elevating qualitative and quantitative data, ultimately confirming the signal generated. Therefore, spontaneous reporting primarily aims to create signals and new safety alerts.

Contrary to the previous intuitive reporting era, the present situation is shaping toward a better path with increased professionalism and government interest. Countries are ADR reporting compulsory reporting by physicians and healthcare professionals. Spontaneous reporting is functional when physicians can associate an adverse reaction with the drug (Hadi et al. 2017; López-Valverde et al. 2021).

On the other hand, spontaneous reporting is used less when there is a high background frequency and doubt or no relationship between the ADR and the drug. Its success is a multiple-factorial phenomenon. Continuous professional programs and training improve reporting rates (Gonzalez-Gonzalez et al. 2013; Pagotto et al. 2013). Advantages include being simple, cheap, can be applied to all the drugs, and a limitless study period. Under-reporting and rate calculation are limitations of this system.

Another system of reporting ADR is consumer reporting. Reports of suspected ADRs toward a medicinal product initiated by consumers and submissions assisted by healthcare professionals are called consumer reporting. Consumer reporting for adverse reactions toward medications is encouraged by various countries to a spontaneous reporting system as consumers are direct participants in pharmacovigilance. "Patient reporting" and "consumer reporting" are used interchangeably in some countries. However, patient reporting is a broader term and is inappropriate for a consumer to use for ADR reporting. The ADR reports are relayed using the WHO international Individual Case Safety Reports (ICSR) database (World Health Organization 2012). The generalized flow of a case reporting process is represented in Fig. 1.4.

1.5.1 The "4 Ws" of Case Reporting

- *Who*: The person who will be reporting the ADRs. It can be a healthcare professional (spontaneous reporting) or a patient (consumer reporting). The reporting form includes patient information, ADR reported, suspected medicine, medical history or ongoing medications information, risk factors, place of purchase, severity of ADR, and seriousness. Confidentiality is ensured during the whole process to protect the patient.
- *What*: The cause of ADR. It could be a single-drug or multiple drug event. The content, dose, dosage form, duration of consumption, and co-medication, if any, are all considered to assess the report. All suspected ADRs are encouraged to report. A rise in ADR frequency can be detected. Along with medicinal products, reports on dietary supplements and cosmetics are also collected (World Health Organization 2012).
- *When*: The timeline of events is of paramount value. The date of starting the medication, the time when ADR first occurred, and the discontinuation date.

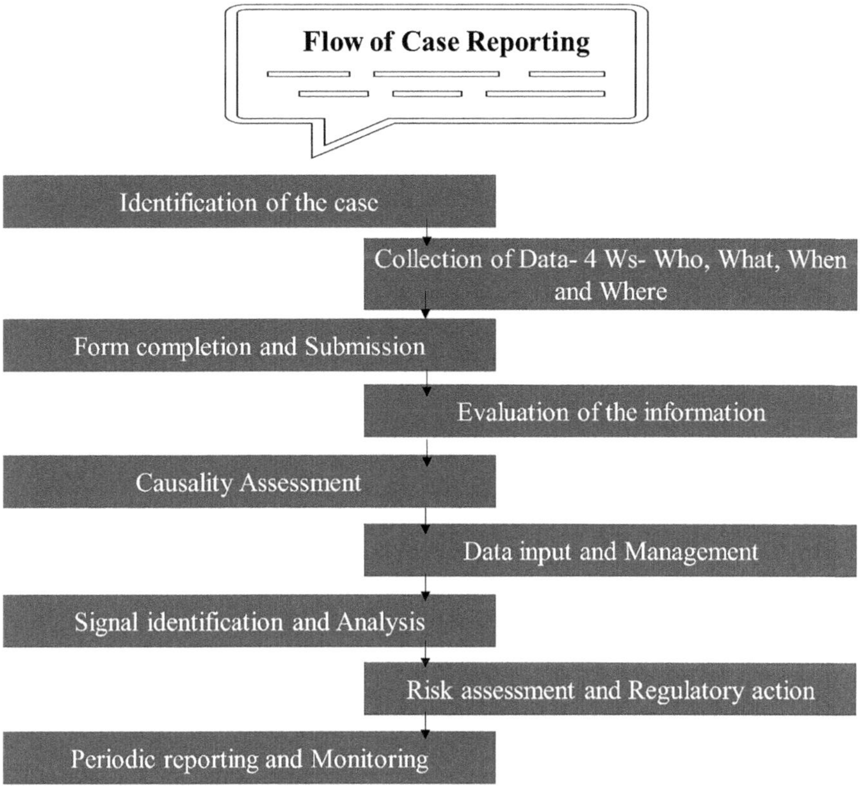

Fig. 1.4 General flow of case reporting

- *Where*: The location details are being reported, where the event occurred, and the relationship between the ADR and the environmental factors is being understood.

1.5.2 Issues and Possible Solutions in Reporting

Spontaneous reporting is generally done using the central pharmacovigilance database. However, this only works if the country has a homogenous population in terms of language and culture. A decentralized consumer reporting system is present for the absence of homogeneity. The reporting needs to be stimulated by educating people about consumer pharmacovigilance, which can be achieved through various means.

- Easy access and user-friendly reporting: This involves ease of reporting the ADRs. The process needs to be user-friendly and maintain the confidentiality of the patient. The form should be multilingual to break the language barrier in a heterogeneous population-oriented country. Providing electronic reporting platforms adds to the convenience of the process.

- Feedback: Providing the user with this encourages and ensures that the report is being added to the database and that the respective authorities will take necessary measures toward them. It also helps in increasing our commitment to reporting.
- Education purpose: Healthcare personnel, the public, and patients are educated about the benefits of reporting, which ultimately assists their engagement.
- Active participation of center staff: Regular meetings are held to share information, train the personnel, monitor, break barriers, work on feedback, and communicate the issues and measures.
- Pharmacist's reporting: The pharmacist is an integral part of the system and acts as a point of contact between the multi-component of ADR reporting. They help to strengthen the ADR report quality.

The reports can be made more reliable by verifying and getting the required supplementary data (lab reports) from healthcare personnel. These are termed "medically confirmed" reports as a healthcare professional confirms the ADRs.

The detailed processing of ADRs is discussed in Chap. 4. In Chap. 5, another form of reporting, i.e., aggregate reporting, has been introduced and discussed in detail. The reporting of ADRs concerning various countries and the protocol followed by each are discussed in Chap. 6 of the book.

1.6 Causality Assessment (CA)

Suspected ADRs are an inherent problem in most case reports, and the chances of adverse reactions being specific to a particular drug or diagnostic test are rare. ADRs can be classified accordingly into "certain" or "unlikely," mostly between "possible" or "probable." A systematic causality assessment system has been established to solve the problem encountered (U. M. Centre 2018). Causality assessment can serve as a helpful tool.

1.6.1 Purpose of Causality Assessment

1. Classify and establish a relationship possibility between the ADR and the drug, thus providing proof to take the necessary actions against the drug.
2. A safety evaluation of a drug, vaccine, or medical device has been done to ensure its safe use.
3. Risk management can occur once the relationship between the ADR and the drug/medical intervention has been established, and accordingly, regulatory authority directs their action.
4. The causality assessment can alter the course of treatment. If the ADR is found to be associated with the ongoing treatment, an alternate treatment plan is being implemented by the physician.

Causality assessment needs to answer two main questions. First, whether the drug can cause an adverse event, and second, is the adverse event caused by the drug? These judgments require sound knowledge and expertise. Causality is associated with six causality terms, according to WHO, which are "certain," "probable," "possible," "unlikely," "unclassified," and "unclassifiable" (Dodd et al. 2018).

1.6.2 Tools

Tools available for causality assessment are primarily categorized into three major types: expert judgment (global inspection), probabilistic method (logistic method), and algorithm methods. Figure 1.5 shows the three primary tools used for the CA, and Fig. 1.6 represents the multiple types of algorithm methods available.

The casualty assessment method by WHO Uppsala Monitoring Center (WHO-UMC) and the Naranjo probability scale are the most used methods since they have a simple methodology. The WHO-UMC system was developed by consulting national vigilance centers, and the Naranjo scale is used to standardize the causality assessment of the ADRs (Naidu 2013).

1.6.3 Measures Taken by Regulatory Bodies

Measures taken by regulatory authority toward the CA include activities like collecting reports of ADRs, documentation, analysis and evaluating the results, ensuring transparent communication with healthcare professionals, industry personnel,

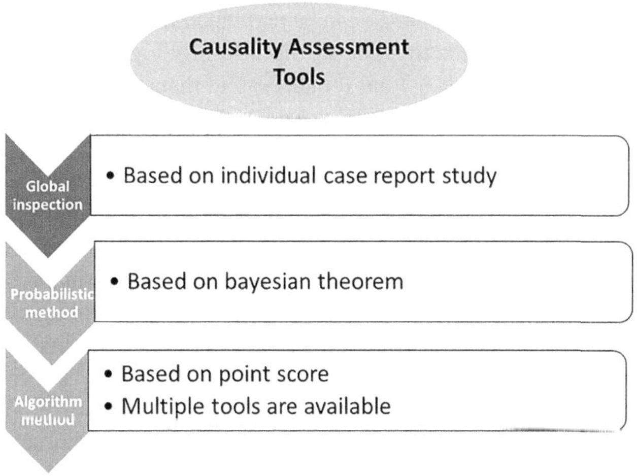

Fig. 1.5 Classification of causality assessment tools

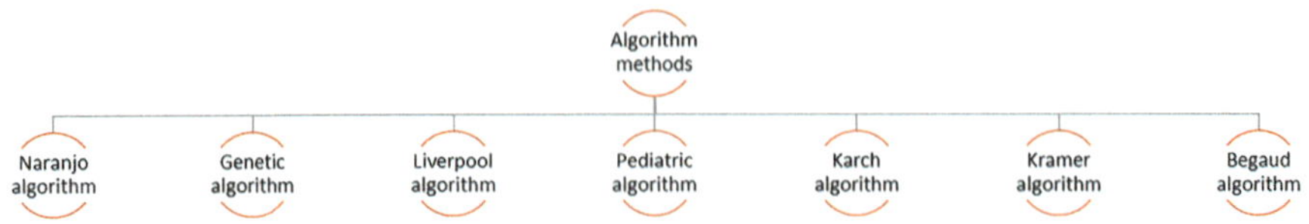

Fig. 1.6 Types of algorithm methods available for causality assessment

and the public., label updates are made periodically, safety reviews are issued, and regulatory actions are taken.

1.6.4 Challenges

A set of challenges accompanies causality assessment. The first step is to find a causal link between the reaction and the drug, followed by hypothesis generation. Clinical suspicion is led by diagnosis to reach a potential cause, thus making it a complex and time-consuming process. The data must be authentic, detailed, and reliable to perform the CA efficiently (Ralph 2017).

1.7 Management of ADRs

Globally, adverse drug reactions are among the top ten causes of death after heart disease, cancer, and stroke, irrespective of age, gender, and geographical distribution (Bates 1998). There are two terms: adverse reaction and adverse effect. The former is used in terms of patients, and the latter is used for drugs. The primary reason behind these deaths is under-reporting and lack of awareness. Nearly 75% of the ADRs are dose-dependent, which can be prevented if care is taken (Bonn 1998). Healthcare facilities costs due to ADR are significantly high yet avoidable. Timely identification of safety signals is vital for successful management of ADRs.

Among the ADRs mentioned above, type A and type B are preventable if taken care of; however, preventable ADRs mainly occur due to incorrect dose/drug/time/prescription to an allergic patient and weak monitoring. Hospital in-patients suffering from ADRs can add to the risk of repeated hospitalization and are subjected to high mortality risk. To evaluate adverse events, a skilled professional with basic knowledge of the pharmacology of the drugs, immunology, and clinical pharmacy is required, as false assessment and reporting can generate incorrect data and future complications. Since spontaneous reporting is the most widely used, under-reporting of the ADRs is a major drawback. According to figures, nearly 94% of cases are under-reported (Hazell and Shakir 2006). The characteristics of ADR reports are another factor of concern. Definitions vary depending on the origin country, healthcare setup, and medication. The quality of ADR reports is of equal importance. The minimum number of datasets required to determine the causality, determines the quality and completeness of the report. The entirety of the information is assessed using the Uppsala Monitoring

Centre developed 'vigiGrade score'. Risk communication includes issuing medical alert cards to patients briefed on hospital discharge summaries. Educating and spreading awareness toward ADRs is essential. Familiarity with symptoms, pathophysiology, and side effect profiles helps in better understanding and management. Education in the form of outreach has improved the reporting rates (Aung et al. 2022).

Management of ADRs occurs at two levels: on an individual level and the population level. The patient level aims to prevent the drug reaction and subsequent reporting of the ADR if it occurs, while the population level implies regulatory processes. The best possible way to deal with ADRs is to prevent them. It is a challenge owing to the complexity of the treatment process. Robust ADR and vigilance programs in the education sector are needed to strengthen the gaps in the ADR management programs.

1.8 Conclusion

In conclusion, the chapter takes the reader through pharmacovigilance and its components. Pharmacovigilance is a very efficient system in terms of patient safety and care. The collaborative work between the healthcare personnel, the public, and the industry can bring changes. ADRs are preventable; thus, spreading awareness is crucial, along with the required regulations. The active participation of PV in multiple sectors, based on the specified niche involved, is being discussed. PV is a robust tool that strengthens the healthcare system and progresses toward its betterment.

References

Agrawal P (2014) Drug discovery and development: an insight into pharmacovigilance. J Pharmacovigil 2(3):e120. https://doi.org/10.4172/2329-6887.1000e120

Amery WK, ISPE (1999) Why there is a need for pharmacovigilance. Pharmacoepidemiol Drug Saf 8(1):61–64. https://doi.org/10.1002/(SICI)1099-1557(199901/02)8:13.0.CO;2-A23

Aung AK, Walker S, Khu YL, Tang MJ, Lee JI, Graudins LV (2022) Adverse drug reaction management in hospital settings: review on practice variations, quality indicators and education focus. Eur J Clin Pharmacol 78(5):781–791. https://doi.org/10.1007/s00228-022-03287-1

Bates DW (1998) Drugs and adverse drug reactions: how worried should we be? JAMA 279(15):1216–1217. https://doi.org/10.1001/jama.279.15.1216

Beninger P (2018) Pharmacovigilance: an overview. Clin Ther 40(12):1991–2004. https://doi.org/10.1016/j.clinthera.2018.07.012

Bonn D (1998) Adverse drug reactions remain a major cause of death. Lancet 351(9110):1183. https://doi.org/10.1016/S0140-6736(98)23016-9

Coleman JJ, Pontefract SK (2016) Adverse drug reactions. Clin Med (Lond) 16(5):481–485. https://doi.org/10.7861/clinmedicine.16-5-481

Dimasi JA (2001) New drug development in the United States from 1963 to 1999. Clin Pharmacol Ther 69(5):286 296. https://doi.org/10.1067/mcp.2001.115132

Dodd C, Pacurariu A, Osokogu OU, Weibel D, Ferrajolo C, Vo DH, Becker B, Kors JA, Sturkenboom M (2018) Masking by vaccines in pediatric drug safety 25 signal detection in the EudraVigilance database. Pharmacoepidemiol Drug Saf 27(11):1249–1256. https://doi.org/10.1002/pds.4623

Edwards IR (2000) The accelerating need for pharmacovigilance. J R Coll Physicians Lond 34(1):48–51
Fornasier G, Francescon S, Leone R, Baldo P (2018) An historical overview over pharmacovigilance. Int J Clin Pharmacol 40(4):744–747. https://doi.org/10.1007/s11096-018-0657-1
From the Centers for Disease Control and Prevention (1999) Ten great public health achievements—United States, 1900–1999. JAMA 281(16):1481
Gonzalez-Gonzalez C, Lopez-Gonzalez E, Herdeiro MT, Figueiras A (2013) Strategies to improve adverse drug reaction reporting: a critical and systematic review. Drug Saf 36(5):317–328. https://doi.org/10.1007/s40264-013-0058-2
Hadi MA, Neoh CF, Zin RM, Elrggal ME, Cheema E (2017) Pharmacovigilance: pharmacists' perspective on spontaneous adverse drug reaction reporting. Integr Pharm Res Pract 6:91–98. https://doi.org/10.2147/IPRP.S105881
Hazell L, Shakir SA (2006) Under-reporting of adverse drug reactions: a systematic review. Drug Saf 29(5):385–396. https://doi.org/10.2165/00002018-200629050-00003
Heininger U, Holm K, Caplanusi I, Bailey SR, CIOMS Working Group on Vaccine Safety (2017) Guide to active vaccine safety surveillance: report of CIOMS working group on vaccine safety—executive summary. Vaccine 35(32):3917–3921. https://doi.org/10.1016/j.vaccine.2017.06.033
Joshi D, Sharma I, Gupta S, Singh TG, Dhiman S, Prashar A, Gulati M, Kumar B, Vishwas S, Chellappan DK, Gupta G, Jha NK, Gupta PK, Negi P, Dua K, Singh SK (2021) A global comparison of implementation and effectiveness of materiovigilance program: overview of regulations. Environ Sci Pollut Res Int 28(42):59608–59629. https://doi.org/10.1007/s11356-021-16345-5
Joshi D, Gupta S, Singh TG, Parashar A, Singh SK (2022) A qualitative evaluation of ADR reporting in India: non-regulatory confronts and their possible solutions. ECS Trans 107(1):6763. https://doi.org/10.1149/10701.6763ecst
Khobragade RS, Paranjape SG, Gadhade JB, Premchand A (2022) Hemovigilance: a momentous step to blood safety. Int J Basic Clin Pharmacol 11(3):267. https://doi.org/10.18203/2319-2003.ijbcp20221043
López-Valverde L, Domènech È, Roguera M, Gich I, Farré M, Rodrigo C, Montané E (2021) Spontaneous reporting of adverse drug reactions in a pediatric population in a tertiary hospital. J Clin Med 10(23):5531. https://doi.org/10.3390/jcm10235531
Martin JH, Lucas C (2021) Reporting adverse drug events to the therapeutic goods administration. Aust Prescr 44(1):2–3. https://doi.org/10.18773/austprescr.2020.077
Montastruc JL, Bondon-Guitton E, Abadie D, Lacroix I, Berreni A, Pugnet G, Durrieu G, Sailler L, Giroud JP, Damase-Michel C, Montastruc F (2016) Pharmacovigilance, risks and adverse effects of self-medication. Therapie 71(2):257–262. https://doi.org/10.1016/j.therap.2016.02.012
Mukherjee S, Maiti R (2016) Haemovigilance: a current update in Indian perspective. J Clin Diagn Res 10(11):EE05–EE09. https://doi.org/10.7860/JCDR/2016/21029.8868
Naidu RP (2013) Causality assessment: a brief insight into practices in pharmaceutical industry. Perspect Clin Res 4(4):233–236. https://doi.org/10.4103/2229-3485.120173
Nuwarda RF, Ramzan I, Weekes L, Kayser V (2022) Vaccine hesitancy: contemporary issues and historical background. Vaccine 10(10):1595. https://doi.org/10.3390/vaccines10101595
Pagotto C, Varallo F, Mastroianni P (2013) Impact of educational interventions on adverse drug events reporting. Int J Technol Assess Health Care 29(4):410–417. https://doi.org/10.1017/S0266462313000457
Pitts PJ, Louet HL, Moride Y, Conti RM (2016) 21st century pharmacovigilance: efforts, roles, and responsibilities. Lancet Oncol 17(11):e486–e492. https://doi.org/10.1016/S1470-2045(16)30312-6
Ralph EI (2017) Causality assessment in pharmacovigilance: still a challenge. Drug Saf 40(5):365–372. https://doi.org/10.1007/s40264-017-0509-2
Saha L (2014) Role of pharmacovigilance in drug development. Enliven: Pharmacovigil Drug Saf 1(1):e002. https://doi.org/10.18650/2378-5411.11e002

Singh A, Kalaivani M, Srivastava S, Goyal RK, Gupta SK (2020) Post-marketing safety of Biosimilars: current status, challenges, and opportunities in the spontaneous reporting system. Ther Innov Regul Sci 54(3):667–680. https://doi.org/10.1007/s43441-019-00101-6
Trifirò G, Crisafulli S (2022) A new era of pharmacovigilance: future challenges and opportunities. Front Drug Saf Regul 2:1. https://doi.org/10.3389/fdsfr.2022.866898
U. M. Centre (2018) The use of the WHO-UMC system for standardised case causality assessment. Uppsala Monitoring Centre, Uppsala
World Health Organization (2002) The importance of pharmacovigilance. Accessed 10 Jul 2023
World Health Organization (2004a) Pharmacovigilance: ensuring the safe use of medicines (No. WHO/EDM/2004.8). World Health Organization. Accessed 10 Jul 2023
World Health Organization (2004b) WHO guidelines on safety monitoring of herbal medicines in pharmacovigilance systems. World Health Organization. Accessed 30 Jul 2023
World Health Organization (2012) Safety monitoring of medical products: reporting system for the general public. Accessed 15 Aug 2023
World Health Organization (2016a) Immunization safety surveillance: guidelines for immunization program managers on surveillance of adverse events following immunization. Accessed 28 Aug 2023
World Health Organization (2016b) A guide to establishing a national haemovigilance system. Accessed 28 Jul 2023
World Health Organization (2017) WHO | WHO department on immunization, vaccines and biologicals. WHO, Geneva. Accessed 22 Aug 2023

History of Pharmacovigilance

2

Muntaha Javid, Mukesh Nandave, and Anoop Kumar

2.1 Introduction

In this chapter, we highlight the critical events, tragedies, and significant milestones in shaping the current practice of pharmacovigilance. The idea of side effects or harmful reactions on administering drugs and monitoring the adverse events by the trial and error method has been in history as human existence. However, the establishment of pharmacovigilance occurred only after a series of unfortunate events, when the death of a young girl occurred on administration of chloroform. Following this, an array of tragic episodes occurred, crafting modern-day pharmacovigilance. As the complexity of drug development increased, new technologies emerged in the twentieth and twenty-first centuries, leading to the development of electronic reporting systems, data mining techniques, and advances in signal detection methods. All these methods culminated in recognizing safety concerns and drug safety issues in real time. Today, pharmacovigilance has become a fundamental part of drug development. Pharmacovigilance includes but is not limited to post-marketing surveillance, risk management strategies, and continuous safety assessment. It involves several parties that cooperate and work together to ensure the safe use of medications, including regulatory bodies, pharmaceutical firms, medical professionals, and patients. This chapter will assess the significant events, regulatory framework, and technological developments that have constructed this field. Knowing the history of pharmacovigilance can help us better comprehend the evolution, difficulties faced, lessons learned, current efforts, and future challenges to safeguard public health and drug development.

M. Javid (✉) · M. Nandave · A. Kumar
Department of Pharmacology, Delhi Pharmaceutical Sciences and Research University, New Delhi, India
e-mail: mukeshnandave@gmail.com; anoopdpsru@dpsru.edu.in

M. Nandave, A. Kumar (eds.), *Pharmacovigilance Essentials*, https://doi.org/10.1007/978-981-99-8949-2_2

2.2 Historical Background

The effect of drugs being beneficial and harmful was talked about long back since the time of Hippocrates. Hippocrates' primum non nocere warned about the side effects of medicines during pregnancy and asserted that the use of medicines should be avoided (Jones and Kingery 2014; Caron et al. 2016). The advice quoted as "leave your drug in the chemist's pot if you can heal the patient with food" is mentioned in the literature of about 370 BC (Stephens 2011). The Book of Medicine by Yellow Emperor, compiled between 800 and 200 B.C., also pointed to the effects of toxic and non-toxic herbs. Preclinical testing on animals was first suggested by Abu Bakr Muhammad Ibn Zakariya al-Razi in his compilation Continens Medicinae. Around 1200 BC, strict regulations were made for physicians to qualify for public examination before practicing medicine and proper certification for preparing and selling drugs and medicine. If usage of any drug caused death, the apothecary was executed.

The need for stringent laws and regulations governing medicinal use started around 1848 and continued until the mid-1900s (Jones and Kingery 2014). The step forward in the field of pharmacovigilance started on 29th January 1848 when a 19-year-old teenager, Hannah Greener, a resident of England, was given chloroform as an anesthetic for toe-nail removal surgery. A year before this incident, chloroform was introduced as a replacement for ether due to its lesser side effects, including nausea and vomiting. Unfortunately, using chloroform led to Hannah Greener's death (Routledge 1998). The actual cause of the death was unknown, but it was concluded to be a lethal arrhythmia or pulmonary aspiration (Fornasier et al. 2018). In the event of this aftermath, The Lancet took the initiative, and a commission was set up in which all the anesthesia-related deaths were reported. The reports were also published in the journal in 1893 (Routledge 1998). Followed by this, in 1901, 13 deaths were reported due to contaminated diphtheria antitoxin (Jones and Kingery 2014). As a result, the Biological Control Act was passed in 1902. This law was established mainly for biological entities such as viruses, therapeutic serums, toxins, antitoxins, or analogous products. Due to various public outcry and publications, the US Federal Food and Drugs Act (USFDA) was passed in 1906 by President Franklin Roosevelt. In this act, only the purity of any drug needed to be tested without knowledge of its efficacy (Routledge 1998). This was only an initial step in the existence of pharmacovigilance. This was followed by an incident during the synthesis of acetylsalicylic acid. Acetylsalicylic acid was synthesized on 12th August 1897. After 2 weeks, along with the synthesis of aspirin, a re-synthesis of diacetylmorphine was done. Within a year, it was concluded to be used in humans for antitussive and analgesic effects. However, within a few years, 500,000 dependent patients were reported in the US (Caron et al. 2016). Also, reports of acetylsalicylic acid causing gastrointestinal diseases were proved in 1955, and therefore, it was contraindicated in gastrointestinal ulcers (Fornasier et al. 2018).

These being the minor incidents, the actual breakthrough of pharmacovigilance occurred after the sulfanilamide tragedy in 1937 when over 107 deaths, including 34 children, appeared as a result of the usage of diethylene glycol for solubilizing the sulfanilamide. In light of this tragedy, the Federal Food and Drugs Act (F&D Act) amendment was passed in 1938 (Routledge 1998). In the amendment, reporting about the safety of medicinal products before their introduction into the market was made necessary. It was the first step where drug monitoring was done (Caron et al. 2016). In 1951, another action was taken to expand the Food and Drug Administration's authority. A Durham–Humphrey Amendment was made in the Food, Drug, and Cosmetics Act (FD&C Act) that classified drugs into two types: one that doesn't need the physician's assistance and these were then known as over-the-counter drugs and the other one being that need prescription by the physician (Jones and Kingery 2014).

During World War II, the need for antibiotics increased. This was associated with the allergic reactions they caused. Chloramphenicol, a broad-spectrum antibiotic, was recognized to have severe adverse effects like bone marrow hypoplasia and aplastic anemia. Several changes in the label and registry were made to report blood dyscrasia events (Jones and Kingery 2014). In 1954, diiodo diethyl by-product of tin was manufactured to be used in the production of Vitamin F. A negligence in the quality production of the tin pearls led to the death of 102 patients primarily due to encephalopathy and more than 100 patients suffered with irreversible neurological side effects (Caron et al. 2016). The visa regulations for marketing products were made tougher after this event and were published by Ordonnance on February 4th, 1959 (Caron et al. 2016).

Another major incident that laid a vital milestone in developing pre-marketing and post-marketing surveillance was the thalidomide disaster (Jones and Kingery 2014). A fetal abnormality called phocomelia was reported on using thalidomide during pregnancy. Thalidomide, in a very short time, was sold as an OTC drug in West Germany, and the impact was worst in that area. Following the event, an amendment, namely Kefauver-Harris, was made to the USFDA Act in 1962. The amendment required the efficacy and safety data of drugs from the FDA before marketing (Routledge 1998). Also, a European council was set up in Europe on 26 January 1965 called European Legislation with the EC Directive 65/65. According to the council, before introducing any drug in the market, the competent authorities of that Member State should issue a marketing authorization by this Directive (Couve de Murville 1966). Furthermore, a resolution was adopted by the Sixteenth World Health Assembly in 1963 to facilitate the spontaneous reporting of ADRs (Surendra and Garlapati 2020). A WHO Program for International Drug Monitoring (PIDM) was launched as a WHO Pilot Research Project in 1968, in which recording all the adverse events taking place internationally was done in a central VigiBase database. The database management was done by the WHO Collaborating Centre for International Drug Monitoring, today known as the Uppsala Monitoring Centre (Surendra and Garlapati 2020). In 1964, a Committee on the Safety of Drugs (CSD) came into existence. This was renamed the Committee on Safety of Medicines (CSM) in 1968. The chairman of the committee suggested using yellow cards to report ADRs. This came to be known as the yellow card system. This was initially started for dentists and physicians, but later on, pharmacists, nurses, and even consumers were added (Jones and Kingery 2014). This was a voluntary reporting system, and therefore, many ADRs went unnoticed. An event where an ADR went unnoticed occurred in 1974 when a cardio-selective beta blocker, practolol, was reported to produce oculomucocutaneous syndrome and sclerosing peritonitis as side effects. The early symptoms were overlooked as common allergic symptoms, and clinical trials for only the possible adverse reaction were done. It was then proposed that all ADRs be monitored, not only the suspected ones. Within 2 years, the drug was withdrawn from the market (Jones and Kingery 2014; Routledge 1998). Prof. Jan Venulet 1968 started a joint program with ten countries to undergo a 3-year feasibility study. Italy became a part of it in 1970 (Fornasier et al. 2018). An international drug monitoring program was established following the success of the feasibility study. It was later relocated to the WHO headquarters in Geneva, Switzerland, and then, in 1978, to Uppsala, Sweden. Today, it is known as the Uppsala Monitoring Centre (UMC) (Jones and Kingery 2014) and consists of 170 full members and associate members (Surendra and Garlapati 2020) and records nearly 99% of adverse reporting (Rahman and Galib 2022). Drug Advisory Response Team (DART) was created as a thesaurus to categorize spontaneous complaints using a standard body-system-based language. DART later changed into COSTART (Coding Symbols for Thesaurus of Adverse Reaction Terms). In the later 1990s, MedDRA (Medical Terminology for Drug Regulatory Authorities) was finally adopted. Diethylstilboestrol (DES) was used as a drug to prevent miscarriage from 1948 up until the 1970s. In young females aged 15–22 years of age, seven cases of vaginal adenocarcinoma were reported, and it was indicated in the study that 7 out of 8 mothers were given DES during pregnancy. Besides cancer, some more effects were also seen in these patients, lasting up to third generation. The results were also seen in men. This implored the fact that the results can last up to several generations. The drug was immediately contraindicated during pregnancy in the USA, but in France, about 160,000 cases of DES exposure were seen (Caron et al. 2016).

France started the pharmacovigilance program very differently from other countries. It was a joint venture that the pharmacologists, toxicologists, physicians, and pharmacists started. Initially, ADR was reported in three special units in Paris, Lyon, and Marseilles. This gradually expanded to about 31 centers nationally (Jones and Kingery 2014). In Japan, in 1979, a pharmacovigilance program was formed by the Ministry of Health and Welfare in which monitoring hospitals were set up, and any severe ADRs were reported from those hospitals to the National Drug Monitoring Center (Jones and Kingery 2014). Similarly, a drug benoxaprofen was brought to market in 1980 and was withdrawn due to hepatoxicity and photosensitivity in 1982. Twelve deaths were published in the British Medical Journal in May 1982, primarily due to liver and kidney failure (Jones and Kingery 2014; Routledge 1998). Following this event, a UK committee named Committee on Safety of Medicines (CSM) set up the Grahame-Smith Working Party to issue recommendations mostly addressing the problem of underreporting adverse drug reactions (Routledge 1998). These recommendations were mentioned in November 1981 in Medicines Act Information Letter No. 32 (Snell 1983). The recommendations mainly emphasized the increasing availability of the yellow card (Jones and Kingery 2014). A second report was published in July 1985, highlighting that post-marketing surveillance on newly marketed drugs should be given utmost importance along with immediate reporting by professionals. Complete information about the drug should be given to the patients, especially the possible ADR (Mann and Andrews 2007). The International Society of Pharmacovigilance evolved from the European Society of Pharmacovigilance in 1992. The safety and proper usage of medicines were ensured by this society (Fornasier et al. 2018). In 1993, a phase 2 clinical trial was set up for fialuridine for the treatment of chronic hepatitis B. Within a few weeks, severe hepatoxicity along with lactic acidosis was reported. This also led to the withdrawal of the drug (McKenzie et al. 1995).

The events along the way of the development of Pharmacovigilance did not stop there and are still happening. All the events and tragedies leading to modern-day pharmacovigilance have been summarized in Table 2.1 and detailed in the upcoming paragraphs.

Table 2.1 Events occurred in the past with regulatory actions taken along with the benefits of the regulatory actions

Year	Event occurred	Action taken
1848	Death of Hannah Greener due to chloroform	Commission for reporting anesthesia-related deaths
1901	13 deaths due to diphtheria antitoxin	Biological Controls Act, 1902
1906	US FDA Act	Mandatory requirement of drug testing before introduction into the market
1937	Over 107 deaths due to sulfanilamide poisoning	Amendment to FDA Act in 1938
1951	Durham–Humphrey Amendment to FDC Act	Classification of prescription and non-prescription drugs
1954	Encephalopathy due to Diiodo diethyl of tin and 102 deaths	Tougher visa regulations for obtaining drugs
1961	Thalidomide disaster	Drug withdrawal
1962	Kefauver-Harris Amendment (USA)	Data on both safety and efficacy was to be submitted to the FDA
1963	Chloramphenicol-induced aplastic anemia	Blood Dyscrasias registry formulated
1964	Committee on the Safety of Drugs	Evaluate the safety and benefit-risk profile of drugs
1964	Yellow card scheme in the UK	Reporting of drug toxicity
1965	Directive 65/65/EEC	Centralized authorization of drugs in Europe
1965	Canada Vigilance Programme	Collected and recorded all suspected ADR
1966	Boston Collaborative Drug Surveillance Programme	Created a comprehensive database, conducted signal detection, and confirmed drug safety through epidemiological studies
1968	WHO Adverse Drug Reaction Monitoring Programme	WHO program for global monitoring of drug safety came into existence
1968	Drug Advisory Response Team	3-year feasibility study

(continued)

Table 2.1 (continued)

Year	Event occurred	Action taken
1970	Poison Prevention Packaging Act (USA)	Requirement for child-resistant packaging for medications
1974	Oculomucocutaneous syndrome and sclerosing peritonitis due to Practolol	Monitoring of all ADRs rather than only suspected ADR
1977	Council for International Organizations of Medical Sciences (CIOMS)	A discussion forum for pharmaceutical businesses and worldwide drug regulatory agencies
1978	Uppsala Monitoring Centre	Support to WHO-PIDM
1982	Hepatotoxicity and photosensitivity due to Benoxaprofen	Withdrawal of the drug
1983	Orphan Drug Act (USA)	Incentives for the development of drugs for rare diseases
1990	Establishment of International Conference on Harmonization of Technical Requirements	Harmonization of pharmacovigilance guidelines globally
1992	Establishment of the FDA database for reporting adverse events	FDA Adverse Event Reporting System (FAERS)
1992	Implementation of the Prescription Drug User Fee Act (PDUFA)	Allowing the FDA for collection of fees from pharmaceutical companies to expedite drug approvals
1993	Hepatoxicity and lactic acidosis due to Fialuridine	Withdrawal of the drug
1993	Establishment of MedWatch	Collection of data for adverse events
1995	European Agency for the Evaluation of Medicinal Products (EMEA)	Centralizing the scientific evaluation and supervision of medicinal products
1998	Agranulocytosis due to sulpyrine	Withdrawal of the drug
2001	EudraVigilance	Database for managing and analyzing suspected ADR for clinical trial
2002	EU Directive 2001/83/EC (EU)	Legal basis for pharmacovigilance in the European Union
2003	Medicines and Healthcare products Regulatory Agency (MHRA) was launched	Government agency responsible for regulating drugs, medical devices, and blood and tissue components for transfusion and transplantation in the UK
2004	Hemorrhagic stroke due to phenylpropanolamine	Withdrawal of the drug
2004	European Medicines Agency (EMA)	Replacement of EMEA with EMA
2004	MedWatch Plus (USA)	Expansion of the FDA's MedWatch program for reporting adverse events
2004	GVP in Canada	Structured framework for the conduct of pharmacovigilance activities, including the collection, evaluation, and reporting of ADRs and other safety-related data

(continued)

Table 2.1 (continued)

Year	Event occurred	Action taken
2005	CIOMS III (Council for International Organizations of Medical Sciences) Guidelines	Updated guidelines for adverse event reporting
2005	National Pharmacovigilance Program of India	Monitoring of drug safety within the country
2005	Introduction of the EU Pharmacovigilance Legislation	Enhanced pharmacovigilance activities and regulations across the EU.
2006	Korean Regional PV Centers (RPVC)	Facilitation of ADR reporting
2006	TGN1412 Tragedy	Expert Scientific Group (ESG)
2007	Amendment of USFDA Act, Risk Evaluation and Mitigation Strategies (REMS)	To facilitate PV of certain high-risk drugs
2008	Volume 9A guidance for human medicinal products	Provided guidance and regulations that promote the safe and efficacious use of medicinal products
2010	Pharmacovigilance Risk Assessment Committee (PRAC) (EMA)	Creation of a dedicated safety committee within the European Medicines Agency
2010	Pharmacovigilance Programme for India (PvPI)	Regulation of ADR reporting
2012	Korea Institute of Drug Safety and Risk Management (KIDS-RM)	Collection, evaluation, and management of ADR
2012	FDA Safety and Innovation Act (USA)	Expanded FDA authority over drug safety and post-market surveillance
2012	Hemovigilance Programme of India (HvPI)	Regulation of blood products
2014	Falsified Medicines Directive (Directive 2011/62/EU)	To combat counterfeit medicines and enhance pharmacovigilance
2014	Launch of the Purple Book by the FDA	Information on biological products, including biosimilars
2015	Materiovigilance Programme of India (MvPI)	Regulation of medical devices
2015	EU Clinical Trials Regulation (Regulation (EU) No 536/2014)	Impacting pharmacovigilance in clinical research
2016	Regional Pharmacovigilance Center extended to 27 centers	Facilitate Pharmacovigilance in Korea
2019	Withdrawal of the UK from the European Union (Brexit)	Regulatory adjustments
2020	Digital transformation of EMA	Modernize pharmacovigilance processes
2021	GVP implemented in China	Structured framework for the conduct of pharmacovigilance activities

2.3 Development of Pharmacovigilance in the USA

2.3.1 Sulfanilamide Tragedy

The history of pharmacovigilance in the USA takes back to the discovery of sulfanilamide, a metabolic product of prontosil that was initially discovered to possess anti-streptococcal activity and was used in humans and animals since 1937 and endorsed by Long and Bliss (Paine 2017). Sulfanilamide was already manufactured in 1906 as tablets and capsules, and no patent was required. Soon, a respectable pharmaceutical company, S.E. Massengill Co., recognized the need for liquid preparation, especially for use in children, and prepared an elixir preparation of sulfanilamide for various streptococcal diseases in the USA (Paine 2017; Kille 2017). While preparing sulfanilamide, Harold Watkins, the company's chief chemist, found it insoluble in water (Kille 2017). Therefore, ethanol was used as the solvent to increase the solubility. However, to make the elixir more palatable and soluble, a formulation with 10% sulfanilamide, 72% diethylene glycol (DEG), and 16% water diethylene glycol was prepared (Paine 2017). The toxicity testing of individual components in the elixir was never performed (Paine 2017). Manufacturing of 240 gallons of the product was done and distributed by early September 1937, and almost 353 patients were exposed to the medication (Paine 2017). This preparation resulted in kidney failure and, therefore, death in more than 100 consumers, including 34 children and 71 adults (Paine 2017; Swaters et al. 2022). The youngest child died at 11 months of age (Gupta and Waldhauser 1997). On 11 October 1937, the first update about the death due to the intake of elixir was brought into notice by the president of the Tulsa (Oklahoma) County Medical Society, namely Dr. James Stevenson, to the American Medical Association. Deaths of eight children and one adult were confirmed by an inspector from the agency's Kansas City Station with the intake of Elixir Sulfanilamide (Carpenter and Sin 2007). Immediately, a team of inspectors was sent to the company headquarters at Bristol, along with other units in Kansas City, New York, and San Francisco. By then, the company was aware of the situation and had already sent telegrams to 1000 distributors, doctors, and salespeople. Due to lack of impact, another telegram was sent on the demand of the FDA stating, "Imperative you take up immediately all elixir sulfanilamide dispensed. The product may be dangerous to life. Return all stocks, our expense" (Ballentine 1981). The early symptoms were nausea, vomiting, stoppage of urine, and stomach ache, which led to the discontinuation of the drug (Paine 2017). Later symptoms included renal failure, starting from polyuria, anuria, and flank pain. Hepatic injury and tubular nephrosis were noted. Seizures were also developed, and sometimes patients entered a coma (Paine 2017). Later on, toxicity studies on rats, rabbits, and dogs were performed for the individual components along with the elixir of Sulfanilamide produced by Massengill and with a synthetic elixir of sulfanilamide compounded by the American Medical Association Chemical Laboratory. It was concluded that DEG, rather than sulfanilamide led to toxic symptoms and deaths (Gupta and Waldhauser 1997) (Figs. 2.1, 2.2 and 2.3).

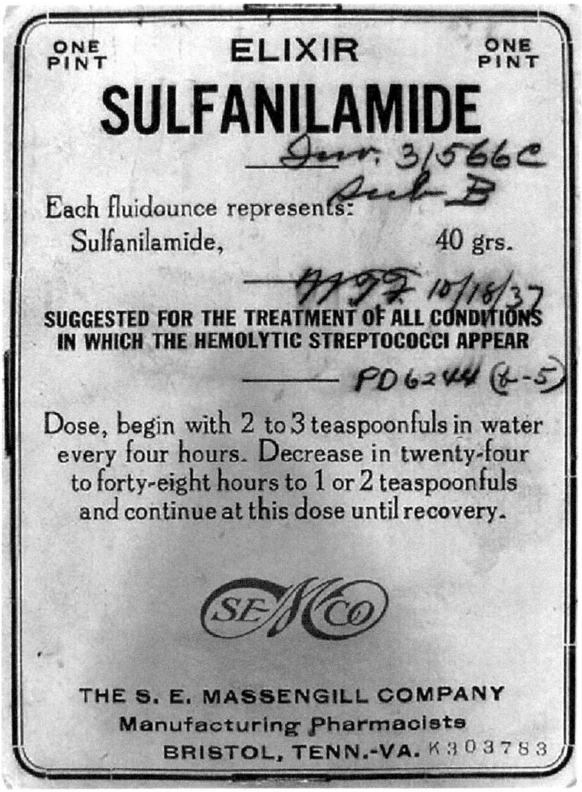

Fig. 2.1 A label on sulfanilamide elixir. (Adapted from RG 246, National Archives)

2.3.2 Regulatory Action Taken After Sulfanilamide Tragedy

2.3.2.1 Federal Food, Drug, and Cosmetic Act (FD&C Act)

Reflecting the event of the sulfanilamide disaster, an investigation with almost 239 FDA inspectors and chemists was initiated by Walter Campbell, the chief of the FDA at that time (Wax 1995). The staff was assigned to check the shipment records of the sales units sold to wholesale and retail drugs. As many as thousands of sales slips were checked within one establishment alone (Ballentine 1981). Tracking of the salesman as well as the purchaser was done. Due to the need for more adequate data on the salesman and purchaser, locating them took much work. Even after finding the person, ingenious questioning had to be done to determine what was done to dispose of the drug (Ballentine 1981). The Pure FDA of 1906 was already implemented under the guidance of President Theodore Roosevelt. This act mainly emphasized adulterated food and drugs. It protected the interstate trade of adulterated and misbranded drugs and food products (Tousley 1941). In case of any violation of purity of drugs, the testing was performed, and no testing was done for the new products in the market (Wax 1995). Until this act, no particular guidelines

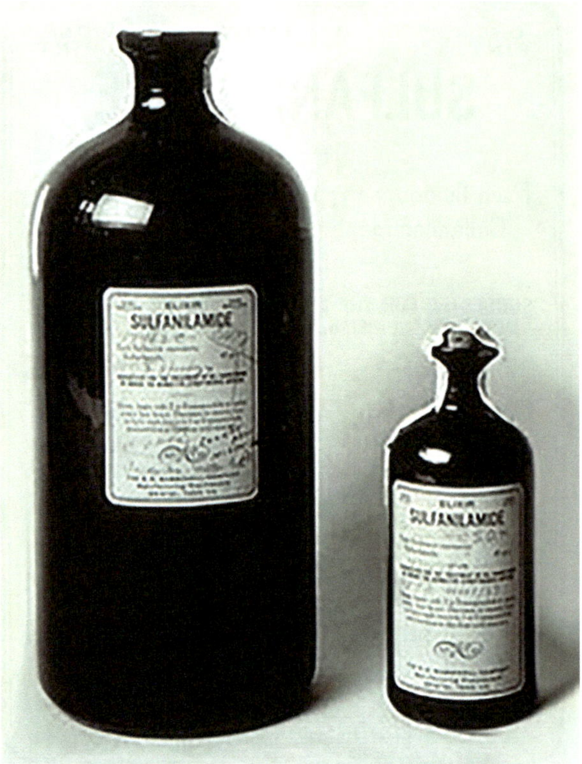

Fig. 2.2 A bottle of sulfanilamide elixir. (Adapted from Paine 2017)

existed for labeling the drugs (Nasr et al. 2011). Furthermore, in 1911, false therapeutic indications were forbidden according to the act (Fornasier et al. 2018). The sulfanilamide tragedy brought the amendment to the Pure F&D Act, which came into existence under the guidance of President Franklin Delano Roosevelt on 25 June 1938 and was named by the U.S. Congress as the Federal FD&C Act (Wax 1995). This act began to regulate the sale, production, and distribution of food, drugs, cosmetics, and medical devices (Lam and Patel 2023). Under this act, the meaning of the term drug was made more specific and concise, and cosmetics and medical devices were also included to be tested (Tousley 1941). The testing of the safety of drugs was made mandatory. Factory inspections were performed. Special directions were ruled for labeling drugs that included mentioning the list of ingredients in the formulation, the effects of drugs, and the storage conditions (Tousley 1941). Small regulatory changes were made before the amendment of 1938, and the act was revised and amended seven times. The amendment of 1912 was necessary to clarify that the falsely labeled drug was not confused with a misbranded drug (Tousley 1941). Another amendment was made in 1951. Before the Durham-Humphrey Amendment, only 25% of the drugs were sold under prescription, and mostly all drugs were sold OTC except for narcotics (Wax 1995). This act made a

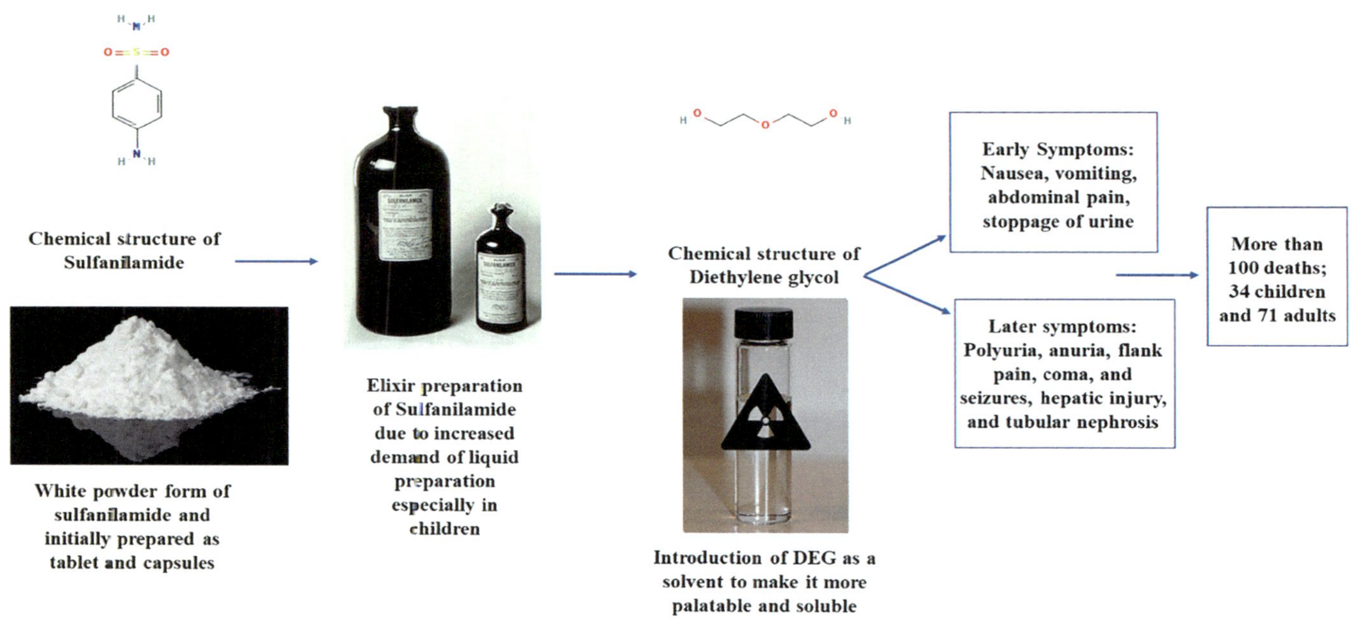

Fig. 2.3 Overview of sulphanilamide tragedy

clear distinction between prescription and non-prescription drugs (Nasr et al. 2011). Three evident points were highlighted in the amendment. First that the habit-forming drugs should only be sold under prescription drugs. Secondly, drugs sold under the responsibility of a licensed healthcare practitioner were also listed as prescription drugs. Lastly, new drugs approved to be used under the supervision of a professional were also mentioned as prescription drugs (Brass 2001). Even after this act, certain limitations existed. The efficacy of the drug was not needed. No proper animal and human testing were performed. New drug applications were not reviewed appropriately, and even the drugs were approved automatically within 60 days if not reviewed by the FDA (Wax 1995). However, if any doubt existed, the FDA could extend the review to 180 days, and the drug approval could be rejected based on the drug's safety (Tousley 1941). Some relaxation was provided for the timeline of labeling requirements (Tousley 1941). The USFDCA was a significant step in the history of pharmacovigilance and drug safety evaluation, but many other incidences and tragedies could form the basis of pharmacovigilance today.

2.3.3 Thalidomide Disaster

Another important event that shaped pharmacovigilance in the USA was the Thalidomide disaster. Thalidomide was discovered by Wilhelm Kunnz in West Germany in 1953 due to its similar structure to that of diazepam and barbital (Moro and Invernizzi 2017; Greek et al. 2011) first manufactured by Chemie Grünenthal as an antibiotic additive and introduced on 1 October 1957 (Moro and Invernizzi 2017; Tuffs 2007). The drug's sedative effect was found within no time, and pregnant women used it to treat nausea and morning sickness (Dally 1998; Kim and Scialli 2011). The product soon gained global importance and was distributed to nearly 46 countries (Swaters et al. 2022; Moro and Invernizzi 2017). The physicians distributed sample packets to pregnant women with morning sickness (Vargesson 2015). Testing of thalidomide in mice, rats, guinea pigs, and rabbits showed promising results. Simple tests like a righting reflex, wheel running, and jiggle cage tests were performed to evaluate the safety of hypnotics (Ridings 2013). However, no effect was studied in the fetus or the offspring (Swaters et al. 2022). Drug teratogenic potential was already established until then, but the compulsion of animal testing was not there (Ridings 2013). Congenital disabilities were found in children within a few years of its use. The first medical report about teratogenicity was reported in 1959 in Germany (Moro and Invernizzi 2017). Two clinicians, Lenz and McBride, in Germany and Australia, respectively, declared thalidomide to be a disaster (Vargesson 2015). The first case of thalidomide adverse effect was reported on 30th May 1962 at Leonor Mendes Barros Maternity Hospital, where a girl child was born with no arms (Moro and Invernizzi 2017). Phocomelia was the primary effect, and about 8000–10,000 children were born with limb deformities (Swaters et al. 2022). Of 2000 babies born with congenital disabilities in the UK, only 466 survived (Lachmann 2012). Other than that, congenital heart disease, inner and outer ear malformations, and eye abnormalities were also seen. Paralysis of the face, respiratory tract and heart impairment, and mental retardation were also reported (Moro and Invernizzi 2017). Around 40% to 45% person died from exposure to thalidomide (Moro and Invernizzi 2017). Soon, a review of the effect of thalidomide on a fetus with 354 references became evident (Dally 1998). In December 1961, a letter was published by the Australian obstetrician William McBride in The Lancet stating the increase in the number of cases of congenital abnormalities due to thalidomide use (Dally 1998). This led to the withdrawal of thalidomide by the manufacturer on 25 November 1961 (Kim and Scialli 2011; Van Grootheest 2003). In the USA, before the drug withdrawal worldwide, Dr. Kelsey put a hold on the medication due to the concern about peripheral neuropathy caused by the drug (Kim and Scialli 2011). He also received an award from President John F. Kennedy for preventing this disaster in the USA (Vargesson 2015). Even though the effects of the drug were so severe that in 1975, the FDA approved the cure for leprosy use (Tantibanchachai 2014). On 16 July 1998, the FDA, along with Celgene Inc., a New Jersey pharmaceutical company, initiated the System for Thalidomide Education and Prescribing Safety (STEPS) (Tantibanchachai 2014). A proper registration of the physician prescribing the medicine and the patient to whom it was prescribed had to be done. As a consequence of the program, valid proof of negative pregnancy tests before treatment, evidence of contraceptive measures, and monthly pregnancy tests were to be provided (Tantibanchachai 2014) (Figs. 2.4a–c and 2.5).

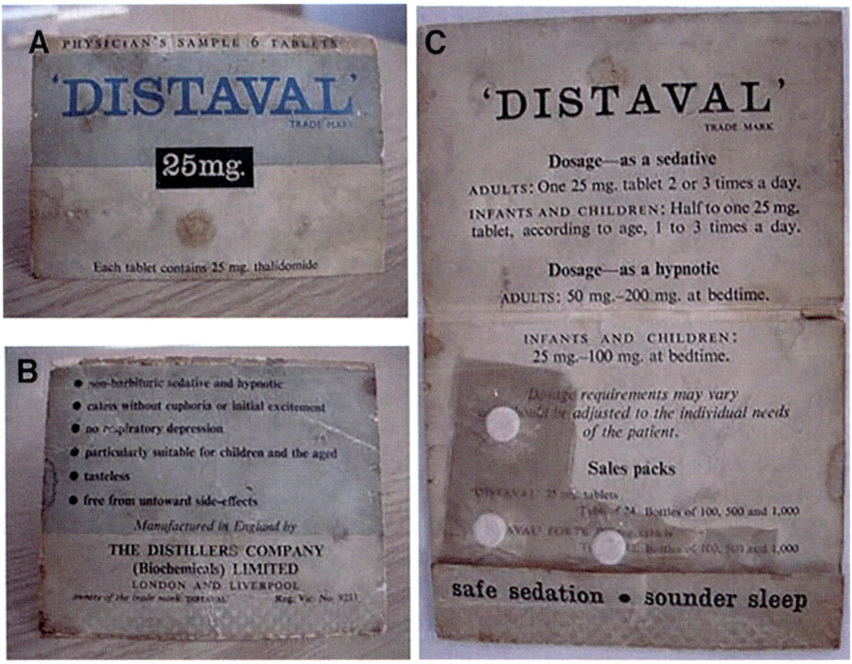

Fig. 2.4 A Packet of thalidomide sold under the UK's trade name "Distaval." (**a**) Front packing. (**b**) Rear packing claiming to be safe and free from side effects. (**c**) Inside the packet indicating dosage regimen and three tablets in a packet. (Adapted from Neil Vargesson, 2009)

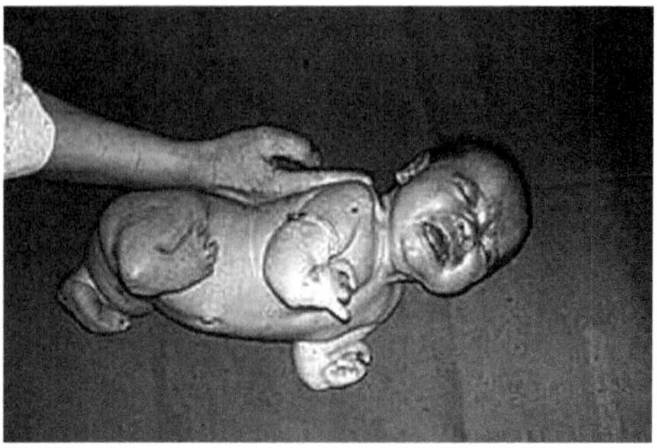

Fig. 2.5 Pictorial representation of deformities caused by Thalidomide. (Adapted from Hormones matter)

Thalidomide is a racemic mixture containing both enantiomers: (S)-thalidomide and (R)-thalidomide. The sedative and teratogenic effects were produced by the (S)-enantiomer, and the (R)- enantiomer was free from these effects (Rajkumar 2004). This fact was a hope for thalidomide to be used as a therapeutic modality in various diseases. Thalidomide was reintroduced as an anticancer drug, and today, it is in use to treat a vast array of medical conditions, including immune disorders such as leprosy, multiple myeloma, cancers such as Crohn's disease, HIV, and others (Vargesson 2015). Thalidomide analogs or immunomodulatory drugs (IMiDs) are used in many types of cancer. An example is Lenalidomide, which has immunomodulatory, antiangiogenic, and antineoplastic properties and is used as the regimen for multiple myeloma and certain types of myelodysplastic syndromes (Cruz 2016) (Fig. 2.6).

2.3.4 Regulatory Actions Taken After the Thalidomide Tragedy

2.3.4.1 Kefauver Harris Amendment

As a result of the thalidomide disaster in the USA, an amendment was passed to the Federal FD&C Act on 10th October 1962, known as Kefauver Harris Amendment by President John F. Kennedy (Greek et al. 2011). This amendment strengthened the FDA's regulation and approval of existing and newly marketed drugs (Kelsey n.d.). This amendment mandated that the drug molecule be safe and effective irrespective of being only safe as per Pure USFDA (Greek et al. 2011). An organized, systemic, and well-regulated reporting of ADRs became evident (Fornasier et al. 2018).

Investigational New Drug Regulations were also implemented. The comprehensive safety data of the drug in animals had to be submitted to the FDA before undergoing human studies. Clinical research was made more exhaustive with the duration of the study. A three-phase clinical trial study was initiated. Consent from the patients participating in the clinical studies was made compulsory (Kelsey n.d.). The time frame for the deposition of new drug applications was also removed (Paine 2017). Teratogenic studies on three animals were made necessary (Fornasier et al. 2018). Accurate and complete knowledge about the medicine should be provided to the user. Selling existing drugs under different trade names at an expensive price was prohibited (Kelsey n.d.).

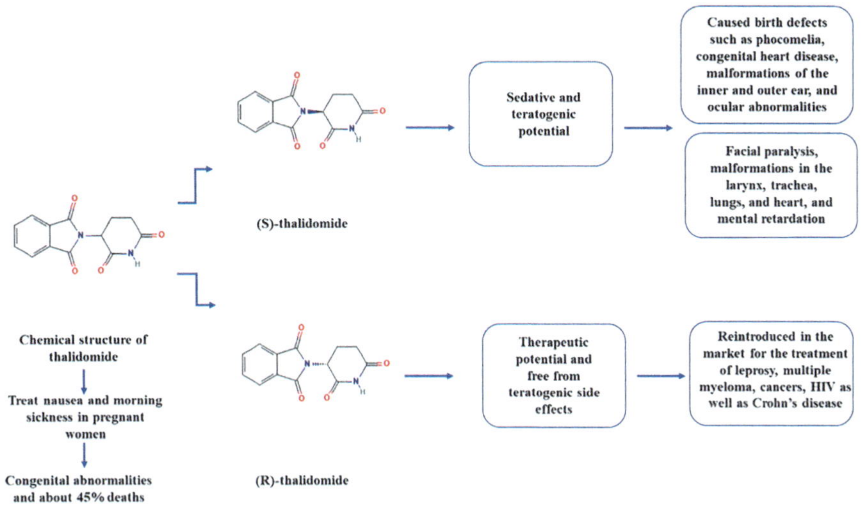

Fig. 2.6 Overview of Thalidomide Tragedy

Even after the beneficial effects of the amendment, it still received criticism as the cost of the drug reaching the market had substantially increased. The drug had to pass various checkpoints, and many failed. Many also suggested that the usage of the medicine should be made autonomous, and the user should decide whether to use the drug (Tantibanchachai 2014).

2.3.4.2 FDA 3-Segment Study Designs

A protocol for a 3-segment study was issued for the safety of foods, drugs, and cosmetics in 1959, and the guidelines were issued by the FDA in 1966. The preclinical studies for animal drug testing were more extensive and followed a 3-step reproductive study design. The study was divided into three phases following three sequential periods of reproductive cycles. The segments were divided into three parts, the first being the fertility and reproductive performance, the in-utero development (teratology), and finally, the perinatal and postnatal effects. In the first phase of the study, emphasis was laid on the behavior of the parent as well as the fetus for the proper functioning of gonads, estrogen cycles, mating behavior, rates for conception, and initial time of gestation. The entire reproductive process was viewed for teratogenesis until parturition and even lactation. Rats were the commonly used experimental animals for this phase. A study duration of 60–80 days before mating and 14 days after was done in both males and females. After performing all the necessary measures, the reproductive performance was studied. In the second phase, teratogenic effects in at least two species of rats, rabbits, and mice were studied. At last, in the third phase, prenatal and postnatal studies were performed (Collins 2006). This study design ensured the prediction of fetal adverse events and prevented a disaster like thalidomide from occurring again.

2.3.4.3 International Drug Monitoring Programme

Six months after the thalidomide tragedy, the WHO's WHA highlighted the issues concerning drug safety and suggested some methods for dealing with these problems (Venulet and Helling-Borda 2010). As a result, the international drug monitoring program was initiated on 7th February 1968 in Alexandria, Virginia, USA by WHO, as a pilot project with ten countries as their member (Australia, UK, USA, Germany, Canada, Ireland, Sweden, Denmark, New Zealand, and the Netherlands) (Venulet and Helling-Borda 2010). All these countries had well-established ADR monitoring programs at a national level (Pal 2013). The first meeting of the representatives of each country was held in September 1968 in Alexandria, Virginia (Venulet and Helling-Borda 2010). It was intended to form an international platform to report adverse reactions that could not be detected during clinical trials (Lindquist and Edwards 2001). Dr. Bruce Royall, the WHO Headquarters Drug Safety Unit's Chief, handled all the essential measures, such as the recruitment of the staff, all the technical details, and administrative support from the WHO Regional Office (Venulet and Helling-Borda 2010). Within 2 years, more than 24,000 case reports were received by the center (Venulet and Helling-Borda 2010). In 1978, WHO headquarters were moved from Geneva to Uppsala, Sweden (Lindquist and Edwards 2001). The main reason for its shift was the use of WHO computer facilities at WHO headquarters in Sweden (Venulet and Helling-Borda 2010). By 1974, ten more countries joined the program, including Japan, Poland, and France. This collaborating center is today called the Uppsala Monitoring Center, and 99% of adverse reactions are reported by this committee only (Lindquist and Edwards 2001).

2.3.4.4 Drug Efficacy Safety Implementation Programme

The Drug Efficacy Safety Implementation Programme was launched to review the effectiveness of active ingredients of drugs marketed between 1938 and 1962. A contract was signed for this on June 17, 1966, and ended on June 30, 1969 (Pritchett 1998). The study was supervised by the National Academy of Sciences and National Research Council for the government. Of the 7000 items still available, the Drug Efficacy Study had authority over around 4000, depicting about 300 different molecular units and, on average, 13 closely related compounds for each. After being reviewed, approximately 600 medicines were removed from the market as being ineffective (Greene and Podolsky 2012). Many were given black box warnings due to their adverse effects (Paine 2017). A list of all the preparations undergoing clinical trial on and after August 8, 1962, was to be submitted by 8th March 1963. A notice about all the drugs under study by 7th June 1963 had to be made. A total of almost 2500 drugs were listed. Following these advances in the regulation, clinical investigation of a few was discontinued. In such a case, a valid reason for discontinuation had to be provided, but no notice had to be filed (Kelsey 1963).

2.3.4.5 Prescription Drug User Fee Act (PDUFA)

To fasten and lower the cost of drug development, the US Congress passed the first PDUFA with the help of then-commissioner David Kessler in 1992. This law allowed the FDA to charge sponsors who submit NDAs or BLAs fees and let the FDA hire more reviewers to allow for a quicker review process. The 1992 PDUFA legislation was updated several times, and the Food and Drug Modernization Act of

1997 (PDUFA II) was one of the updates. Similarly, the Bioterrorism Preparedness and Response Act of 2002 (PDUFA III) also was an update for the existing PDUFA. The FDA is required by law to "review and act on" NDA /BLA filings under PDUFA, but not necessarily to approve them more quickly in return for user fees being collected. In this law, it was necessary to issue a comprehensive action letter and a thorough review of a fully submitted application. If the letter was not approved, it will outline the specific defects and, if necessary, the steps that must be taken to make the application ready for approval. PDUFA requires letters of action and responses, not approvals (Berndt et al. 2005).

2.3.4.6 MedWatch

In 1993, a program called MedWatch was initiated. It was a database for the voluntary reporting of ADRs. The goal of MedWatch was to clarify what ADR should be reported and what should be excluded. It was a systemic and organized way of writing ADRs. It also increased awareness about adverse reactions caused by the drugs (Martin 2008).

2.3.4.7 US FDA Modernization Act (FDAMA)

In 1997, a law called the US FDA Modernization Act was signed by President Clinton. The act was the renewal of the PDUFA User Fees Act. It was a measure taken to improve regulatory actions of biological products. This was done by collaborating the evaluation procedure with that of chemical drugs, thereby excluding the need for an establishment license for biologicals. For deadly diseases, hasty authorization procedures and substitute endpoints in clinical studies were permitted. Additionally, the FDAMA had a pediatric exclusivity provision that gave sponsors who carried out studies on drugs to be administered to children, 6 months of market exclusivity. In 2002, a revision of the terms of this provision was made and declared as the Best Pharmaceuticals for Children Act (Marshall and Baylor 2011).

2.3.4.8 USFDA Amendment of 2007

The US FDA Amendments Act of 2007 (FDAAA) gave the FDA new powers by forcing application holders to provide a proposed Risk Evaluation and Mitigation Strategy (REMS). FDA-approved labeling was sufficient for most medicines to guarantee that the advantages outweigh the hazards. However, in some cases, risk mitigation strategies beyond labeling were required. A REMS is a risk management strategy that uses resources other than the labeled information of the prescribed drug. The possible components of REMS are the patient package inserts, a medication guide, and a communication strategy (Wu and Juhaeri 2016).

2.3.4.9 Purple Book

The US FDA released a list that includes the licensed biological products with either the exclusive product or the biosimilar or interchangeable products, often known as the 'Purple Book, on 9 September 2014. The Purple Book contains all approved biologics along with their BLA numbers, as well as any interchangeable or biosimilar drugs that may be available. The Purple Book also includes a withdrawal notice for the biological product (Kelly and Onoe 2015) (Fig. 2.7).

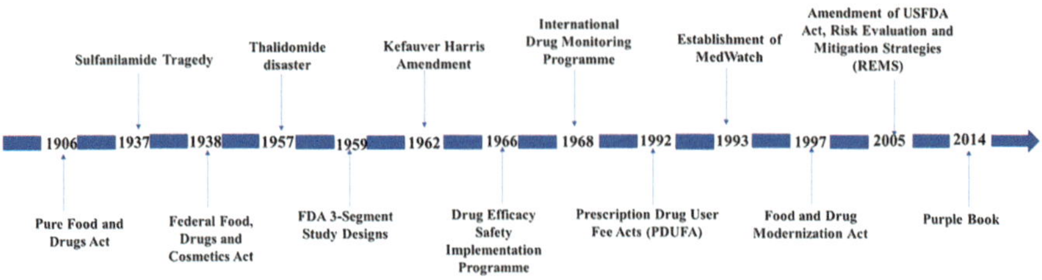

Fig. 2.7 Development of Pharmacovigilance in USA

2.4 Development of Pharmacovigilance in Europe

2.4.1 Thalidomide Disaster

As already discussed, the thalidomide disaster originated in Germany and soon spread worldwide. European PV underwent significant change after the thalidomide disaster. The thalidomide tragedy revealed various concerns and major issues, such as how reliable the testing of animals could be, the working of the industries, and the significance of drug monitoring after being introduced. The pharmacovigilance system has developed substantially since this system of reporting adverse drug reactions became systematic, coordinated, and controlled due to this tragedy. The event also established the Yellow card in the UK in 1964 (Fornasier et al. 2018). All the drug toxicity reports were registered in this yellow card. Also, a committee for the safety of drugs was formed in 1963 (Griffin 1972).

2.4.2 Regulatory Action Taken After the Thalidomide Disaster

2.4.2.1 Committee for Safety of Drugs

Along with the FD&C Act amendment, a separate committee was set up in June 1963 by the health minister. This committee was named the Committee for the Safety of Drugs. The committee was established in the presence of medical and pharmaceutical professionals and the British Pharmaceutical Industry. No legal powers were provided to the committee, but it was a mutual agreement between the Association of British Pharmaceutical Industry and the Proprietary Association of Great Britain. The company's role was to provide reports on any newly formulated drug to be marketed on the drug's safety. This committee decided whether the drug needs any further tests on toxicity or may initiate the clinical testing. They also regulated the clinical trial results. They also oversaw the management of each drug's safety and effectiveness and the indication for usage and safety precautions. General advice to the manufacturers and others concerned was provided. Finally, the reports received were assembled and evaluated, followed by submitting the messages to the doctors prescribing the drug. After the emergence of the Medicines Act of 1968, the Committee on Safety of Drugs translated into the Committee on Safety of Medicines in 1971 (Griffin 1972).

2.4.2.2 EC Directive 65/65

The EC Directive 65/65 was developed due to the destruction caused by thalidomide in Europe in 1965. The directive played a pivotal role in shaping the regulatory landscape for medicinal products within the European Economic Community (EEC) when it was adopted in 1965. This directive was instrumental in harmonizing pharmaceutical regulations among EEC member states, fostering the free movement of medicinal products across borders. It introduced standardized procedures for marketing authorization, emphasizing rigorous scientific evaluation to ensure the safety and efficacy of pharmaceuticals. Furthermore, Directive 65/65/EEC set forth requirements for labeling, packaging, and pharmacovigilance, contributing to higher standards of quality and safety in the pharmaceutical industry (Couve de Murville 1966). In 1966, a pilot experiment for the Boston Collaborative Drug Surveillance Programme was launched. It was the first organization to employ in-hospital monitoring to conduct epidemiologic studies to estimate probable side effects of pharmaceuticals, and it was significant in developing and implementing tools for drug epidemiology (Fornasier et al. 2018). A European Society of Pharmacovigilance was formed in 1992 with the aim of promoting pharmacovigilance and maintaining patient safety, which later developed into the International Society of Pharmacovigilance.

2.4.2.3 European Medicines Agency

In 1995, the European Medicines Agency was established. It was a new administrative organization to serve as a coordination hub for the latest advisory committees and licensing procedures. About 150 employees, primarily administrative and support workers, were responsible for human and veterinary products (Jefferys and Jones 1995). According to this, any new medicine could only be marketed, prescribed, and utilized after a scientific evaluation by the European Medicine Agency. Only medications with a favorable risk–benefit profile were given marketing authorizations (Bighelli and Barbui 2012). EMA's decision had to be accepted by all European member states (Bighelli and Barbui 2012). EMA would approve or reject any drug based on Randomized Clinical Trials (RCT). Once the reports were published, a European Public Assessment Report led to the decision to grant marketing authorization (Bighelli and Barbui 2012) The information consisted of a document containing a detailed description of the RCT results and a summary of the preclinical and clinical data recorded by the manufacturer. In 2001, EudraVigilance was formed and was first operated on 10 December 2001. EudraVigilance oversees the gathering and examination of alleged adverse responses to drugs approved in the European Economic Area (Postigo et al. 2018).

2.4.3 Theralizumab (TGN1412) Tragedy

Another tragedy in the UK includes the TGN1412 tragedy. A humanized (IgG4κ) monoclonal antibody specific for CD28 T cell, called TGN1412 (Theralizumab), was developed by Thomas Hünig, working in a German pharmaceutical company,

TeGenero (Lemoine 2017). The molecule was evaluated for autoimmune disorders like rheumatoid arthritis and B cell lymphocytic leukemia and put under a double-blind, randomized, placebo-controlled phase I clinical trial conducted on 13th March 2006 at Northwick Park Hospital, London, in Parexel's clinical pharmacology research unit (Lemoine 2017). TGN antibody binds to the C″D loop near the T cell membrane. Therefore, it does not require co-stimulatory agents and can stimulate T regulatory cells, initiating specific immediate immune responses (Sandilands et al. 2010). The UK's Medicines and Healthcare Products Regulatory Agency (MHRA) and Germany's Paul-Ehrlich Institute raised a query about the toxicology and immunotoxicity of the molecule. After the successful submission of reports, the preclinical testing in cynomolgus and rhesus monkey (Macaca fascicularis) was approved (Schneider et al. 2006). Both in vivo and in vitro studies showed that this antibody could initiate an immune response and generate a flush of anti-inflammatory cytokines and, therefore, could treat autoimmune disorders (Sandilands et al. 2010). The safest dose of the drug was 50 mg/kg for four consecutive weeks (Dowsing and Kendall 2007; Attarwala 2010). Eight male healthy volunteers were selected, of which six were given the TGN1412, and two were controls and received a placebo. The average age of the volunteers participating in the clinical trial studies was 26 years (Dowsing and Kendall 2007). The administration dose was 0.1 mg/kg, 500 times less than the safe dose in animals, and was given intravenously. As a result, within 9 h, six men who were given the treatment started to develop headaches, lumbar myalgia, rigors, pyrexia, hypotension, and tachycardia (Lemoine 2017). All six volunteers were immediately shifted to the ICU (Dowsing and Kendall 2007). After 12–16 h, multisystem failure like lung injury, renal failure, and disseminated intravascular coagulation developed. After 1 day, severe and unexpected depletion of lymphocytes and monocytes occurred (Lemoine 2017). The two volunteers who received the placebo were unharmed (Goodyear 2006). Luckily, none of them died, and they were monitored for 3 months and fortunately recovered. However, residual effects like memory loss, inability to concentrate, and headaches remained (Dowsing and Kendall 2007). One individual had dry gangrene of the fingers and toes, and the other had recurrent aphthous ulcers (Dowsing and Kendall 2007). Initially, it was believed that due to the binding of TGN1412 to CD28 T cell surface receptors, a cytokine storm was created by TNF-α, leading to the multiorgan failure. However, this fast-acting response that took only 2 h did not fit with the classical T cell immune response. Therefore, a study was conducted to find out the actual cause of this disaster (Sandilands et al. 2010). In a 2-h study, only monocytes were upregulated, and it was proposed that monocytes, rather than the T cells, were responsible for the failure. Furthermore, it was suggested that the formation of an array of antibodies occurred on the vascular endothelium. The suspension form of TGN1412 could not elicit an immune reaction. Only when immobilized or tagged with an anti-IgG antibody could it create an immune response, but a delay in response, i.e., 16–24 h, was seen (Sandilands et al. 2010). It was believed to be possible by an interaction between TGN1412 and CD64 (FcγRI) (Sandilands et al. 2010). In 2015, the drug was again put under clinical trials with at least 20 times less dose than the original one. The drug was renamed as TAB08 (TheraMab) (Figs. 2.8 and 2.9).

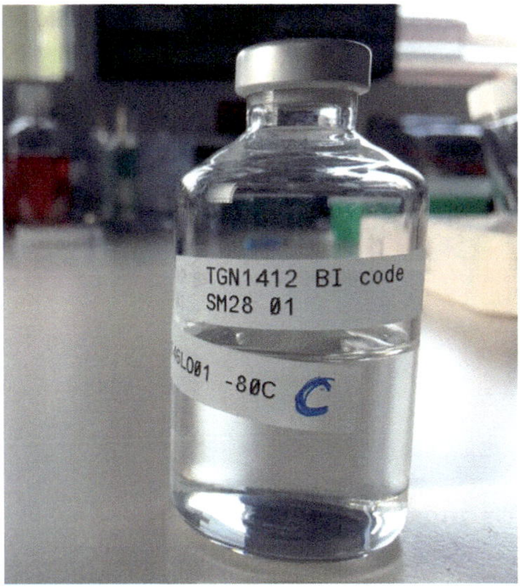

Fig. 2.8 TGN1412 formulation

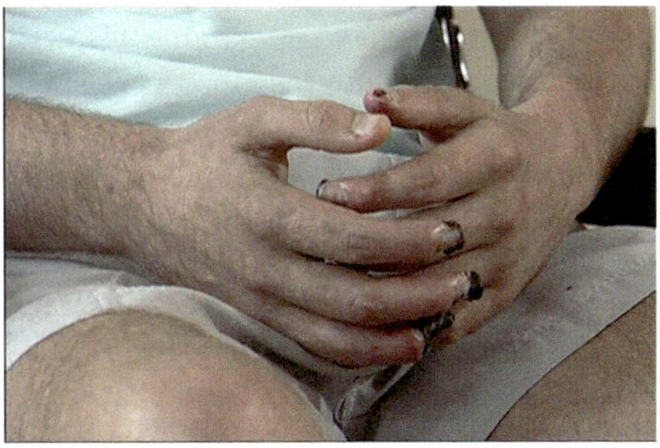

Fig. 2.9 Pictorial representation of the development of gangrene in TGN1412 volunteer. (Adapted from The Sun, 2017)

A tragedy of such type could be prevented if only a single patient were put on trial rather than all six. Also, a dose escalation protocol could be better designed, followed, and monitored after every escalated dose. A patient in these trials should be selected based on age, medical history, and other relevant health factors. A transparent data sharing, independent ethics review, post-trial patient monitoring, and early reporting and response plan should always be followed while conducting clinical trials (Fig. 2.10).

2.4.4 Regulatory Action Was Taken After the TGN1412 Tragedy

After the episode of TGN1412, immediately in April 2006, the Secretary of State for Health, under the leadership of Sir Gordon Duff, the Chairman of the Commission on Human Medicines and Medical Research, Dean at Sheffield University at that time, founded an Expert Scientific Group (ESG). The role of

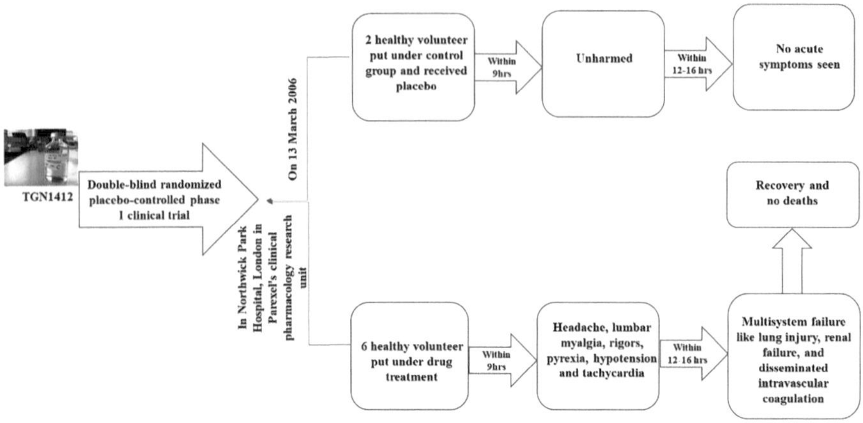

Fig. 2.10 Overview of the TGN1412 Tragedy

this group was to make up a report on the incident and give some recommendations on how this disaster could be prevented. The group had to reshape the preclinical to human trial studies (Dowsing and Kendall 2007). A final report was presented within less than a year on 30th November 2006 (Dowsing and Kendall 2007). The report comprised a total of 106 pages with 521 pages of appendices (Dowsing and Kendall 2007). The committee made 22 recommendations. It was clear that all the preclinical and clinical studies should have a solid theoretical background for such studies. The animal-to-human dose conversion should be done very keenly, and the safety of human exposure should always be kept in mind. While calculating the starting dose in humans, the novelty, potency, mechanism of action, species selected, DRC on animal and human cells, and in-vivo studies in animals should be considered along with the no observable adverse effect level (NOAEL) (Dowsing and Kendall 2007). Other than that, it was necessary to communicate with experts in that area and maintain proper communication at the early stage of development, like phase 1 (Dowsing and Kendall 2007). An Expert Advisory Group of the Commission on Human Medicines was set up to study the high-risk-causing drugs and their targets (Dowsing and Kendall 2007). A proper dosing interval between dosing and all the necessary measures with the antidote for possible adverse effects should always be available (Dowsing and Kendall 2007).

Other than the ESG, reports were also issued by MHRA, the Early Stage Clinical Trial Taskforce, and the Royal Statistical Society (Milton and Horvath 2009). In January 2007, it was suggested that a guideline should be created by the European Medicines Agency (EMEA) for the high-risk medicinal products to be evaluated by the clinical trials. The guidelines were finally titled "Guideline on Strategies to Identify and Mitigate Risks for First-in-Human Clinical Trials with Investigational Medicinal Products." The Committee for Medicinal Products for

Human Use (CHMP) of EMEA started to implement these guidelines on 19th July 2007, which finally came into effect on 1st September 2007 (Milton and Horvath 2009). The guideline suggested the study design for clinical studies, informed consent, safety reporting, Good Manufacturing Practices, and ADR reporting (Milton and Horvath 2009).

Some European Directives and regulations, such as 2010/84/EU and Regulation EC No. 1235/2010, were implemented to strengthen the pharmacovigilance system in Europe. The revised directive and regulation went into effect in July 2012, changing the requirements for marketing authorization by requiring all new products to have a risk management plan and introducing a pharmacovigilance system master file (PSMF) in place of a detailed description of the pharmacovigilance system. Post-authorization measures were also improved with the addition of post-authorization safety studies and post-authorization efficacy studies. Additionally, the EMA (for centrally authorized products) and national competent authorities (for nationally authorized products) must evaluate company reporting on its risk minimization measures (RMMs) and assess drug utilization studies and health outcomes for significant benefit–risk issues to determine the effectiveness of RMMs. The new EU regulations also defined who oversaw national noninterventional study oversight. In cases involving multiple member states, the EMA and its Pharmacovigilance and Risk Assessment Committee (PRAC) regulated protocol agreements and evaluated results. PRAC's primary focus areas were the referral of PSURs, post-authorization safety study (PASS), and detection and assessment of signals. PRAC was regarded as the primary advisory body on safety matters in reference to goods or applications centrally authorized through the centralized procedure and for national authorities through their coordination group, the CHMP, a division of the EMA. If appropriate, the coordination group or CHMP received recommendations from PRAC for adoption. The new regulation also mandated the establishment of an EU database listing all medications that had received EU approval. Listings for goods identified as requiring "additional monitoring" in the package leaflet were to be listed in this database by marketing authorization holders (MAHs).

Along with this, good vigilance practices (GVP) came in formation. The Rules that govern Medicinal Products in the European Union for Human Use Volume 9A were effectively replaced by the GVP modules. The creation and execution of a GVP guideline were critical directive deliverables. These procedures comprised a collection of policies to control how pharmacovigilance was carried out in the EU. This guideline comprised many chapters that diverged into two categories: one where major pharmacovigilance processes were defined and product- or population-specific considerations. It applied to MAHs and EU regulators. GVP Modules I through XVI, available on the EMA website, covered the critical pharmacovigilance processes (Borg et al. 2015).

In 2017, EudraVigilance was updated with new functionalities to give access to data on ADRs and involve academic research institutions in gathering extensive and detailed information on ADRs (Postigo et al. 2018) (Fig. 2.11).

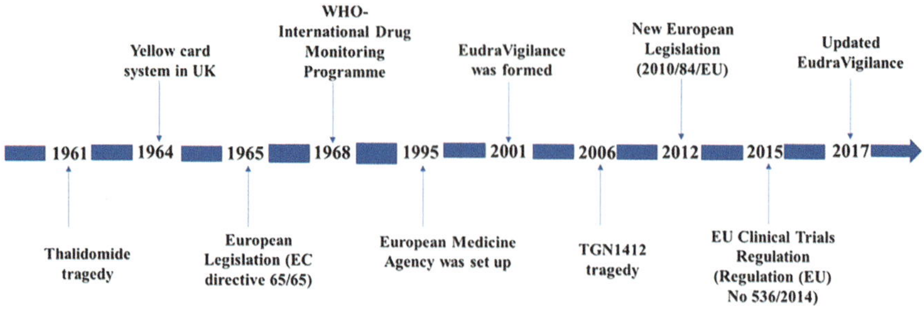

Fig. 2.11 Development of Pharmacovigilance in Europe

2.5 Development of Pharmacovigilance in India

The pharmacovigilance reporting system in India existed in 1983 when a pharmacologist from Christian Medical College, Dr. Molly Thomas, trained about 1650 doctors to report ADRs. In 1 year, she received about 600–900 reports (Thatte et al. 2018). In 1986, a program was initiated by the Drugs Controller General of India (DCGI) where reporting of ADRs was done with 12 main centers in Mumbai, Delhi, Chandigarh, Lucknow, Pondicherry, Kolkata etc. Along with this, India became a part of the WHO Program for International Drug Monitoring in 1997, with its main centers in Mumbai, New Delhi, Kolkata, Lucknow, Pondicherry, Chandigarh, and Aligarh. However, neither of the two initiatives provided efficient reporting. After that, an initiative was taken by the Indian Council of Medical Research (ICMR) in 1989 to launch their adverse reactions monitoring project at the Department of Pharmacology, Jawaharlal Nehru Medical College, and Aligarh Muslim University. Up to 58,000 ADRs were reported through a specially designed ADR Form and submitted to the ICMR (Rahman and Galib 2022). This program had different centers across India, and by 1992, it became the ICMR task force. The task force collapsed in 1999, but the areas to improve became quite evident (Thatte et al. 2018). Along with the ICMR project, another program by the Ministry of Health and Family Welfare (MoHFW), New Delhi, called Multicentric Monitoring of New Drugs (Rahman and Galib 2022). The first scientific conference on adverse drug reporting, prevention, and treatment was held in January 1997, led by Prof. Neelima Kshirshagar and Prof. Urmila Thatte (Rahman and Galib 2022). An agreement was signed between the WHO Headquarters, Geneva, and DCGI in 1997 to collaborate with the WHO Collaborating Centre for International Drug Monitoring, Uppsala-Sweden WHO-UMC. Prof. K. C. Singhal and Prof. Neelima Kshirsagar were appointed Honorary Consultants to WHO-UMC (Agrawal et al. 2022). The three central centers were selected to submit the report on ADRs to the drug regulatory authority of India (Agrawal et al. 2022). The selected centers included the Department of Pharmacology, All India Institute of Medical Sciences, New Delhi, Department of Pharmacology, Jawaharlal Nehru Medical College,

Aligarh Muslim University, Aligarh, and Department of Clinical Pharmacology, Seth GS Medical College and KEM Hospital, Mumbai (Agrawal et al. 2022).

On November 9–12, 1998, the first international conference was organized at JNU Auditorium, New Delhi, under the supervision of K. C. Singhal (Rahman and Galib 2022). During this conference, training was provided to the young pharmacologists and allied health scientists, regarding ADR. In light of this, the Society of Pharmacovigilance, India' (SoPI) was constituted under the leadership of Prof. K.C Singhal and was registered in 1999 (Rahman and Galib 2022).

A significant step in India's pharmacovigilance history was when India received funding from the WHO and World Bank in 2004/2005. The National Pharmacovigilance Program (NPVP) was launched in India on 1 January 2005 under the supervision of the National Pharmacovigilance Advisory Committee at the Central Drugs Standard Control Organization (CDSCO) office. The reports from all over the country were submitted to and compiled by two main centers, i.e., the Department of Clinical Pharmacology, King Edward VII Memorial Hospital, Mumbai, and the Department of Pharmacology, AIIMS, New Delhi. However, due to improper organization, the funding was ceased in mid-2009 (Thatte et al. 2018). During this time, many drugs like the antibiotic Gatifloxacin, COX 2 Inhibitors like Rofecoxib and Valdecoxib, and Diclofenac in veterinary practices were banned (Rahman and Galib 2022).

The fourth attempt was made by the MoHFW of the Government of India in 2010 when the Pharmacovigilance Programme for India (PvPI) was launched with its national center in AIIMS (Madhur et al. 2018). The program was planned to have four phases: initiation, consolidation, maintenance, and optimization (Thatte et al. 2018). Then, in 2011, The Indian Pharmacopeia Commission became India's National Coordinating Centre (NCC) for Pharmacovigilance activities. By 2018, about 250 Reactions Monitoring Centers were set up throughout India. The Hemovigilance Programme of India (HvPI) was launched by the National Institute of Biologicals (NIB) on 10 December 2012 to regulate blood products (Madhur et al. 2018). The launch of a toll-free helpline service for reporting ADR was done on 11 October 2013 by the NCC. Furthermore, to make reporting easier, an app was launched on Android devices in May 2015 in collaboration with NSCB Medical College, Jabalpur, and reporting could be done in ten vernacular languages (Thatte et al. 2018). A Materiovigilance Programme of India (MvPI) was introduced on July 6, 2015, to track unfavorable outcomes brought on by the use of medical devices (Madhur et al. 2018). IPC, the National Health System Resource Centre (NHSRC), the Sree Chitra Tirunal Institute for Medical Sciences & Technology (SCTIMST), and CDSCO are all involved in the program's direction (Madhur et al. 2018). Under the Drugs and Cosmetics Act, it became necessary for manufacturing and importing enterprises to create pharmacovigilance centers in 2016. The PSUR and Post-Marketing Surveillance were highlighted in Schedule Y of this Act (Madhur et al. 2018). The Indian Pharmacopoeia Commission (IPC) announced a guidance document with the title "Pharmacovigilance Guidance Document for MAHs of Pharmaceutical Products," which went into force in January 2018 (Jose and Rafeek 2019) (Fig. 2.12).

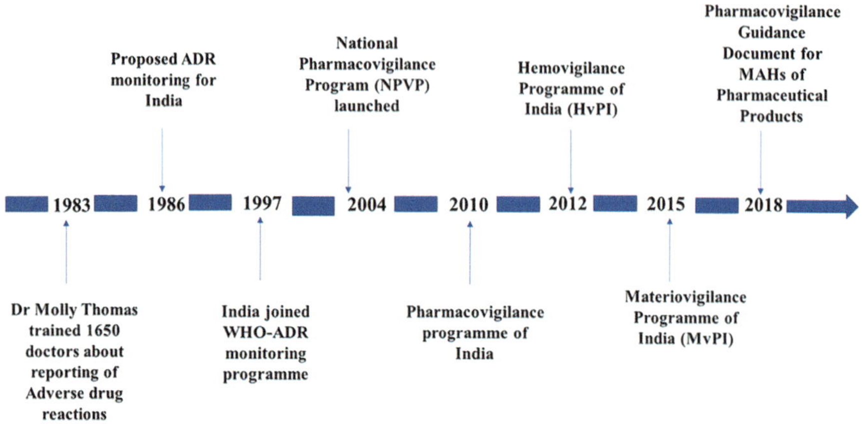

Fig. 2.12 Development of Pharmacovigilance in India

2.6 Development of Pharmacovigilance in Non-European Countries

2.6.1 Pharmacovigilance in Korea

In Korea, sulpyrine was used as an analgesic drug, but it was withdrawn in 1998 due to the risk of agranulocytosis (Shin et al. 2014). Similarly, various other interactions were reported with the use of drugs in different parts of the world. Phenylpropanolamine was approved for cold and cough use in 2001. Within a year, it was suggested that it might lead to hemorrhagic stroke. Therefore, it was withdrawn from the market in 2004 (Domingue 2007). Since 1977, the approved and marketed drugs have been re-evaluated in Korea. Later, in 1988, a reporting system was launched under the supervision of the Korea Ministry of Food and Drug Safety (Shin et al. 2014). Korea also became a member of WHO-UMC in 1992. For the newly approved drugs, a re-examination was conducted in 1995. In 2000, an online ADR reporting system was initiated. Furthermore, by the end of 2003, ADR reporting was made mandatory for pharmacists and manufacturers. The list of all contraindicated drugs was issued in 2004. In 2006, Korean Regional PV Centers (RPVCs) were introduced to facilitate ADR reporting, which included 15 centers by the end of 2009 that PVNet connected and 22 centers by 2013. A nationwide drug utilization review was started for clinicians and pharmacists in 2010. Furthermore, in April 2012, the Korea Institute of Drug Safety and Risk Management (KIDS) was formed to collect, evaluate, and manage ADRs (Shin et al. 2014). The KIDS established an ADR call center, the Korea Adverse Event Reporting System (KAERS), in November 2012 to collect ADR reports and give drug information. In 2013, KIDS was finally responsible for safety evaluation in the re-examination system, allowing for a more complete study of these new medications (Fig. 2.13).

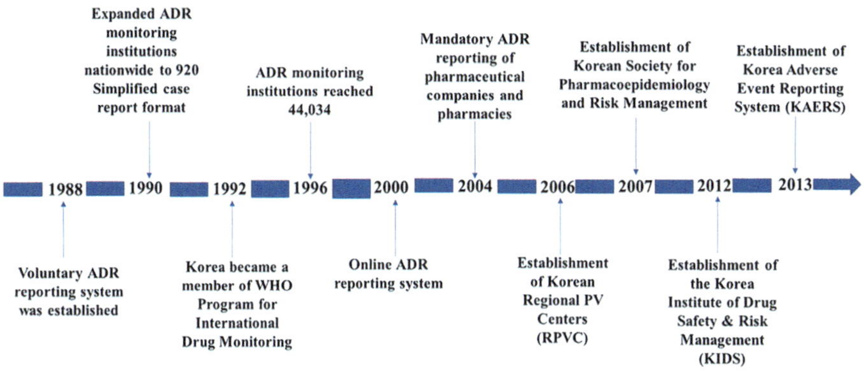

Fig. 2.13 Development of Pharmacovigilance in Korea

2.6.2 Pharmacovigilance in China

The history of pharmacovigilance in China is nearly 35 years old and can be divided into four stages from 1989 till now. The phases include the preparatory phase (1989–1999), the developmental phase (1999–2004), the expansion phase (2004–2011), and the stability phase (2011–till now) (Song et al. 2023). In 1988, 14 hospitals in Beijing, Guangzhou, Shanghai, and other cities initiated a small project on voluntary reporting on ADR. As a result of this, MoH established a national ADR monitoring center. This was followed by the establishment of ten provisional monitoring centers. In 1998, China officially became the 68th member of WHO-PIDM and formed the State Food and Drug Administration. Various laws and regulations have been passed in China over the years. The Measures for Monitoring and Management of ADRs (for Trial Implementation) were published by the National Medical Products Administration (NMPA) in 1999. After these regulatory measures, a law known as the Drug Administration Law was formulated in 2001, making reporting the ADR according to a state reporting system mandatory. As a result, the China ADR Monitoring System (CADRMS) was established in 2003. It was an online platform to connect four-level PV networks. Finally, in 2004, a publication was made for reporting and monitoring ADR measures. The first national PV conference was held in 2007, and a national PV system was established in China. By 2008, ten PV stations were made in tertiary hospitals, and a municipal PV platform was made (Zhao et al. 2018). A guideline for reporting adverse events after immunization was formed in 2010, named the National Guideline for the Surveillance of Suspected Adverse Events following Immunization. According to the guidelines, accountable reporting units and reporters must notify their county's Centers for Disease Control and Prevention, providing the location of the patients of any suspected cases of adverse events following immunization. By 2011, rapid progress in PV reporting occurred, and a total of 34 provisional monitoring centers and 333 regional monitoring centers were established, along with a national monitoring center. Additionally, an update in measures for ADR reporting was made in 2011. The national ADR monitoring platform was officially launched in 2012 that collects and analyses the information about the safety of drugs. In 2013, the State Food and Drug Administration was renamed to the China Food and Drug Administration (CFDA). The CFDA had also established the National Adverse Drug Reaction Monitoring Sentinel Alliance program to improve drug post-marketing safety oversight and ADR monitoring capabilities. This program was established in 2016 for active surveillance based on electronic health records. With intentions to expand to 300 hospitals across China, the Alliance has been operating in more than 60 hospitals. The Alliance also established the China Hospital Pharmacovigilance System (CHPS). With CHPS, information on adverse drug reactions could be easily gathered to encourage responsible medication use, reduce drug risks as soon as feasible, and improve the public safety of medicines. Within 1–2 years, CHPS was expanded over to 60 hospitals. In 2017, a series of reforms were introduced by the CFDA to increase regulatory transparency (Zhao et al. 2018). The International Conference on Harmonisation of Technical Requirements for Registration of Pharmaceuticals for Human Use was joined by the CFDA in August 2017. NMPA announced the reporting of ADR (No. 66 of 2018) on September 30, 2018. According to this principle, based on the suspicion, MAHs could directly and immediately report the observed or confirmed ADRs with the help of the China Adverse Drug Reaction Monitoring System (CADRMS). With the change of circumstances in China, new guidelines were issued by the Centre for Drug Evaluation (CDE) while keeping in view the ICH E2A, E2B, and E2F guidelines. On April 26, 2019, CDE allowed the submission of development safety update reports (DSUR) on its official website so drug registration sponsors could submit their DSUR. The NMPA implemented Good Pharmacovigilance Practices in 2021. According to the guidelines, The MAH and the applicants for Drug Registration who have been approved to conduct clinical drug trials in China must adhere to all 134 items and nine chapters of the GVP of China. It served as a manual for the parties on how to set up a PV system and carry out PV operations. Shenzhen became home to China's first municipal pharmacovigilance institute in May 2019. Several institutions were opened in Inner Mongolia, Shanxi, Hebei, Linyi, and other regions and cities (Song et al. 2023) (Fig. 2.14).

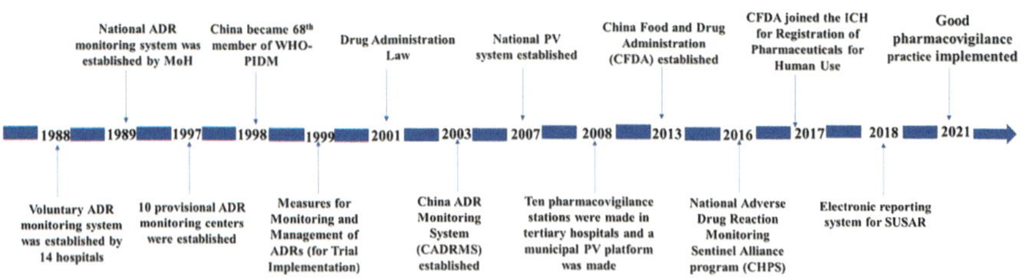

Fig. 2.14 Development of Pharmacovigilance in China

2.7 Some Recent Tragedies

2.7.1 Heparin Contamination

Heparin, a sulfated carbohydrate derivate, is used as an anticoagulant in particular infections, cell growth, and inflammation (Liu et al. 2009). Out of all the animal-derived heparin, only porcine-derived is approved by the FDA. In late 2007 and 2008, allergic reactions were reported with pediatric dialysis on intravenous heparin sodium injections. These allergic reactions were associated hypotension, nausea, shortness of breath, urticaria, and tachycardia that appeared within 30 minutes of administration. Till 31st January 2008, 113 patients showed 152 adverse reactions. On 17 January 2008, Baxter Healthcare Company, the manufacturer, issued a voluntary recall of the nine lots of multidose heparin vials. Finally, the FDA approved withdrawing all the products from the market on 28 February 2008 (Chess et al. 2012). After various analytical, chemical, and biological screening, it was found that an oversulfated chondroitin sulfate (OCSC) was present as an adulterant in heparin and caused direct activation of the kinin–kallikrein vasoactive mediator, leading to acute hypotension (Blossom et al. 2008). In response to this outbreak, the FDA created test procedures for identifying the contaminant and made them available to the public, started a program of product sampling to identify contaminated goods as they crossed U.S. borders, and increased the inspection coverage of all heparin manufacturers. To stop the import of tainted heparin into the USA, the FDA was allowed to place companies on Import Alert (automatic detention without physical examination). Additionally, the FDA collaborated with the United States Pharmacopoeia (USP) to incorporate the improved test procedures in the June 2008 Heparin Sodium API monograph update (McMahon et al. 2010).

2.7.2 Counterfeit Avastin

In 2012, a counterfeit Avastin (Bevacizumab) was introduced into the US market. Avastin is a prescription drug administered by i.v. route. It is a biological antibody that shows binding properties to a protein called vascular endothelial growth factor (VEGF). It is crucial for developing and maintaining angiogenesis. The FDA initially authorized bevacizumab to manage metastatic colorectal cancer in 2004. It was then allowed to treat conditions like glioblastoma, renal cell carcinoma, and non-small cell lung cancer. On February 10, 2012, the FDA delivered letters of warning to 19 medical practices as it was reported that fake Avastin had entered the market. The counterfeit medications were distributed in the US and entered the markets of Turkey, Switzerland, Denmark, the UK, and Canada (Mackey et al. 2015). FDA was informed of the supply chain breach in December 2011 by MHRA. On 14 February 2012, the FDA told healthcare professionals and patients about this incident. Roche Pharmaceuticals, the manufacturer of Avastin, and Genentech, the drug's distributor, were informed about this introduction (Anagnostiadis and Chatterjee 2018). The counterfeit drug did not contain the active pharmaceutical ingredient and, therefore, was not safe and effective. They had common materials like corn starch and acetone as solvents (Mackey et al. 2015). The chemical testing also confirmed the absence of API. The company soon recognized specific differences in the label and packaging of the medications, and the public was informed of the same. A few differences were the brand names of Avastin and Genentech, a different expiry date format, the 6-digit lot number with no alphabet, and all the text on vails was in English. Helpline numbers were circulated to report any side effects and receiving of counterfeit drugs (Anagnostiadis and Chatterjee 2018). Nearly 1000 FDA warning letters were sent to medical professionals in almost 48 states and two US territories after additional batches of counterfeit Avastin were discovered. Despite so many warnings, the supply of counterfeit drugs was still ongoing, and various counterfeit drugs were detected, and the FDA notified about the same on 5 February 2013 (Mackey et al. 2015). This time, it was sold under the Turkish name Altuzan. This led to an understanding of the importance of purchasing medications from a reliable and regulated source to maintain the patient's well-being at all times and costs. The discovery of fake Avastin ultimately emphasized the value of constant watchfulness, strict procurement procedures, and the continual commitment to maintaining the safety and authenticity of the pharmaceutical supply chain.

2.7.3 Ranitidine Tragedy

Ranitidine (Zantac), a GlaxoSmithKline (GSK) product, was used in various conditions of heart burn, acid reflux, and ulcers and to treat gastroesophageal reflux disease (GERD). On 1 April 2020, the FDA requested all the manufacturers to remove the prescription and OTC Ranitidine drugs from the market. It was noted that when ranitidine was stored at higher temperatures and longer duration, it caused an increase in the concentration of a contaminant known as N-Nitrosodimethylamine (NDMA) due to the rapid breakdown of ranitidine into dimethylamine and nitrites. NMDA is a carcinogen ordinarily present in foods and water in a low quantity. It is also naturally present in the body. In 2019, Valisure Pharmacy confirmed the presence of NMDA in ranitidine, but it could not be stated whether or not the drug would be safe to use. In September 2019, a warning was issued about this effect, and it was recommended that other alternatives be used. Some third-party laboratories focused that there was an increase in NMDA and significantly higher at elevated temperatures even under normal storage conditions. The presence of NMDA was nine times more than the daily intake limit of NMDA, i.e., 96 nanograms (Adamson and Chabner 2020). As a result, a letter was sent to all manufacturers to remove ranitidine from the markets immediately. It was advised to stop using the already purchased liquid or tablet preparations and adequately dispose of them. Due to the COVID-19 pandemic, it was asked to dispose of the medication with proper disposal instructions mentioned on the label or follow FDA guidelines. Also, the patients receiving ranitidine as a prescription drug were suggested to take a doctor's consultation before stopping the medication. Alternate medicines from different manufacturers that did not have any indication of NMDA were recommended (US Food and Drug Administration 2020).

2.7.4 Digene Recall

In the drug testing list for June 2023, issued by CDSCO, out of 1273 drugs tested, 48 were declared not to be of standard quality. One pill was reported as spurious. Likewise, the DCGI warned against using the antacid Digene Gel after Abbott India voluntarily recalled numerous batches of the medication. According to the FDA, the product made at the company's Goa facility may be dangerous and have adverse effects. On 9th August 2023, DCGI received a complaint that the antacid had a harsh taste and offensive scent. The customers provided feedback about the discoloration of liquid in the bottle, which changed from pink to white, with a bitter taste and pungent smell. Usually, the syrup tasted sweet (Dutt 2023). In addition, the government has instructed medical professionals to warn patients about potential side effects before prescribing the medication.

Adverse events linked to pharmaceutical interventions still happen despite significant improvements in PV over time. Pharmacovigilance has significantly improved in identifying, reporting, and managing adverse events, yet it still cannot eliminate the hazards connected with medicinal interventions. Even after all the efforts made, adverse events continue to occur due to various factors, including the complex nature of human biology, the diversity of patient groups, the advances in developing new medicines, and the constraints of clinical trials. However, the advancement of PV has resulted in more proactive monitoring, quicker reactions to safety issues, and improved stakeholder communication. In the ever-changing healthcare and drug development environment, constant monitoring, teamwork, and ongoing research are essential to reducing risks and ensuring patient safety remains a top priority.

2.8 Conclusion

The history of PV discussed in this chapter underlines the cruciality of the safety and security of pharmaceutical preparations. It serves as a reminder of the development in the monitoring and assessing of drug quality for safe disposal in animals and man. The progress made by man over these years, keeping in view the catastrophic events, evolution, and changes in regulation, technical advancements, and international partnerships, is worth emphasizing. This chapter describes how the development followed a cascade from reactive responses to adverse medication events to a proactive discipline intended to identify, evaluate, and manage drug-related risks. With the possibility of various standardized procedures and legislation, as well as national and international pharmacovigilance systems, a systemic and synchronized approach toward monitoring adverse reactions for safety is possible. The efficiency and impact of the computerized reporting of the events for collection, analysis, and signal detection have been possible only after technological advancement. The need for such technological advancements was highlighted only after past disasters. Taking lessons from the past, improvements have come along the way. The calamities can never be predicted to the fullest, but we have evolved with the highest possible safety of patients.

References

Adamson RH, Chabner BA (2020) The finding of N-Nitrosodimethylamine in common medicines. Oncologist 25(6):460–462. https://doi.org/10.1634/theoncologist.2020-0142

Agrawal P, Kushwaha V, Siddiqui S, Khan NF, Tripathi M (2022) History of pharmacovigilance and drug safety. World J Pharmaceut Res 12:575–586

Anagnostiadis E, Chatterjee SV (2018) The dangers of buying prescription drugs from rogue wholesale distributors. J Med Regul 104(1):13–16. https://doi.org/10.30770/2572-1852-104.1.13

Attarwala H (2010) TGN1412: from discovery to disaster. J Young Pharm 2(3):332–336. https://doi.org/10.4103/0975-1483.66810

Ballentine C (1981) Sulfanilamide disaster. FDA Consumer Magazine, p 5

Berndt ER, Gottschalk AH, Philipson TJ, Strobeck MW (2005) Industry funding of the FDA: effects of PDUFA on approval times and withdrawal rates. Nat Rev Drug Discov 4(7):545–554. https://doi.org/10.1038/nrd1774

Bighelli I, Barbui C (2012) What is the European medicines agency? Epidemiol Psychiatr Sci 21(3):245–247. https://doi.org/10.1017/S2045796012000170

Blossom DB, Kallen AJ, Patel PR, Elward A, Robinson L, Gao G, Langer R, Perkins KM, Jaeger JL, Kurkjian KM, Jones M, Schillie SF, Shehab N, Ketterer D, Venkataraman G, Kishimoto TK, Shriver Z, McMahon AW, Austen KF, Kozlowski S, Sasisekharan R et al (2008) Outbreak of adverse reactions associated with contaminated heparin. N Engl J Med 359(25):2674–2684. https://doi.org/10.1056/NEJMoa0806450

Borg JJ, Tanti A, Kouvelas D, Lungu C, Pirozynski M, Serracino-Inglott A, Aislaitner G (2015) European Union pharmacovigilance capabilities: potential for the new legislation. Therapeut Adv Drug Saf 6(4):120–140. https://doi.org/10.1177/2042098615591802

Brass EP (2001) Changing the status of drugs from prescription to over-the-counter availability. N Engl J Med 345(11):810–816. https://doi.org/10.1056/NEJMra011080

Caron J, Rochoy M, Gaboriau L, Gautier S (2016) The history of pharmacovigilance. Therapie 71(2):129–134. https://doi.org/10.1016/j.therap.2015.12.007

Carpenter D, Sin G (2007) Policy tragedy and the emergence of regulation: the food, drug, and cosmetic act of 1938. Stud Am Polit Dev 21(2):149–180. https://doi.org/10.1017/S0898588X0700020X

Chess EK, Bairstow S, Donovan S, Havel K, Hu P, Johnson RJ, Lee S, McKee J, Miller R, Moore E, Nordhaus M, Ray J, Szabo C, Wielgos T (2012) Case 41 study: contamination of heparin with oversulfated chondroitin sulfate. Handb Exp Pharmacol 207:99–125. https://doi.org/10.1007/978-3-642-23056-1_6

Collins TF (2006) History and evolution of reproductive and developmental toxicology guidelines. Curr Pharm Des 12(12):1449–1465. https://doi.org/10.2174/138161206776389813

Couve de Murville M (1966) Directive 65/65 EEC. Council directive of 26 January 1965 on the approximation of provisions laid down by law, regulation or administrative action relating to medicinal products(OJL no 22 of 9.2). 1965: 369. 8 Krantz JC Jr. new drugs and the Kefauver-Harris amendment. J New Drugs 6:77–79

Cruz MP (2016) Lenalidomide (Revlimid): a thalidomide analogue in combination with dexamethasone for the treatment of all patients with multiple myeloma. P & T 41(5):308–313

Dally A (1998) Thalidomide: was the tragedy preventable? Lancet (Lond) 351(9110):1197–1199. https://doi.org/10.1016/S0140-6736(97)09038-7

Domingue JN (2007) Phenylpropanolamine contained in cold remedies and risk of hemorrhagic stroke. Neurology 69(3):320–321. https://doi.org/10.1212/01.wnl.0000275291.02789.b3

Dowsing T, Kendall MJ (2007) The Northwick Park tragedy—protecting healthy volunteers in future first-in-man trials. J Clin Pharm Ther 32(3):203–207. https://doi.org/10.1111/j.1365-2710.2007.00808.x

Dutt A (2023) Digene gel used for acidity and gas relief recalled in India: doctors answer all queries. The Indian Express [Internet]. https://indianexpress.com/article/health/wellness/digene-gel-used-for-acidity-and-gas-relief-recalled-in-india-8927359/. Accessed 20 Aug 2023

Fornasier G, Francescon S, Leone R, Baldo P (2018) An historical overview of pharmacovigilance. Int J Clin Pharmacol 40(4):744–747. https://doi.org/10.1007/s11096-018-0657-1
Goodyear M (2006) Learning from the TGN1412 trial. BMJ (Clin Res Ed) 332(7543):677–678. https://doi.org/10.1136/bmj.38797.635012.47
Greek R, Shanks N, Rice MJ (2011) The history and implications of testing thalidomide on animals. J Philos Sci Law 11(3):1–32. https://doi.org/10.5840/jpsl20111133
Greene JA, Podolsky SH (2012) Reform, regulation, and pharmaceuticals—the Kefauver-Harris Amendments at 50. N Engl J Med 367(16):1481–1483. https://doi.org/10.1056/NEJMp1210007
Griffin JP (1972) Drug surveillance: the role of the committee on safety of medicines. Ulster Med J 41(2):111–120
Gupta A, Waldhauser LK (1997) Adverse drug reactions from birth to early childhood. Pediatr Clin North Am 44(1):79–92. https://doi.org/10.1016/s0031-3955(05)70464-8
Jefferys DB, Jones KH (1995) EMEA and the new pharmaceutical procedures for Europe. European medicines evaluation agency. Eur J Clin Pharmacol 47(6):471–476. https://doi.org/10.1007/BF00193696
Jones JK, Kingery E (2014) History of pharmacovigilance. In: Mann's pharmacovigilance, pp 11–24. https://doi.org/10.1002/9781118820186.ch2
Jose J, Rafeek NR (2019) Pharmacovigilance in India in comparison with the USA and European Union: challenges and perspectives. Ther Innov Regul Sci 53(6):781–786. https://doi.org/10.1177/2168479018812775
Kelly RD, Onoe Y (2015) The FDA purple book: black and blue all over. Biotechnol Law Rep 34(3):75–80. https://doi.org/10.1089/blr.2015.29000
Kelsey FO (1963) Government: the Kefauver-Harris amendments and investigational drugs. Am J Hosp Pharm 20(10):515–517. https://doi.org/10.1093/ajhp/20.10.515
Kelsey FO (n.d.) Kefauver Harris amendment. https://www.chemeurope.com/en/encyclopedia/Kefauver_Harris_Amendment.html. Accessed 20 Aug 2023
Kille JW (2017) Regulatory toxicology. In: A comprehensive guide to toxicology in nonclinical drug development. Academic Press, New York, pp 499–539. https://doi.org/10.1016/B978-0-12-803620-4.00019-0
Kim JH, Scialli AR (2011) Thalidomide: the tragedy of birth defects and the effective treatment of disease. Toxicol Sci 122(1):1–6. https://doi.org/10.1093/toxsci/kfr088
Lachmann PJ (2012) The penumbra of thalidomide, the litigation culture and the licensing of pharmaceuticals. QJM 105(12):1179–1189. https://doi.org/10.1093/qjmed/hcs148
Lam C, Patel P (2023) Food, drug, and cosmetic act. In: StatPearls. StatPearls, Treasure Island, FL. https://pubmed.ncbi.nlm.nih.gov/36251824/. Accessed 20 Aug 2023
Lemoine M (2017) Animal extrapolation in preclinical studies: an analysis of the tragic case of TGN1412. Stud Hist Philos Biol Biomed Sci 61:35–45. https://doi.org/10.1016/j.shpsc.2016.12.004
Lindquist M, Edwards IR (2001) The WHO Programme for international drug monitoring, its database, and the technical support of the Uppsala monitoring center. J Rheumatol 28(5):1180–1187
Liu H, Zhang Z, Linhardt RJ (2009) Lessons learned from the contamination of heparin. Nat Prod Rep 26(3):313–321. https://doi.org/10.1039/b819896a
Mackey TK, Cuomo R, Guerra C, Liang BA (2015) After counterfeit Avastin®—what have we learned, and what can be done? Nat Rev Clin Oncol 12(5):302–308. https://doi.org/10.1038/nrclinonc.2015.35
Madhur G, Preeti K, Kalaiselvan V, Shridhar M, Singh GN, Nilima K, Shanthi P (2018) Pharmacovigilance programme of India: the journey traveled and the way forward. WHO Drug Inform 32(1):10–17
Mann RD, Andrews EB (eds) (2007) Pharmacovigilance. Wiley, Hoboken, NJ. https://doi.org/10.1002/9780470059210
Marshall V, Baylor NW (2011) Food and Drug Administration regulation and evaluation of vaccines. Pediatrics 127(Suppl 1):S23–S30. https://doi.org/10.1542/peds.2010-1722E

Martin RP (2008) Postapproval marketing practices regarding drug safety and pharmacovigilance. In: The pharmaceutical regulatory process. CRC, Boca Raton, FL, pp 237–248. https://doi.org/10.3109/9781420070439-13

McKenzie R, Fried MW, Sallie R, Conjeevaram H, Di Bisceglie AM, Park Y, Savarese B, Kleiner D, Tsokos M, Luciano C (1995) Hepatic failure and lactic acidosis due to fialuridine (FIAU), an investigational nucleoside analogue for chronic hepatitis B. N Engl J Med 333(17):1099–1105. https://doi.org/10.1056/NEJM199510263331702

McMahon AW, Pratt RG, Hammad TA, Kozlowski S, Zhou E, Lu S, Kulick CG, Mallick T, Dal Pan G (2010) Description of hypersensitivity adverse events following administration of heparin that was potentially contaminated with oversulfated chondroitin sulfate in early 2008. Pharmacoepidemiol Drug Saf 19(9):921–933. https://doi.org/10.1002/pds.1991

Milton MN, Horvath CJ (2009) The EMEA guideline on first-in-human clinical trials and its impact on pharmaceutical development. Toxicol Pathol 37(3):363–371. https://doi.org/10.1177/0192623309332997

Moro A, Invernizzi N (2017) The thalidomide tragedy: the struggle for victims' rights and improved pharmaceutical regulation. A tragédia da talidomida: a luta pelos direitos das vítimas e por melhor regulação de medicamentos. Hist Cienc Saude Manguinhos 24(3):603–622. https://doi.org/10.1590/S0104-59702017000300004

Nasr A, Lauterio TJ, Davis MW (2011) Unapproved drugs in the United States and the Food and Drug Administration. Adv Ther 28(10):842–856. https://doi.org/10.1007/s12325-011-0059-4

Paine MF (2017) Therapeutic disasters that hastened safety testing of new drugs. Clin Pharmacol Ther 101(4):430–434. https://doi.org/10.1002/cpt.61

Pal S (2013) WHO programme for international drug monitoring. Clin Ther 35(8):e123. https://doi.org/10.1016/j.clinthera.2013.07.381

Postigo R, Brosch S, Slattery J, van Haren A, Dogné JM, Kurz X, Candore G, Domergue F, Arlett P (2018) EudraVigilance medicines safety database: publicly accessible data for research and public health protection. Drug Saf 41(7):665–675. https://doi.org/10.1007/s40264-018-0647-1

Pritchett EL (1998) Evolution and revolution in drug labeling: Regulation of antiarrhythmic drugs by the Food and Drug Administration 1962-1996. Pacing Clin Electrophysiol 21(7):1457–1469. https://doi.org/10.1111/j.1540-8159.1998.tb00218.x

Rahman SZ, Galib R (2022) History of pharmacovigilance in India (1983-2022). J Pharmacovigil Drug Saf 19(1):6–17. https://doi.org/10.21276/jpds.2021.19.01.02

Rajkumar SV (2004) Thalidomide: tragic past and promising future. Mayo Clin Proc 79(7):899–903. https://doi.org/10.4065/79.7.899

Ridings JE (2013) The thalidomide disaster, lessons from the past. Methods Mol Biol 947:575–586. https://doi.org/10.1007/978-1-62703-131-8_36

Routledge P (1998) 150 years of pharmacovigilance. Lancet (Lond) 351(9110):1200–1201. https://doi.org/10.1016/S0140-6736(98)03148-1

Sandilands GP, Wilson M, Huser C, Jolly L, Sands WA, McSharry C (2010) Were monocytes responsible for initiating the cytokine storm in the TGN1412 clinical trial tragedy? Clin Exp Immunol 162(3):516–527. https://doi.org/10.1111/j.1365-2249.2010.04264.x

Schneider CK, Kalinke U, Löwer J (2006) TGN1412—a regulator's perspective. Nat Biotechnol 24(5):493–496. https://doi.org/10.1038/nbt0506-493

Shin JY, Jung SY, Ahn SH, Lee SH, Kim SJ, Seong JM, Chung SY, Park BJ (2014) New initiatives for pharmacovigilance in South Korea: introducing the Korea Institute of Drug Safety and Risk Management (KIDS). Pharmacoepidemiol Drug Saf 23(11):1115–1122. https://doi.org/10.1002/pds.3715

Snell ES (1983) Regulatory authorisation of clinical trials. Br J Clin Pharmacol 15(6):625–627. https://doi.org/10.1111/j.1365-2125.1983.tb01543.x

Song H, Pei X, Liu Z, Shen C, Sun J, Liu Y, Zhou L, Sun F, Xiao X (2023) Pharmacovigilance in China: evolution and future challenges. Br J Clin Pharmacol 89(2):510–522. https://doi.org/10.1111/bcp.15277

Stephens MD (2011) Review of the "the dawn of drug safety". Pharmacoepidemiol Drug Saf 20(3):327. https://doi.org/10.1002/pds.2107

Surendra E, Garlapati R (2020) Development of pharmacovigilance culture. Int J Pharmacy Res Technol 10(1):1–4. https://doi.org/10.31838/ijprt/10.01.01

Swaters D, van Veen A, van Meurs W, Turner JE, Ritskes-Hoitinga M (2022) A history of regulatory animal testing: what can we learn? Altern Lab Anim 50(5):322–329. https://doi.org/10.1177/02611929221118001

Tantibanchachai C (2014) US regulatory response to thalidomide (1950-2000). In: The Embryo Project Encyclopedia, p 1. https://embryo.asu.edu/handle/10776/7733. Accessed 20 Aug 2023

Thatte UM, Chaudhari NL, Gogtay NJ (2018) Pharmacovigilance program of India: history, evolution and current status. Adverse Drug React Bull 312(1):1207–1210. https://doi.org/10.1097/fad.0000000000000036

Tousley RD (1941) The federal food, drug, and cosmetic act of 1938. J Mark 5(3):259–269. https://doi.org/10.1177/002224294100500312

Tuffs A (2007) Thalidomide: the true story? BMJ (Clin Res Ed) 334(7600):933. https://doi.org/10.1136/bmj.39199.637986.59

US Food and Drug Administration (2020) FDA requests removal of all ranitidine products (Zantac) from the market. https://www.fda.gov/news-events/press-announcements/fdarequests-removal-all-ranitidine-products-zantac-market. Accessed 20 Aug 2023

Van Grootheest K (2003) The dawn of pharmacovigilance: an historical perspective. Int J Pharmaceut Med 17(5–6):195–200. https://doi.org/10.2165/00124363-200317050-00006

Vargesson N (2015) Thalidomide-induced teratogenesis: history and mechanisms. Birth Defects Res C Embryo Today 105(2):140–156. https://doi.org/10.1002/bdrc.21096

Venulet J, Helling-Borda M (2010) WHO's International Drug Monitoring—the formative years, 1968–1975: preparatory, pilot and early operational phases. Drug Saf 33(7):e1–e23. https://doi.org/10.2165/11532410-000000000-00000

Wax PM (1995) Elixirs, diluents, and the passage of the 1938 federal food, drug and cosmetic act. Ann Intern Med 122(6):456–461. https://doi.org/10.7326/0003-4819-122-6-199503150-00009

Wu J, Juhaeri J (2016) The US Food and Drug Administration's risk evaluation and mitigation strategy (REMS) program - current status and future direction. Clin Ther 38(12):2526–2532. https://doi.org/10.1016/j.clinthera.2016.11.007

Zhao Y, Wang T, Li G, Sun S (2018) Pharmacovigilance in China: development and challenges. Int J Clin Pharmacol 40(4):823–831. https://doi.org/10.1007/s11096-018-0693-x

Databases Used in Pharmacovigilance Across the Globe

3

Vipin Bhati, Mukesh Nandave, Anoop Kumar, and Deepti Pandita

3.1 Introduction

As per the WHO, PV is defined as the science and activities relating to the detection, assessment, understanding, and prevention of adverse effects and other drug-related safety problems. Several adverse drug reactions (ADRs) are noticed when medicine first enters the market, leading to the need for post-market surveillance (Javed and Kumar 2023).

PV is tightly controlled in key global regions involved in drug development. The primary regulatory bodies overseeing worldwide PV standards are the EMA, the FDA, and the PMDA.

3.2 Databases Used in Pharmacovigilance

Pharmacovigilance databases are used to record and monitor individual case safety reports (ICSRs) for a company's pharmaceutical products from all sources worldwide (Lindquist 2008). These databases, which include ICSRs as well as analysis, visualization, and reporting options, are an essential component of a PV system. There are several commercially accessible databases to select from, each with its own set of features and benefits (Suke et al. 2015). The main regulatory

V. Bhati (✉) · M. Nandave · A. Kumar · D. Pandita
Department of Pharmacology, Delhi Pharmaceutical Sciences and Research University, New Delhi, India
e-mail: mukeshnandave@gmail.com; anoopdpsru@dpsru.edu.in

M. Nandave, A. Kumar (eds.), *Pharmacovigilance Essentials*,
https://doi.org/10.1007/978-981-99-8949-2_3

organizations responsible for supervising global standards in PV are the European Medicines Agency, the Food and Drug Administration, and the Pharmaceuticals and Medical Devices Agency. Some countries have their own PV system which have describe below and compiled in Table 3.1 and commercially used database also compiled in Table 3.2.

3.3 National Pharmacovigilance Databases Used by the Different Countries

Various databases are being used by regulatory authorities, pharmaceutical companies, CRO to handle the data related to PV across the globe.

3.3.1 VigiBase

The VigiBase (https://who-umc.org/vigibase/) is created by the Uppsala Monitoring Centre (UMC), a worldwide database of reported possible adverse effects of pharmaceutical products and it is controlled by the WHO Programme for International Drug Monitoring (WHO PIDM). With over 30 million suspected ADR reports filed by WHO PIDM member nations since 1968, it is the biggest database of its type in the world. Incoming reports are regularly updated in VigiBase, which is also connected to databases for medical and pharmaceutical categories including WHODrug, MedDRA, WHO ICD, and WHO-ART. Through VigiBase, it is possible to analyse potential patient damage and consider ways to avoid it. Its objective is to provide the proof from which perspective medication safety risks (signals) may be identified and shared. The speed, accuracy, and quality of reports generated by the VigiBase system rely on national centres, and it also heavily depends on the cooperation of the participating PV centres (VigiBase 2023). The screenshot of VigiBase is presented in Fig. 3.1.

3.3.1.1 Advantages

1. **Worldwide Coverage:** VigiBase gathers data from a different variety of sources globally, providing a comprehensive overview of ADRs across diverse populations and regions. This enables the detection of rare or previously unreported adverse events.
2. **Signal Detection:** The big amount of data in VigiBase permits for effective signal detection, where the possible safety alarms or a series of possible adverse reactions can be recognized. This helps to regulatory bodies and healthcare experts in making decisions about medication safety.
3. **Longitudinal Analysis:** The database contains data collected over long period of time, simplifying longitudinal analysis. This helps in understanding the progression of adverse events over time and detecting probable trends.
4. **Supports Regulatory Decisions:** After the evaluation of the VigiBase data the regulatory bodies are able to make decision on drug withdrawal from the market, label changes, and any serious warning.

Table 3.1 National Pharmacovigilance databases used by different countries

Sr. no.	Database name	Country	Application	Advantage	Disadvantage	Company name	Access link	Cost
1	VigiBase	WHO	VigiBase is the unique WHO global database of reported potential side effects of medicinal products	It ensures that early signs of previously unknown medicines-related safety problems are identified as rapidly as possible	Underreporting, lack of completeness, and potential reporting biases	UMC has developed and maintained VigiBase since 1978	https://who-umc.org/vigibase/	Free
2	EudraVigilance	Europe	To provide public access to reports of suspected side effects *To provide information on suspected adverse events following administration of veterinary medicines as well	Providing information related to an individual case of a suspected side effect due to a medicine') and less duplication	Possible risk of false negatives in case of reporting of orphan drugs suspected ADRs and as well as signal detection of orphan drugs	This database owned and administered by the European Medicines Agency (EMA)	https://eudravigilance.ema.europa.eu/human/index.asp	Paid

(continued)

Table 3.1 (continued)

Sr. no.	Database name	Country	Application	Advantage	Disadvantage	Company name	Access link	Cost
3	FDA Adverse Event Reporting System (FAERS)	USA	FAERS is a database that contains adverse event reports, medication error reports and product quality complaints resulting in adverse events that were submitted to FDA regarding drugs and therapeutic biologics	The FAERS Public Dashboard is specifically designed for the public to access and view FAERS data in a customizable, searchable format. It allows users to view a summary of adverse event reports received from 1968 to the present or for a specific timeframe	*Duplicate and incomplete reports are in the system *Rates of occurrence cannot be established with reports	US-FDA	https://fis.fda.gov/sense/app/95239e26-e0be-42d9-a960-9a5f7f1c25ee/sheet/7a47a261-d58b-4203-a8aa-6d3021737452/state/analysis	Free

4	Indicator-Based Pharmacovigilance Assessment Tool (IPAT)	African country	Indicator-Based Pharmacovigilance Assessment Tool: Manual for Conducting Assessments in Developing Countries	The tool focuses on significant issues related to health systems that are recognized as the key factors in the overall capacity and sustainability of a medicine safety system	*The sensitivity and specificity of the indicators are not established *Non-medication-related patient safety indicators are not included	USAID	https://pdf.usaid.gov/pdf_docs/PNADS167.pdf	Free
5	Database of Adverse Event Notifications (DAEN)	Australia	Provides information about adverse events and incidents related to therapeutic goods used in Australia			Govt. of Australia	https://daen.tga.gov.au/medicines-search/	Free
6	Canada Vigilance Adverse Reaction Online Database	Canada	It contains information about suspected adverse reactions			Govt. of Canada	https://cvp-pcv.hc-sc.gc.ca/arq-rei/index-eng.jsp	Free

(continued)

Table 3.1 (continued)

Sr. no.	Database name	Country	Application	Advantage	Disadvantage	Company name	Access link	Cost
7	Korea Adverse Event Reporting System (KAERS)	Korea	The database includes the data collected through spontaneous reports, reports from studies (re-examination, post-marketing studies, individual case studies, etc), and literature information			Korea Institute of Drug Safety & Risk Management (KIDS)	https://www.mfds.go.kr/eng/search/searchEn.do	Free

Table 3.2 Details information about the commercial PV databases

Sr. no.	Database name	Application	Company name	Cost	Access link
1	AB Cube: Safety Easy	It is a multiVigilance management solution which integrates automation with existing drug safety processes	AB Cube	Paid	https://www.ab-cube.com/pharmacovigilance/
2	Argus Safety Database	It is used for intake, case prioritization, field validations, letters, action items, coding, listedness, narratives, case lock, submission, and archiving—can reduce manual work by 50% or more	Oracle	Paid	https://www.oracle.com/in/life-sciences/pharmacovigilance/argus-safety-case-management/
3	ARISg/ LifeSphere Safety	An automated end-to-end Drug Safety system, LifeSphere MultiVigilance saves time, ensures compliance, and aligns global teams	Aris Global	Paid	https://lifesphere.arisglobal.com/platform/safety/
4	SafetyBase Interchange	SafetyBase Interchange is an intuitive secure web-based pharmacovigilance and drug safety software that allows the receipt, sending and management of electronic adverse event reports reliably and in accordance with compliance standards	BaseCon	Paid	https://basecon.com/basecon/safetybase-interchange/

5. **Research and Analysis:** Researchers can use VigiBase to conduct epidemiological studies, explore patterns of adverse reactions, and assess the comparative safety of different drugs. This contributes to advancing drug safety knowledge.

3.3.1.2 Limitations

1. **Underreporting:** One major limitation of VigiBase, like many PV databases, is underreporting. Not all adverse events are reported, leading to an incomplete picture of the true safety profile of a medication.
2. **Reporting Bias:** The adverse events reporting is subject to bias. Healthcare professionals and regulatory authorities may be more likely to report severe or unexpected events, while milder events may be underreported. This can skew the representation of adverse reactions.

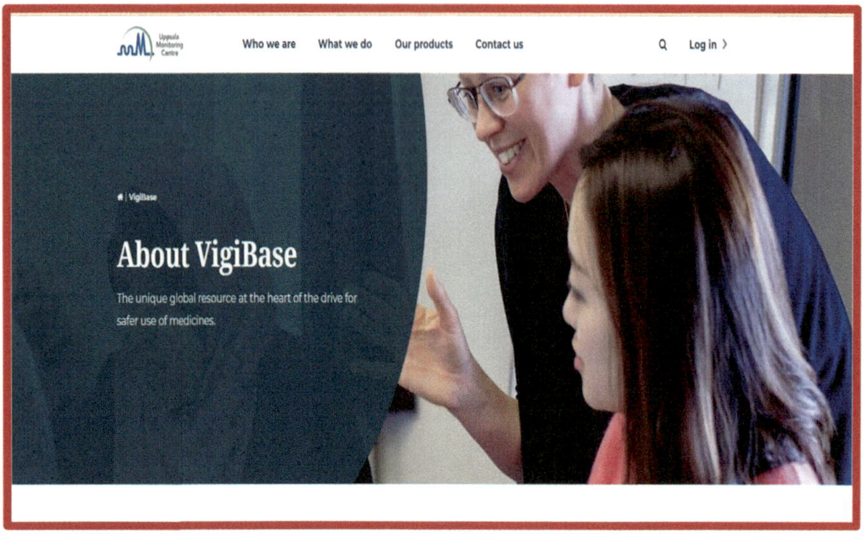

Fig. 3.1 Homepage of VigiBase

3. **Causality Assessment:** VigiBase data alone may not create a direct causality relationship between a medication and side effect and adverse event. Further investigation and analysis are often required to determine the causal link.
4. **Data Quality:** The accuracy and comprehensiveness of the data is based on the quality of reporting from various sources. Inconsistencies or errors in data entry can impact the reliability of analyses.
5. **Confounding Factors:** The database may not always account for confounding factors, such as patients' underlying health conditions or concurrent medications, which can influence the occurrence of adverse events.
6. **Language and Reporting Variability:** The data in VigiBase come from various sources, potentially leading to language-related challenges and variability in reporting standards and terminologies.

3.3.2 EudraVigilance

EudraVigilance (https://eudravigilance.ema.europa.eu/human/index.asp) is a system which is developed and managed by the European Medicines Agency to supervise and assess data regarding potential adverse reactions related with medicines that have either been granted authorization or are under investigation in clinical trials within the European Economic Area. This database allows the identification of new signals related to the potential side effects. Reports that are submitted to the EudraVigilance comprehend suspected adverse reactions to medications reported in both the pre-authorization and post-authorization phases. This system can manage the electronic transfer of Individual Case

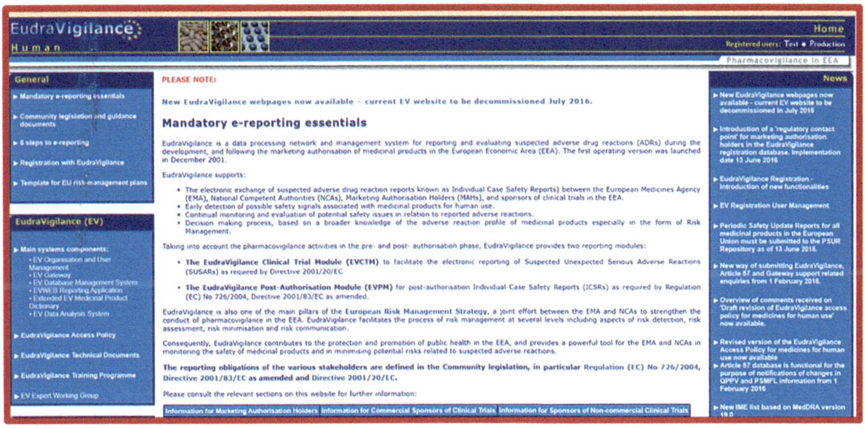

Fig. 3.2 Homepage of EudraVigilance

Safety Reports following the ICH E2B standards. This database consists of two modules of collection of data, one is EudraVigilance Clinical Trial Module (EVCTM) and another one is EudraVigilance Post-Authorization Module (EVPM) (EudraVigilance 2023). The screenshot of EudraVigilance is presented in Fig. 3.2.

3.3.2.1 Advantages

1. **Regulatory Oversight:** EudraVigilance supports the regulatory bodies in the European union as well as in European Economic Area nations with the investigation of drug safety. It helps in the rapid identification of new safety issues.
2. **Comprehensive Data:** The data is obtained from different sources and sources such as national regulatory agencies, pharmaceutical industries and other healthcare professionals.
3. **Signal Detection:** EudraVigilance uses advanced signal detection algorithms to identify possible safety indicators, and patterns within the reported adverse events, contributing to the early identification of safety concerns.
4. **Timely Communication:** The system enables rapid communication between regulatory authorities, which is essential for addressing safety concerns promptly and implementing necessary measures to protect patient safety.
5. **Collaboration:** EudraVigilance promotes cooperation among European Union and European Economic Area nations by offering a unified platform for exchanging safety information and sharing experiences concerning medications.

3.3.2.2 Limitations

1. **Underreporting:** Like many other PV systems, EudraVigilance encounters the issue of underreporting, where not all adverse events get reported. This can result in an incomplete depiction of a medication's actual safety profile.

2. **Data Quality:** The precision and excellence of the data rely on the sources of reporting. Inconsistent or inadequate reporting can influence the dependability of the information stored within EudraVigilance.
3. **Causality Assessment:** The system's data by itself may not definitively establish a direct cause-and-effect link between a medication and an adverse event. In many cases, a comprehensive examination and inquiry are required to ascertain the causal connection.

3.3.3 FDA Adverse Event Reporting System (FAERS)

The FDA Adverse Event Reporting System (FAERS) (https://fis.fda.gov/sense/app/95239e26-e0be-42d9-a960-9a5f7f1c25ee/sheet/7a47a261-d58b-4203-a8aa-6d3021737452) is a database covering records of adverse drug event reports and medication errors reports to the US-FDA. This database is designed to assist the FDA's post-market safety monitoring effort for pharmaceuticals and therapeutic biologics.

It encompasses adverse event reports furnished by manufacturers as mandated by regulations, as well as reports directly submitted by consumers and healthcare practitioners. Within FAERS, there are adverse event reports that manufacturers are obligated to submit to the FDA as stipulated by regulations, in addition to reports coming directly from consumers and healthcare professionals. FAERS serves as a valuable resource for the FDA in tasks like identifying potential new safety issues associated with marketed products, assessing manufacturers' adherence to reporting requirements, and satisfying external requirements for information. After that the reports are available in FAERS, are analyse and evaluated by the clinical reviewers who are working in Center for Drug Evaluation and Research (CDER) and the Center for Biologics Evaluation and Research (CBER), to monitor the safety of medicinal products or drugs which are approved by the US FDA. The dashboard of the FAERS database is highly user-friendly and interactive. The main purpose of the FAERS database to allow individual to find out the information related to adverse events submitted by pharmaceutical companies, consumers, and other health care professionals. As an illustration, the presence of reports in FAERS related to a specific drug or biologic does not necessarily indicate a causal relationship between the drug and the adverse event. It is important to know that that the FAERS data alone do not serve as a reliable parameter for the safety information of the drugs (FDA Adverse Event Reporting System (FAERS) 2023). The screenshot of webpage of FAERS is presented in Fig. 3.3.

3.3.3.1 Advantages

1. **Regulatory Oversight:** FAERS plays a pivotal role for the FDA in overseeing the post-market safety and efficacy of medications and medical devices. It assists in the detection of emerging safety issues and facilitates the implementation of necessary regulatory measures.

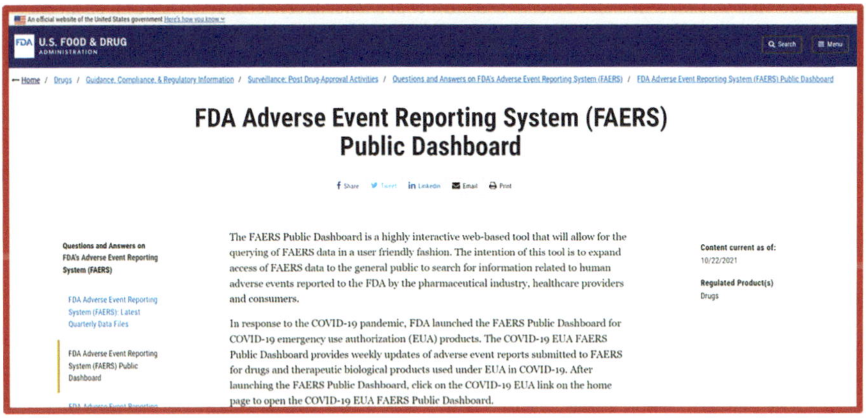

Fig. 3.3 Homepage of FAERS database

2. **Diverse Data Sources:** The system gathers information from a variety of origins, including healthcare practitioners, patients, and manufacturers. This diversity broadens the scope of safety data and enables a more thorough evaluation.
3. **Signal Detection:** FAERS utilizes sophisticated data analysis methods to identify potential safety indicators, patterns, and trends within reported adverse events, aiding in the early recognition of safety concerns.
4. **Rapid Response:** FAERS facilitates prompt communication between the FDA and pertinent parties, enabling swift responses to address safety worries and reduce potential risks.
5. **Data Sharing:** FAERS data is accessible to the public and researchers, fostering transparency and making it easier for independent assessments of medication safety to take place.
6. **Research and Analysis:** Researchers have the opportunity to employ FAERS data for conducting epidemiological investigations, assessing drug safety characteristics, and adding to the body of scientific knowledge within the PV domain.

3.3.3.2 Limitations

1. **Underreporting:** One major drawback of FAERS, similar to other PV systems, is the issue of underreporting. This occurs when not all adverse events get reported, resulting in an incomplete portrayal of the genuine safety profile of medications.
2. **Reporting Bias:** Reports of adverse events in FAERS may be vulnerable to reporting bias, where there is a greater probability of severe or unexpected events being reported in comparison to milder ones. This has the potential to skew the assessment of safety data.

3. **Causality Assessment:** FAERS data on its own may not definitively establish a direct causality relation between a medication and an adverse event. Often, a thorough analysis and additional investigation are necessary to establish causation.
4. **Data Quality:** The accuracy and reliability of FAERS data depend on the quality of reporting, data entry, and coding. Inaccurate or incomplete information can affect the integrity of analyses.

3.3.4 Indicator-Based Pharmacovigilance Assessment Tool (IPAT)

The indicator-Based PV Assessment Tool (IPAT) (https://pdf.usaid.gov/pdf_docs/PNADS167.pdf) is an extensive measurement tool used to evaluate the performance of PV and medication safety. It consists of 43 indicators in which 43, 26 considered core indicators and rest 17 are supplementary indicator, which collectively assess various aspects of PV systems. The tool was created to assess the effectiveness of PV systems, pinpoint deficiencies, and areas requiring enhancement. The IPAT is employed for evaluations in less developed nations. The tool is administered by interviewers and serves to assess the entire PV system within a country. The IPAT is a crucial instrument for nations to assess their PV systems and enhance medication safety (Jha et al. 2021). The screenshot of webpage of IPAT is presented in Fig. 3.4.

3.3.4.1 Advantages

1. **Standardized Assessment:** The IPAT provides a standardized framework for assessing PV systems, allowing for consistent evaluation across different countries and regions.

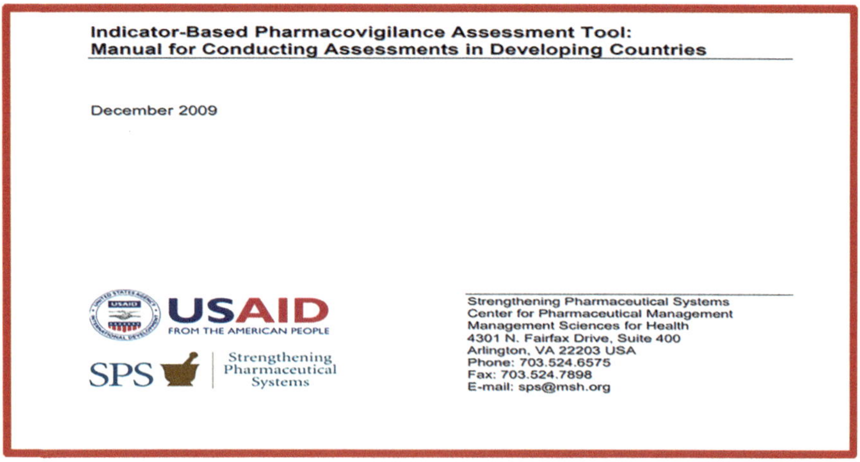

Indicator-Based Pharmacovigilance Assessment Tool: Manual for Conducting Assessments in Developing Countries

December 2009

USAID FROM THE AMERICAN PEOPLE

SPS Strengthening Pharmaceutical Systems

Strengthening Pharmaceutical Systems
Center for Pharmaceutical Management
Management Sciences for Health
4301 N. Fairfax Drive, Suite 400
Arlington, VA 22203 USA
Phone: 703.524.6575
Fax: 703.524.7898
E-mail: sps@msh.org

Fig. 3.4 Homepage of IPAT

2. **Comprehensive Evaluation:** The tool covers various aspects of PV, including inputs, processes, outputs, outcomes, and impacts, providing a comprehensive assessment of the system.
3. **Identifying System Gaps**: By using the IPAT, stakeholders can identify areas where the PV system may be lacking or needs improvement, allowing for targeted interventions and resource allocation.
4. **Monitoring and Evaluation:** The IPAT enables ongoing monitoring and evaluation of the PV system, helping to track progress over time and assess the impact of interventions (Javed and Kumar 2023).

3.3.4.2 Limitations

1. **Lack of Sensitivity:** Certain research has voiced doubts regarding the sensitivity of the IPAT as an evaluation tool, proposing that it might not precisely capture the intricacies and intricacies of PV systems.
2. **Limited Specificity:** The IPAT may not provide detailed insights into specific weaknesses or areas of improvement within a PV system.
3. **Lack of Established Sensitivity and Specificity**: Due to the lack of sensitivity and specificity of IPAT it may limits to reliability and validity of the IPAT.

3.3.5 Database of Adverse Event Notifications (DAEN)

The Database of Adverse Event Notifications (DAEN) (https://daen.tga.gov.au/medicines-terms-condition/) is an internet-based platform that offers details concerning adverse events and occurrences linked to therapeutic products employed in Australia. It comprises information derived from reports of adverse events, which are also referred to as side effects or adverse reactions, associated with prescription medications, over-the-counter remedies, complementary medicines, and medical devices. Reports can originate from healthcare practitioners, individuals, and pharmaceutical corporations. The DAEN might include a larger proportion of reports detailing severe rather than mild adverse events, as well as infrequent rather than frequent reactions. However, the data provided by the DAEN is unable to give information about how the ADR is severe or also unable to provide the information about the dose, dose strength and time period of drug use (Martin and Lucas 2021). The screenshot of webpage of DAEN is presented in Fig. 3.5.

3.3.5.1 Advantages

1. **Community Access:** The DAEN provides community access to information about adverse events, allowing individuals to make informed decisions about their health.
2. **Early Detection**: The DAEN allows for early detection of safety issues related to therapeutic goods, which can lead to take appropriate action on time by the regulatory bodies to protect public health.

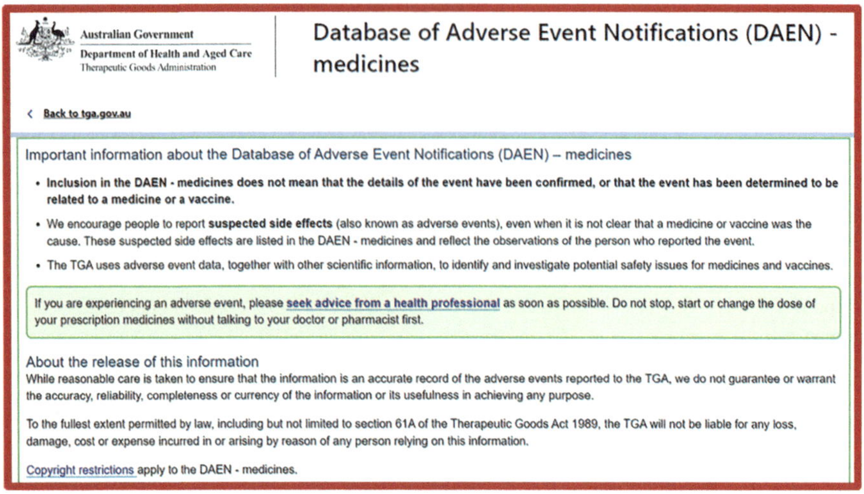

Fig. 3.5 Homepage of DAEN database

3.3.5.2 Limitations

1. **Reporting Bias:** In DEAN database large number of reporting is related to the serious events which can bias the reporting data and results in the high difference between the ratio of serious to non-serious adverse events.
2. **Limited Information:** It unable to provide information about how the ADR is serous means severity of ADR have not explained by DEAN.

3.3.6 Canada Vigilance Adverse Reaction Online Database

The Canada Vigilance Adverse Reaction Online Database (https://cvp-pcv.hc-sc.gc.ca/arq-rei/index-eng.jsp) is a resource provided by Health Canada that comprises data regarding suspected ADRs of medicines or drugs. The database consists of data from 1965-01-01 to 2023-04-30. The data was extracted and compressed in ASCII text files that include full dataset found in the Canada Vigilance Adverse Reaction Online Database. All the reports regarding adverse reactions are voluntarily submitted in the database by the consumers and healthcare professionals, along with reports mandated by the Food and Drugs Regulations from Market Authorization Holders, which include manufacturers and distributors. The database contains patient information, details about medication usage, adverse reactions, and their subsequent outcomes. Users can conduct searches by choosing particular health products and adverse reaction descriptions. Researchers utilize this database for various purposes, including conducting pharmacoeconomic studies and to understand the prevalence and frequency of adverse drug reactions in Canada (Maity and Longo 2020). The screenshot of webpage of Canada Vigilance Adverse Reaction Online Database is presented in Fig. 3.6.

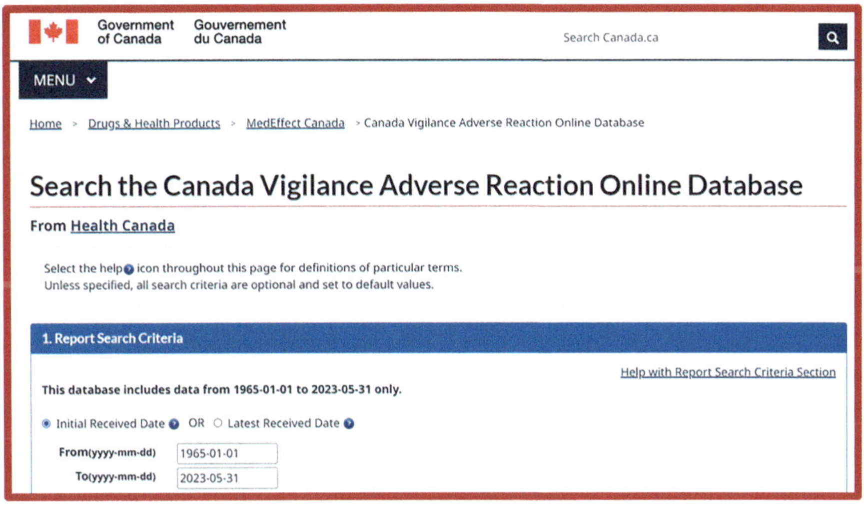

Fig. 3.6 Homepage of Canada Vigilance Adverse Reaction Online Database

3.3.6.1 Advantages

1. **Comprehensive Data**: It consist of all ADRs that are reported in Canada by pharmaceutical companies, consumers, and healthcare professionals.
2. **Longitudinal Data:** The database includes data from 1965 to the present. This longitudinal data allows for the analysis of trends and patterns in adverse reactions over time.
3. **Patient Reporting:** The database includes ADR reports that are reported directly by patients. This allows for the inclusion of patient perspectives and experiences, which can provide valuable insights into the safety and effectiveness of health products.
4. **Source of Post-Market ADR Data:** This database is used as important tool of post-market ADR information for research and analysis. This data can be used for pharmacoeconomic analyses, evaluating the safety of specific drugs, and identifying potential risks and benefits.

3.3.6.2 Limitations

1. **Voluntary Reporting**: The data in the database is collected principally through a spontaneous surveillance system, where all the ADRs regarding health products are reported by the reporter on voluntary basis. This means that not all adverse reactions may be reported, leading to potential underreporting and incomplete data.
2. **Data Quality:** The accuracy and completeness of the data in the database depend on the quality of the reports submitted by HCPs, patients, and pharmaceutical companies. There may be variations in the quality of the data, including missing or incomplete information.

3. **Limited Search Options:** The database has limitations in terms of search options. It may not be possible to search for all health products and all adverse reaction terms simultaneously.

3.3.7 The Korea Adverse Event Reporting System (KAERS)

The Korea Adverse Event Reporting System (KAERS) (https://www.mfds.go.kr/eng/search/searchEn.do) is an adverse drug event (ADE) reporting system created by the Korea Institute of Drug Safety and Risk Management (KIDS) in 2012. KAERS is regulated and managed by the Ministry of Food and Drug Safety (MFDS) and is used to detect the unlisted ADRs that have not detected during the clinical trials and also help to identified rare ADRs occurs during the marketing of the drug. It also helps to monitor the vaccine safety in Korea. It is a complete database of adverse drug reactions and adverse drug events reported by patients, pharmaceutical companies, and healthcare professionals. KAERS is used for signal detection and PV activities. Machine learning algorithms have been applied to KAERS to detect early safety signals of drugs such as fluoroquinolones and infliximab. KAERS is an important tool for drug safety monitoring in Korea (Kim et al. 2023). The screenshot of webpage of KAERS is presented in Fig. 3.7.

3.3.7.1 Advantages

1. This database helps to detect rare ADRs that occurs after post-marketing.
2. It helps to detect those side effects or adverse event that have not detected during clinical trials.
3. Reliable research results.

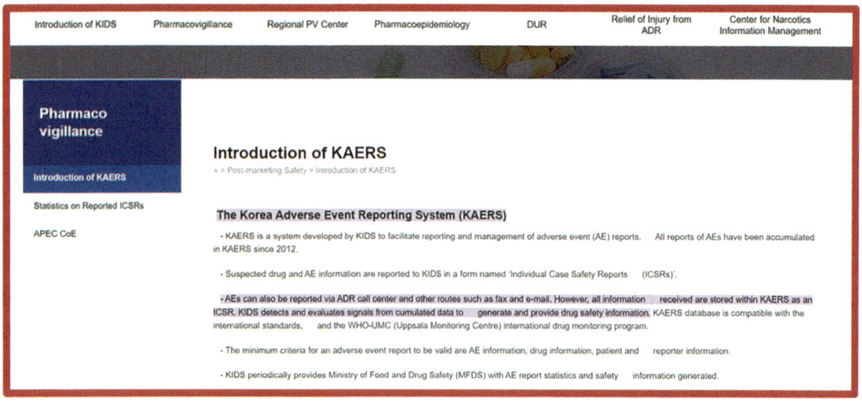

Fig. 3.7 Homepage of KAERS

3.3.7.2 Limitations

1. Underreporting of ADEs.
2. Incomplete data on patient characteristics, such as underlying diseases and concomitant medications.

3.4 Commercially Used Pharmacovigilance Database

3.4.1 AB Cube: Safety Easy

AB cube (https://www.ab-cube.com/pharmacovigilance/) is a safety software firm which offered, a cloud-based PV programme. It was introduced in 2006 as the first PV programme on the cloud, offering an alternative to on-premise software. AB Cube's cloud-based technology attempts to make medication safety simple and help to complete the case processing very easily by the help of SafetyEasy® Suite. A multiVigilance management tool called SafetyEasy® Suite is intended to speed up the procedures involved in PV, medical device vigilance, and nutrivigilance, cosmetovigilance. The programme improves productivity and lowers costs by tracking submission deadlines, ensuring data dependability and quality, and ensuring compliance. It offers a direct connection to regulatory bodies, removing the requirement for manual report filing (SAFETYEASY® SUITE 2023). The Homeage of AB Cube: Safety Easy is presented in Fig. 3.8.

3.4.1.1 Characteristics of AB Cube: Safety Easy

- **MultiVigilance management**: SafetyEasy® Suite is a unified solution for managing all vigilances in one place.
- **Automation:** The solution integrates automation with existing drug safety processes.

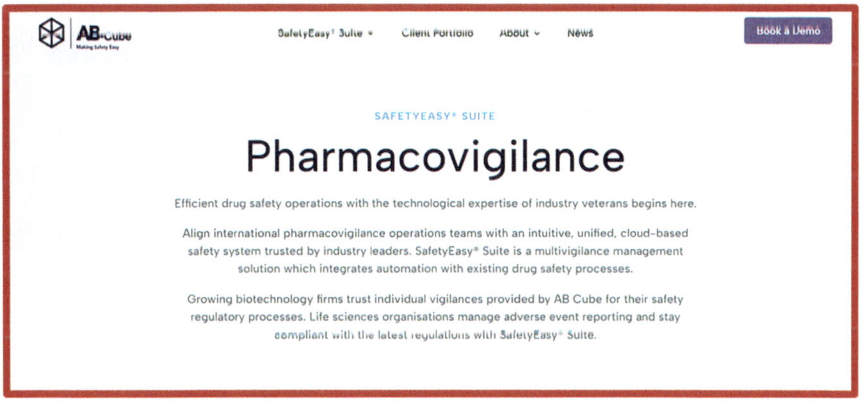

Fig. 3.8 Homeage of AB Cube: Safety Easy

- **Regulatory compliance:** SafetyEasy® Suite is designed to support and obey the E2B(R3) EudraVigilance system and MedDRA coding standards.
- **Streamlined workflows:** SafetyEasy® Suite enables users to generate, review, submit, and maintain PV, medical device vigilance, cosmetovigilance, and nutri-vigilance data and event reports by the help of single application.

3.4.2 Oracle: Argus Safety Database

Oracle Argus Safety Database (https://www.oracle.com/in/life-sciences/pharmacovigilance/argus-safety-case-management/) is a complete PV platform that helps pharmaceutical businesses and clinical trial organizations to improve worldwide compliance, quickly integrate risk management, and make safer safety choice (Kumar and Khan 2015). The Homepage of Oracle: Argus Safety Database is presented in Fig. 3.9.

3.4.2.1 Characteristics of AB Cube: Safety Easy

- **Global case processing:** A huge volume of cases including pre- and post-market pharmaceuticals, biologics, vaccines, and medical devices may be processed effectively thanks to the automated worldwide case processing offered by the Argus database.
- **Signal detection:** Signal detection capabilities in the Argus database make it possible to spot potential trends and safety hazards.
- **Adverse Event Case Management:** Argus Safety is a market-leading system for processing, assessing, and disclosing adverse event cases originating in pre- and post-market medications, biologics, vaccines, and medical devices.
- **Data Entry and Intake:** Utilize Argus Safety to input and receive cases of adverse events, code medical and product terminology, carry out medical and

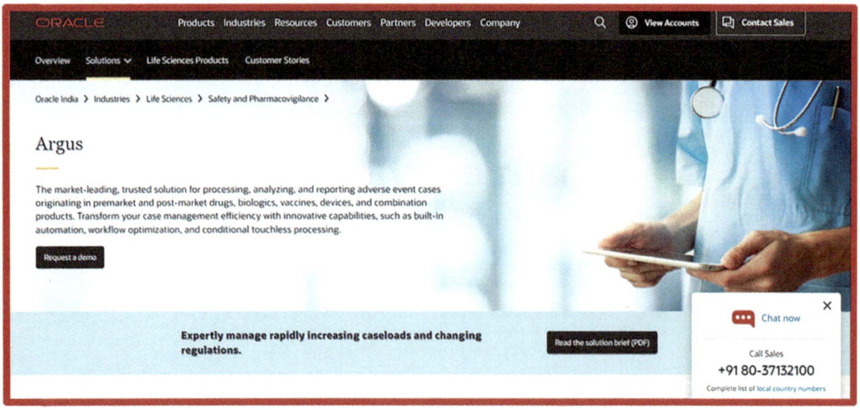

Fig. 3.9 Homepage of Oracle: Argus Safety Database

quality evaluations, and produce periodic and fast reports for partners and health regulators.

- **Schema Creation**: Installing the Argus Safety Schema Creation Tool will enable you to use the interactive user interface (Oracle.com).
- **Training and Certification**: You can implement, configure, browse, and operate Oracle Argus products after completing Oracle Argus Training.
- **Safety Process Automation**: Deep and integrated safety capability that expands to millions of instances is provided out of the box by Argus Safety, and it is simple to match with your business and safety procedures. By automating worldwide case processing, periodic reporting, E2B input and submission, complete reporting, thorough analytics, and Japanese safety operations, the platform allows a highly scalable end-to-end safety process.

3.4.3 Aris Global: ARISg/LifeSphere Safety

ArisGlobal provides LifeSphere Safety suite (https://lifesphere.arisglobal.com/platform/safety/), an end-to-end pharmaceutical safety platform. The main goal of the LifeSphere Safety is to allow PV or drug safety teams throughout all over the world to save time and effort while guaranteeing regulatory compliance in medication safety. It is built is a way that all types of firms such as large biopharma to small and emerging firms can use it with flexible licencing and it help to provide high quality services to the pharmaceutical industries. The software is working on the principle of artificial intelligence and machine learning. Additionally, LifeSphere Safety has Signal and Risk Management, Reporting and Analytics, and other features. To aid PV teams in locating, assessing, and managing safety signals and hazards, the field of signal and risk management was created (Aris Global 2023). The Homepage of Aris Global: ARISg/LifeSphere Safety is presented in Fig. 3.10.

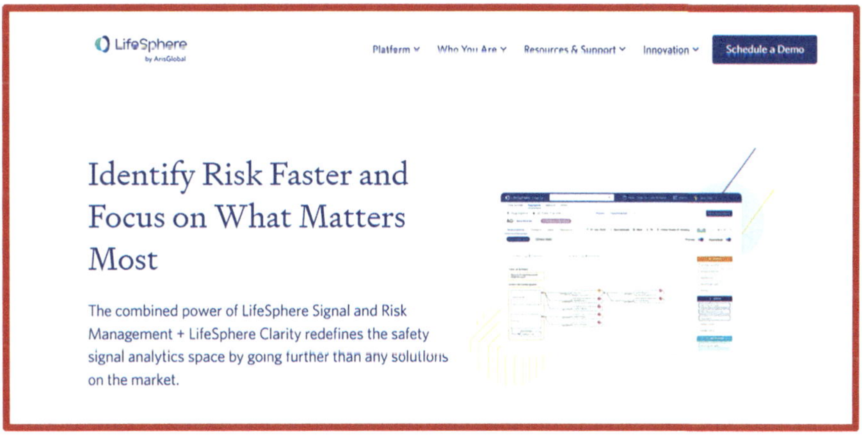

Fig. 3.10 Homepage of Aris Global: ARISg/LifeSphere Safety

3.4.3.1 Characteristics of Aris Global: ARISg/LifeSphere Safety

- **Unified platform:** It is work on integrated and next-generation SaaS safety platform which helps to provide a standardized PV workflow globally.
- **AI/ML and analytics capabilities**: The AI/ML, cognitive automation, and analytics abilities of LifeSphere Safety, which were created and tested with industry leaders, provide the tools that you have to need or manage the highly complex operations efficiently without affecting the quality or compliance of the data.
- **Reporting and analytics:** LifeSphere Reporting offers robust data to support your decision-making.
- **Signal and risk management**: It is a safety risk management tool that analyses data to find pertinent signals and systematically manages them.
- **Safety document distribution**: LifeSphere Safety Document Distribution allows you use automated procedures to guarantee that your reports, such as SUSAR, are filed correctly and on time (Lifesphere.arisglobal.com).

3.4.4 Ennov Pharmacovigilance Suite

Ennov PV Suite (https://en.ennov.com/solutions/pharmacovigilance/) is software that developed to aids in collecting, managing, analysis, and reporting of adverse drug reactions in human and animals in a single database. The suite includes data collection, signal identification and analysis of PV activities. It maintains the flexibility, quality, and supports. Ennov PV Suite is software created to assist in the gathering, managing, evaluating, and reporting of adverse events in humans or animals in a single database. The suite covers data collection, signal identification and analysis, core and extended PV activities, flexibility, quality, support, and price. The suite's capabilities, such case intake and triage, make it possible to analyse cases quickly and identify those that need more inquiry. Ennov PV Suite, have another application called PV-Works Vet, uses adaptable and compliant PV software to assure veterinary safety (Ennov Pharmacovigilance Suite 2023).

The PV Suite from Ennov is intended to make data management simple and help you fulfil important reporting deadlines. Additionally, the suite contains signal detection and management capabilities, which allow proactive risk management by assisting in the identification of possible safety hazards (Ennov Pharmacovigilance Suite 2023). The screenshot of Homepage of Ennov software is presented in Fig. 3.11.

3.4.4.1 Characteristics of Ennov Pharmacovigilance Suite

- **A single authoritative source:** It is a single unified database which optimize the PV operations with compliance, manage and maintain all PV data.
- **Ensure compliance:** It complies with the requirements for establishing and maintaining regulatory compliance, including electronic reporting.
- **Increased visibility:** It helps to get a real-time overview of your safety database as it have dynamic metrics and dashboards.

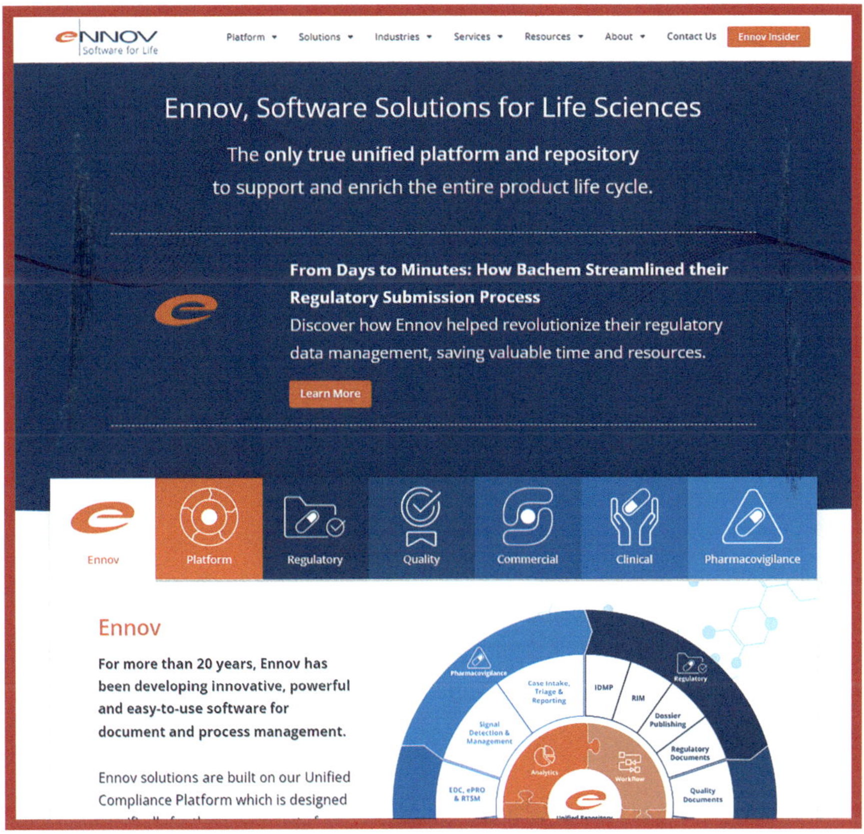

Fig. 3.11 Homepage of Ennov software

3.4.5 BaseCon

BaseCon (https://basecon.com/basecon/safetybase-interchange/) is a corporate firm that provides PV software solutions and it was founded in 1999. It is an easily accessible PV and drug safety tool that obeys with E2B R3 standards and reliably handles electronic adverse event reports. The BaseCon work with experts and drug safety professionals who are dedicated for the development and implementation of verified solutions and who are familiar with the commercial requirements of the pharmaceutical sector (BaseCon 2023). The Homepage of BaseCon is presented in Fig. 3.12.

3.4.5.1 Characteristics of BaseCon

- It is a very user-friendly system developed to process electronic adverse event reports swiftly.
- BaseCon3 is used to control and manage the evaluation of cases which helps to achieve compliance and update reporting to authorities.

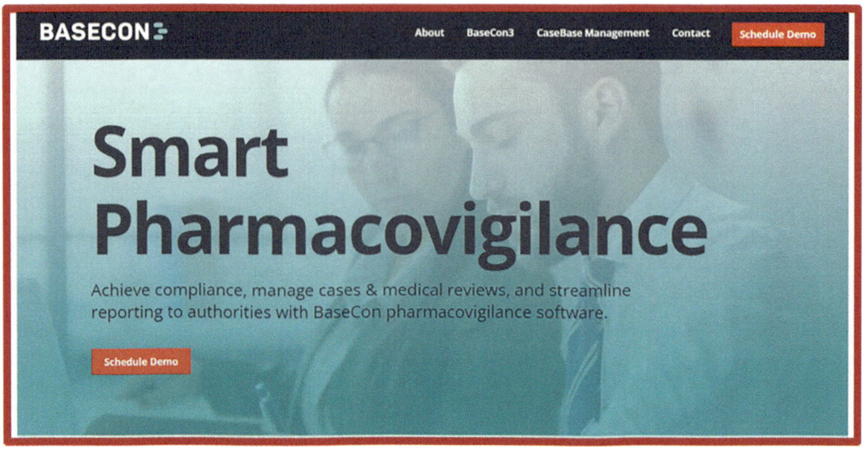

Fig. 3.12 Homepage of BaseCon

- It is a cloud-based tool that helps to users to receive or mange the invoices, receipts, and other financial papers to keep track of financial information.
- It can be access through the mobile phone at is have a mobile application.

3.5 Conclusion

In conclusion, the use of databases in PV is critical on a worldwide scale, allowing medication safety monitoring and evaluation. These databases enable the identification of probable adverse drug responses, the early detection of safety signals, and enhanced patient care through comprehensive and systematic data collection, analysis, and reporting. While various databases are utilized worldwide, such as the LifeSphere Safety MultiVigilance, (ARISg) from ArisGlobal, Oracle's Argus Safety, AB Cube: Safety Easy, Ennov PV Suite, VigiBase and BaseCon, they all share the common goal of enhancing pharmacovigilance efforts by providing valuable insights into the safety profiles of medications. Continuous advancement and integration of sophisticated technologies, such as artificial intelligence and machine learning, improves the efficacy and efficiency of these databases, ultimately contributing to the overall improvement of public health and patient safety.

References

Aris Global: ARISg/LifeSphere safety; available at LifeSphere Signal & Risk Management | Safety AI | ArisGlobal. Accessed 1 Sept 2023

BaseCon.: BaseCon.com. Accessed 1 Sept 2023

Ennov Pharmacovigilance Suite. Ennov Pharmacovigilance Suite—Ennov Software for Life. Accessed 1 Sept 2023

EudraVigilance.: Available at EudraVigilance | European Medicines Agency (europa.eu). Accessed 1 Sept 2023

FDA Adverse Event Reporting System (FAERS). https://open.fda.gov/data/faers. Accessed 1 Sept 2023

Javed F, Kumar A (2023) Identification of signal of clindamycin associated renal failure acute: a disproportionality analysis. Curr Drug Saf 19:123–128

Jha N, Palaian S, Shankar PR, Santosh KC, Kshetry PB (2021) Situation analysis of the pharmacovigilance system in Nepal using the indicator-based pharmacovigilance assessment tool (IPAT). J Pharm Health Serv Res 12(4):485–491

Kim S, Kang T, Chung TK, Choi Y, Hong Y, Jung K, Lee H (2023) Automatic extraction of comprehensive drug safety information from adverse drug event narratives in the Korea adverse event reporting system using natural language processing techniques. Drug Saf 46:781–795

Kumar A, Khan H (2015) Signal detection and their assessment in pharmacovigilance. Open Pharmaceut Sci J 2(1):66

Lindquist M (2008) VigiBase, the WHO global ICSR database system: basic facts. Drug Inf J 42(5):409–419

Maity TS, Longo CJ (2020) Adverse drug reactions in Canada (2009–2018): insights from the Canada Vigilance Database. Healthc Q 23(1):40–46

Martin JH, Lucas C (2021) Reporting adverse drug events to the therapeutic goods administration. Aust Prescr 44(1):2

SAFETYEASY® SUITE. https://www.ab-cube.com/pharmacovigilance/. Accessed 1 Sept 2023

Suke SG, Kosta P, Negi H (2015) Role of pharmacovigilance in India: an overview. Online J Publ Health Inform 7(2):e223

"VigiBase: Uppsala monitoring centre." https://who-umc.org/vigibase. Accessed 1 Sept 2023

Processing of ADRs

4

Sweta Roy, Mukesh Nandave, and Anoop Kumar

4.1 Processing of ADRs

ADRs can range from mild and transient side effects to severe and life-threatening events. They are a significant concern in pharmacovigilance (PV), as they can impact patient safety, treatment adherence, and overall healthcare costs. Understanding ADRs is crucial for ensuring the safe and effective usage of medications (Montané and Santesmases 2020).

4.2 Collection of ADRs

The collection of ADRs is a critical process in PV, which involves systematic monitoring, identification, assessment, and reporting of adverse events or reaction related to the usage of medications and medical products. Proper collection of ADR data is essential to ensure patient safety, detect potential safety signals, and inform regulatory judgments and risk management strategies. Detailed overview of the collection of adverse drug reactions is as follows:

1. **Spontaneous Reporting System:** The most common method used to gather ADRs is through spontaneous reporting systems. Consumers (patients or their carers) and healthcare professionals can voluntarily report any potential adverse effects they see or experience while receiving medication, including doctors, nurses, chemists, and consumers. These reports are often submitted to national regulatory or to PV regulatory agencies (Asiamah et al. 2022).

S. Roy (✉) · M. Nandave · A. Kumar
Department of Pharmacology, Delhi Pharmaceutical Sciences and Research University, New Delhi, India
e-mail: mukeshnandave@gmail.com; anoopdpsru@dpsru.edu.in

M. Nandave, A. Kumar (eds.), *Pharmacovigilance Essentials*,
https://doi.org/10.1007/978-981-99-8949-2_4

2. **Reporting Through Healthcare Programmes**: In some nations, like the US FDA runs programs like MedWatch, which allow consumers and medical experts to file reports about ADRs directly to regulating body (MedWatch 2023).
3. **Clinical Trials:** The gathering of ADR data depends heavily on clinical trials. The investigational medicine may cause adverse effects or reactions; thus, researchers constantly monitor participants throughout these trials. Each incident that is noticed is carefully recorded, and its seriousness and connection to the drug are measured (Allen et al. 2018).
4. **Electronic Health Records (EHRs):** EHRs provide helpful information for ADR collection. Direct entry of adverse event information into the patient's electronic medical records allows for analysis of the documents for safety signals (Feng et al. 2019).
5. **Literature Surveillance:** PV specialists conduct systematic medical literature reviews to find published case reports, clinical trials, and other pertinent sources that offer details on probable ADRs. Safety assessments then take into account these findings (Inácio et al. 2017).
6. **Patient Support Programmes and Social Media:** Pharmaceutical companies may encourage patients to report any adverse effects that occur while undergoing treatment through patient support programs they have established. Patients can also formally report ADRs and share their experiences on social media sites and online forums (Omar and Harris 2016).
7. **Reporting from Healthcare Facilities:** In some countries, healthcare facilities must report adverse events associated with medication use to national regulatory authorities. These reports are valuable for gathering data on ADRs in real-world clinical settings (Katusiime et al. 2015).
8. **Active Surveillance Programmes:** Several countries may adopt active surveillance programs to systematically monitor extensive healthcare databases or electronic health records for suspected ADRs (Huang et al. 2014).
9. **Vaccine Adverse Event Reporting System (VAERS):** For collection of adverse event of vaccines, the VAERS in the USA and similar systems in other countries are used to collect reports related to the vaccination (Chen et al. 1994).

4.3 Processing of Adverse Drug Reactions (ADRs)

The processing of ADRs consists of a systematic approach to collecting, assessing, and managing data about the safety of drugs and medical devices.

The processing steps of ADRs are discussed below:

4.3.1 Case Identification and Collection

Medical professionals, patients, and consumers report adverse events to regulatory agencies, drug manufacturers or PV centers. Cases can be gathered from various sources including literature, clinical trials, and unprompted reporting.

4.3.2 Data Entry

Information from the reported cases is entered into a PV database.

4.3.3 Quality Checks

Severe quality checks are performed to ensure the accuracy and fullness of data entry. Data validation, consistency checks, and reconciliation of discrepancies are carried out to maintain data integrity.

4.3.4 Individual Case Safety Reports (ICSRs) Creation

ICSRs are created, compiling all relevant details of a single AE case. These reports are the foundation for analyzing and assessing ADRs.

4.3.5 Signal Detection and Analysis

PV databases are analyzed for potential safety signals, unexpected patterns, or associations between drugs and adverse events. Quantitative methods, such as disproportionality analysis, are used to identify signals.

4.3.6 Signal Evaluation and Refinement

Detected signals are evaluated further through case series analysis, literature reviews, and clinical expertise. False positives are ruled out, and potentially significant signals are investigated in-depth.

4.3.7 Reporting to Regulatory Authorities

Regulatory authorities require timely reporting of ADRs. Electronic transmission of ICSRs in compliance with international standards [such as the E2B (R3) format] is used for efficient communication with regulatory agencies.

4.3.8 Risk Communication and Management

Regulatory agencies and pharmaceutical companies communicate ADRs possibilities to healthcare professionals and the community through safety alerts, label updates, and other relevant means. Risk management strategies may also be implemented.

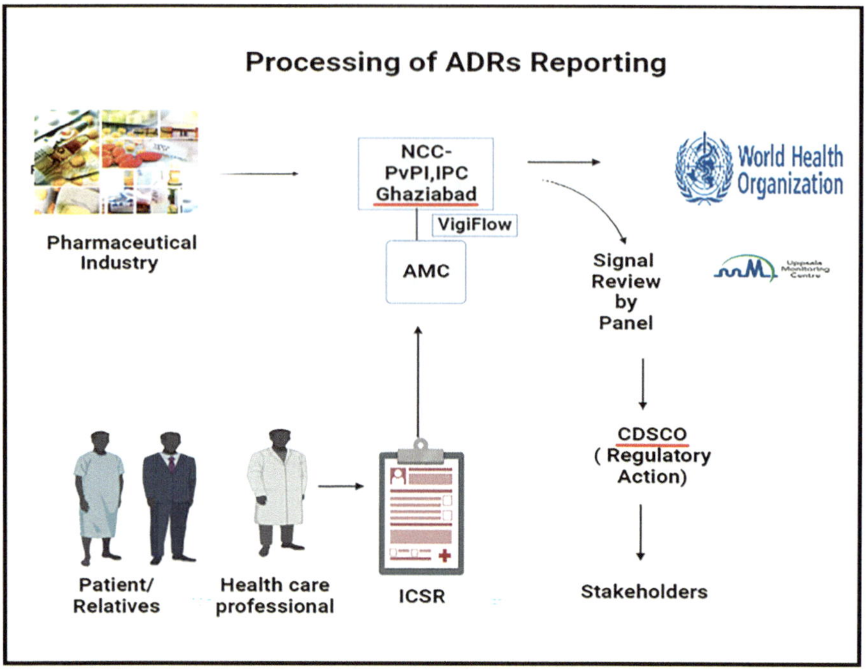

Fig. 4.1 Processing of ADRs

4.3.9 Continuous Monitoring and Assessment

The pharmacovigilance process is on-going. Additional cases, new information, and emerging signals are continuously monitored, and risk–benefit assessments are updated as needed (Indian Pharmacopoeia Commission (IPC) 2023) (Fig. 4.1).

4.4 Reporting of ADRs in India

Drugs must be under surveillance through a PV system to enhance human health and safety. Indian Pharmacopeia Commission (IPC), which is located in Ghaziabad, working as a National Coordination Centre (NCC) for Pharmacovigilance Programme of India (PvPI). Various ADR monitoring centers (AMCs) were established in medical college/hospitals in India. Currently, there are a total of 760 AMCs who are working on ADR reports under NCC-PvPI there is a specific form for reporting in India (Indian Pharmacopoeia Commission (IPC) 2023) (Annexures 4(a) and 4(b)).

ADR reporting is a critical component of pharmacovigilance, which aims to monitor and confirm the safety of medications and other medical products. Specific forms are available for their respective countries (CIOMS I FORM 2023; MedWatch Forms for FDA Safety Reporting 2023) (Annexures 4(c)).

4.4.1 Reporting Requirements

PvPI promotes reporting all suspected ADRs, whether there is a proven causal link between the suspected ADRs and a drug. This includes known, unknown, severe, non-serious, frequent, or infrequent reactions. You can report ADRs associated with the use of allopathic medications, vaccinations, conventional medications, medical equipment, contrast media, etc.

4.4.2 Where to File a Report

ADRs can be reported to NCCs or AMCs by all healthcare providers (doctors, dentists, chemists, and nurses), patients, and consumers. The pharmaceutical industry can also give NCC individual case safety data related to its product.

4.4.3 How to File a Report

ADRs reporting is available in various languages across India, i.e., English, Hindi, Assamese, Bengali, Gujarati, Kannada, Malayalam, Marathi, Oriya, Tamil, and Telugu. The IPC website provides forms for reporting suspected ADR for consumers and healthcare practitioners. ADRs can also be reported by calling the PvPI helpline at (18001803024) on weekdays between 9:00 a.m. and 5:30 p.m. The public can now access the android mobile ADR reporting application (Fig. 4.2).

4.4.4 To Whom Report is Submitted

Reporters can send their completed ADR reporting form directly to NCC or their local AMC. These reports are verified by medical experts in the case of AMC, this information entered into VigiFlow and sent to NCC for additional evaluation. After a final NCC evaluation, these findings are submitted to the WHO-Uppsala Monitoring Centre. Received data is entered into a drug safety database. These data are analyzed and evaluated via experts to find new signals. No legal action is taken against the reporter. The identification of patients is confidential and protected (Indian Pharmacopoeia Commission (IPC) 2023).

4.5 Selection of Database

Choosing the appropriate database for ADR reporting is crucial in ensuring accurate and comprehensive data collection.

EudraVigilance is being used by EU (European Medicines Agency (EMA) 2023).

FDA Adverse Event Reporting System (FAERS) is used in the USA (FDA Adverse Event Reporting System 2023).

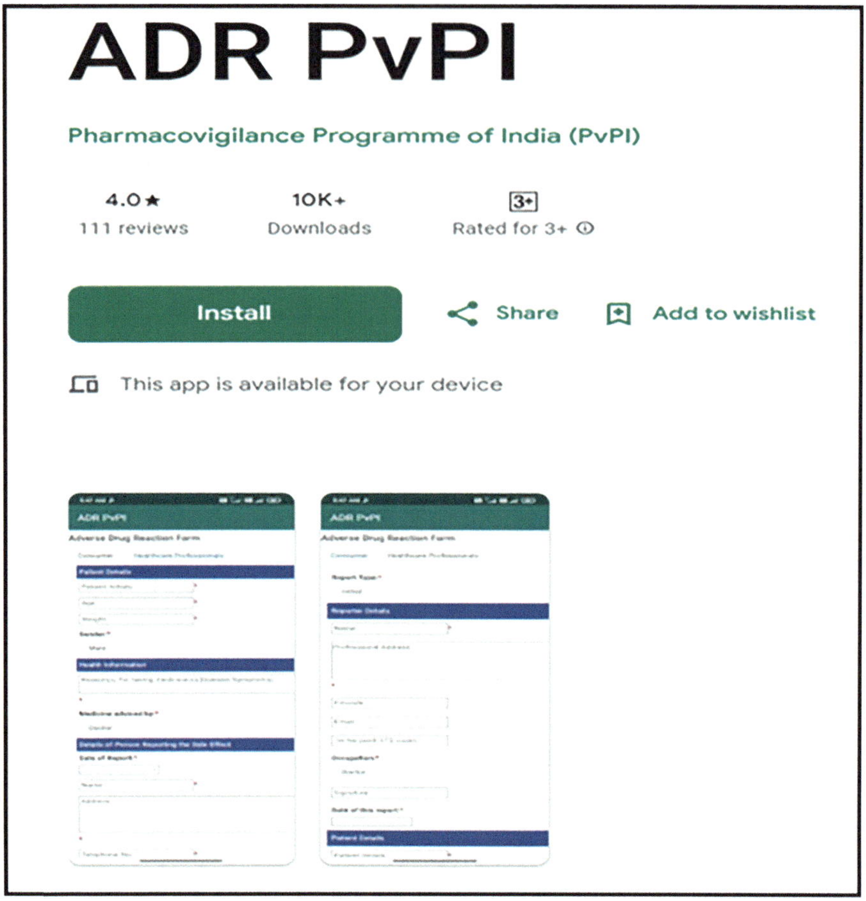

Fig. 4.2 ADR application for online reporting

VigiFlow used across the globe (VigiFlow|UMC 2023).
Argus used in pharma industries (Argus 2023).

4.6 Validity of ADRs

The validity of ADR forms, often called adverse event reporting forms or ICSRs, are crucial for ensuring the accuracy, reliability, and usefulness of the data collected in PV. Valid forms play important role in identifying, evaluating and managing the safety of drugs and medical products. Detailed exploration of the factors that contribute to the validity of ADR forms are as follows:

1. **Data Completeness:** Valid ADR forms should capture all relevant information about the adverse event. This includes patient demographics, medical history,

concomitant medications and details about the suspected drugs, AE description, timeline and outcome. Only complete forms can lead to complete assessments and ensure accurate causality determination.

2. **Standardized Terminology:** Standardized medical terminology like MedDRA (Medical Dictionary for Regulatory Activities), ensures that the AE description is consistent and interpretable across different reports. This aids in data analysis and aggregation.
3. **Timeliness:** Reporting adverse events promptly after they occur improves the accuracy of the information. Delays in reporting can lead to memory bias and missing critical details.
4. **Source Documentation:** Valid ADR forms should be based on source documents such as medical records, laboratory reports, and patient interviews. Relying on accurate source documentation ensures the credibility of the reported information.
5. **Transparent and Detailed Description:** ADR forms should provide a clear and detailed narrative of the AE. This includes information about the symptoms, severity, context, and relevant medical interventions. The description should be comprehensive enough for a thorough assessment.
6. **Relationship to the Drug:** A valid ADR forms should include information about the suspected drug, including its name, dosage, frequency, route of administration, start and stop dates. This information is essential for determining the causal connection among the drug and the AE.
7. **Patient Information:** Detailed patient information, including age, gender, weight, and relevant medical history is critical for understanding the context of the AE and assessing its significance.
8. **Healthcare Professional Details:** In cases where a healthcare professional completes the ADR forms, their contact information, specialty, and affiliation provide credibility to the report and facilitate follow-up if needed.
9. **Concomitant Medications:** Other medications the patient takes concurrently can help identify potential interactions or underlying medical conditions that may contribute to the AE.
10. **Follow-Up Information:** If available details about the patient's progress and any subsequent interventions or outcomes should be included. This helps in evaluating the evolution of the AE.
11. **Data Integrity and Validation:** Data validation checks and quality control measures should be implemented to identify discrepancies or errors in the reported data.
12. **Confidentiality and Privacy:** The form should adhere to data protection and patient privacy regulations to maintain the confidentiality of patient information.
13. **Electronic Systems and Automation:** Electronic ADR reporting systems can enhance validity by providing structured data entry, auto-population of specific fields, and validation checks to ensure completeness and accuracy (Indian Pharmacopoeia Commission (IPC) 2023).

4.6.1 Validity of ADRS Form

For the validity of case, four data are required, i.e., patient identification, a reaction, a potential drug, and a reporter with a known identity (Coleman and Pontefract 2016).

4.6.2 Seriousness of ADRs

It is an unfavorable reaction that leads to a fatality, poses a life-threatening risk, hospitalization or an extension of on-going hospital stays leads to long-lasting or notable disability or inability or results in a congenital anomaly (EMA 2023).

4.7 Triage of Case

In PV, triage is prioritizing incoming reports based on several factors. The goal of triage is to place a potential AE report into one of three categories: non-serious case, serious case, or no case. The factors considered during triage include the receiving date, seriousness, causality, and predictability assessment. The chronology or association in time (or place) among drug intake and the event and the recent information of the nature and rate of reoccurrence of adverse events are also considered. Triage is a crucial step in the PV process, because it helps to identify and prioritize cases that require further investigation and analysis. By prioritizing issues, pharmacovigilance professionals can ensure that they focus on the most critical cases and take appropriate action to minimize the risk of harm to patients (Bhangale et al. 2017).

4.7.1 The Triage Procedure Is Described in Detail Below

1. **Receiving Adverse Event Reports:** Various sources including healthcare workers, patients, clinical trial investigators, electronic health records, literature surveillance and mechanisms for spontaneous reporting are used to gather AE reports. Important details regarding the patient, the suspected drug or medical device and the description of the adverse event are all included in these reports.
2. **Initial Severity Assessment:** One of the main goals of triage is to identify and prioritize major AE that require quick care. AE are rated according to severity based on factors including congenital abnormalities, hospitalization, impairment or life-threatening conditions. Serious adverse events are escalated for more analysis and suitable action.
3. **Categorization by Clinical Significance:** Apart from severity cases are also triaged based on their clinical significance. AE that are well-known side effects of the medication or medical product may be categorized as less urgent than events that suggest new or unexpected safety concerns. This categorization ensures that potential safety signals are noticed.

4. **Signal Detection and Clustering:** As part of the triage process it may be necessary to use signal detection techniques to spot patterns or groups of adverse events that could be signs of possible safety issues. To find new or uncommon ADR occurrences that need further research data mining and statistical methods can be used to uncover signals of disproportionate reporting.
5. **Expert Review:** In some cases AE reports may call for a pharmacologist or a specialist in a particular therapeutic field to conduct an expert review. Making informed decisions regarding the importance and priority of the reported adverse occurrences can significantly benefit from expert perspectives.
6. **Follow-up and timeliness:** The triage procedure emphasizes the significance of timeliness. AE reports are quickly assessed and categorized to guarantee no crucial safety signals are missed due to a delayed assessment. Furthermore, instances may be tracked down and followed up on to gather fresh information that might affect their classification.
7. **Documentation and Reporting:** All actions and decisions to prioritize AE reports are meticulously documented throughout the triage process to maintain transparency and accountability. The triage results are reported to relevant stakeholders including regulatory authorities and pharmaceutical companies to facilitate appropriate risk management strategies (Bhangale et al. 2017).

4.8 Listedness of Cases

Listedness of cases in PV refers to a classification of reported ADRs based on their presence in the product labeling or prescribing information of a particular drug. It is a critical aspect of PV for determining the strength of the link between a medication and an AE. When a case is classified as listed, the reported ADR is explicitly mentioned in the drug product labeling as a potential adverse effect. This listing is typically based on a comprehensive evaluation of clinical trial data, post-marketing surveillance and scientific literature indicating a recognized and established association among the drug and the specific adverse event. On the other hand cases classified as unlisted suggest that reported ADR is not currently mentioned in the drug product labeling or prescribing information. This could be due to various reasons including the rare event, recently discovered or lack of sufficient evidence to establish a definitive causal relationship.

The listedness of cases plays a crucial role in PV signal detection and risk management. A listed ADR indicates a known and acknowledged safety concern requiring continued monitoring and potential regulatory actions. On the other hand, unlisted ADRs may signify emerging safety signals or the need for further investigation to assess their significance and potential impact on patient safety. Regularly assessing and updating drug product labeling is essential to accurately reflect new safety information through continuous monitoring and evaluation PV systems strive to ensure that the listedness of cases remains up to date facilitating the effective communication of known risks associated with medications and supporting informed decision-making by healthcare professionals and patients (18.i. Listedness/ Expectedness assessment 2019).

4.8.1 Categories of Listedness

Company's Common Core Data Sheet (CDS) or Company's Core Sheet Information (CCSI), and serves as the comprehensive "Global Reference Safety Information" document managed by a sponsor which is an entity holding the marketing authorization for medicinal products. CCSI or CDS contains the entirety of safety information about a medicinal product gathered from global patient experiences and is regularly updated as needed.

When it comes to categorizing adverse reactions:

"Listed" refers to adverse reactions thoroughly documented in the CDC/CCSI.
"Unlisted" pertains to adverse reactions that lack comprehensive documentation in the CDC/CCSI.

Depending on the type of therapeutic product (in development or already on the market) and the specific Reference Safety Information (RSI) document (e.g., CCDS, CCSI, USPI, and SmPC) different terms are used to describe adverse events during the assessment.

Well Documented: An AE, Serious Adverse Event (SAE), or ADR is considered "Well Documented" when it is entirely known and its "Nature, Seriousness, Specificity, and Conclusion" align through the existing safety information found in the Reference Safety Information (RSI) document.

Not Well Documented: If an AE, SAE, or ADR reported for a patient is entirely "new" or represents a "new aspect" of a previously known event or reaction according to the RSI. It is categorized as "Not Well Documented."

If the reported event is entirely new, it is automatically classified as "unexpected," "unlabelled," or "unlisted" (depending on the RSI type referred to for assessment).

Suppose the reported event is already documented in the RSI but does not align with the available information, such as a new fact involving a change in nature, severity, specificity or outcome for a known reaction. In that case, it falls under the "Not Well Documented" (Assessing Labelling, Listedness, Expectedness in Pharmacovigilance 2023).

4.9 Medical Coding

It is done to correctly classify the reported medical terminology so that they can be examine and analyzed. Data Collection Instruments (DCIs) also known as Case Record Forms/Report Forms (CRFs) for paper-based trials or electronic Case Record/Report Forms (eCRFs) for web-based trials, data generated during clinical trials is recorded. These studies gather and record data on AE, medical histories

(MH) and concurrent medications (CM) administered in addition to the study drug on the appropriate DCIs. A multi-center clinical study consists of numerous trial sites with investigators from various ethnic backgrounds. All of the trial data is eventually subjected to additional analysis. Consequently, the use of standard medical dictionaries is necessary for medical coding. The above information including AE, SAEs, MH, CM, and other categories is typically coded (Babre 2010).

4.9.1 Most Commonly Used Medical Dictionaries

- MedDRA stands for Medical Dictionary for Regulatory Activities.
- SMQs stands for Standardized MedDRA Queries.
- WHODrug Global stands for World Health Organization Drug Global.
- WHO-ART stands for World Health Organization Adverse Reactions Terminology.
- WHO-DDE stands for World Health Organization Drug Dictionary Enhanced.
- COSTART stands for Coding Symbols for Thesaurus of Adverse Reaction Terms.
- ICD9M stands for International Classification Of Disease, Ninth Revision, Clinical Modification.
- WHO Herbal Dictionary (WHO-HD) (Babre 2010; Nair 2013).

4.9.2 Medical Dictionary for Regulatory Activities (MedDRA)

In 1990s, MedDRA was established by the International Council for Harmonisation (ICH) of Technical Requirements for Pharmaceuticals for Human Use to enhance the global sharing of regulatory data concerning medical products intended for human use. It is a comprehensive and precise standardized medical terminology. Everyone has access to ICH's potent tool MedDRA for the purpose of registering, recording and overseeing the safety of medical products both prior to and following their approval for commercial distribution. These days improved global patient health protection is possible because of its expanding use by regulatory agencies, pharmaceutical corporations, clinical research organizations, and health care professionals (MedDRA 2023). Medical conditions, manifestations, clinical indicators, undesired drug responses, and recommended treatment uses. Names of investigations, qualitative findings, surgical and medical techniques, and medical/social histories are all covered by MedDRA. The terms study design, patient demographics, numerical numbers, and qualifiers such as those characterizing illness severity or frequency are not included in the MedDRA nomenclature for drugs or devices. MedDRA can record AE and MH in clinical trials, analyze and tabulate the data from these and accelerate the process of sending safety information to governmental regulatory authorities. The ICH MedDRA Maintenance and Support Services Organization (MSSO) are charged with maintaining, developing, and disseminating MedDRA is under the general control of the ICH MedDRA

Management Committee which oversees the organization's operations. ICH also created the Japanese Maintenance Organization (JMO) to assist users in Japan which collaborates closely with MSSO. The ICH MedDRA Management Committee oversees the continuing improvement of MedDRA to satisfy the changing demands of its users across the globe. MedDRA has been used for over 20 years and has amassed a wealth of expertise. MedDRA serves for both entering data (coding) and retrieving/analyzing data, and a set of documents on its use are created and updated by the present ICH M1 Points to Consider Working Group. All MedDRA subscribers receive additional crucial supporting documents from the ICH as an added advantage of their membership. There are also exploratory guides for Standardised MedDRA Queries (SMQs) and MedDRA as well as a guide for using the electronic MedDRA files that explains the file format with each new MedDRA version; the MSSO updates these documents which are accessible in all MedDRA languages (MedDRA 2023).

4.9.3 MedDRA Employs a Hierarchical Framework Comprising Five Primary Tiers

4.9.3.1 System-Organ Class (SOC)

Positioned at the apex of the hierarchy. SOCs serve as the highest level of classification, organizing related medical conditions or symptoms. Examples of SOC encompass categories like "Infections and Infestations," "Cardiac Disorders," and "Nervous System Disorders."

4.9.3.2 High-Level Group Term (HLGT)

Each SOC is further subdivided into HLGTs offering more refined groupings of associated terms. As an illustration, within the "Cardiac Disorders" SOC one can encounter HLGTs such as "Cardiac arrhythmias" or "Myocardial disorders."

4.9.3.3 High-Level Term (HLT)

HLGTs are further broken down into HLTs, providing even more specific groupings. For example, beneath the "Myocardial disorders" HLGT one may discover HLTs like "Myocardial infarction" or "Myocarditis."

4.9.3.4 Preferred Term (PT)

PT represents the most granular level within the hierarchy. These are precise medical terms describing particular conditions, symptoms or medical events. Examples of PTs encompass terms like "Atrial fibrillation" or "Chest pain."

4.9.3.5 Lowest Level Term (LLT)

The LLT represents the most intricate level, furnishing synonyms, abbreviations, and specific language variations for PT. LLT are employed for purposes such as coding and indexing. The hierarchical structure of MedDRA facilitates the standardized classification and encoding of medical data, simplifying the task of regulatory bodies and healthcare professionals in reporting and analyzing adverse events and medical information.

4.9.3.6 Advantage

1. **Standardization:** MedDRA offers an internationally recognized language that is standardized for recording, coding, and analyzing medical data. It allows for uniform and consistent reporting of adverse events in various healthcare settings, clinical studies, and regulatory agencies.
2. **The degree of detail and flexibility:** The MedDRA system provides a hierarchical framework that precisely calculates adverse occurrences. Its several levels of words enable accurate and detailed classification of diverse medical illnesses, symptoms, and therapies. This level of specificity makes it easier to pinpoint individual safety issues and allows for thorough study.
3. **Support for Multiple Languages:** MedDRA provides multilingual support essential for international coordination and cooperation in drug safety monitoring and regulatory processes. It improves global PV collaboration by enabling the consistent reporting and analysis of adverse events across various language areas.
4. **Integration with Other Systems:** MedDRA is compatible with several healthcare databases, electronic health records (EHRs), and PV systems allowing easy data sharing and interoperability. The capabilities for data analysis are improved signal detection is made more accessible and this integration supports post-marketing surveillance.
5. **For correct use of MedDRA:** Free training is given to all subscribers on different subjects are covered in a variety of formats including in-person training, online sessions like webinars and pre-recorded video presentations. MSSO personnel also provide training in numerous languages including but not limited to English, French, Spanish, German, Korean, Russian, and Chinese.
6. **ICH has established a governance framework to foster and safeguard the integrity of MedDRA**. The ICH MedDRA MSSO, which is in charge of maintaining, developing, and disseminating MedDRA reports to the ICH MedDRA Management Committee which is responsible for the general direction of MedDRA. To help users in Japan. ICH has also created a Japanese Maintenance Organization (JMO) which closely collaborates with MSSO (MedDRA 2023).

4.9.4 Standardized MedDRA Queries (SMQs)

It is an essential part of MeDRA. SMQs were created to make it easier to evaluate and compare adverse events recorded in clinical trials uniformly, to conduct post-marketing observation and PV activities. They make it easier to analyze and assess safety data in a variety of healthcare settings by enabling the grouping of similar medical terminology into clinically relevant categories (Standardised MedDRA Queries 2023).

SMQs are tools designed to make it easier to retrieve data that has been MedDRA-coded as a preliminary stage in examining remedy safety concerns in PV and clinical development after a thorough examination, testing, analysis, and expert discussion. SMQs are validated and predetermined MedDRA terms are compiled. The MedDRA particular SMQ function is a powerful tool for supporting investigation and reporting on safety. The SMQ themes are designed to cover the crucial PV issues required by governing and company users. Every time a release of a new version of MedDRA, the MSSO updates the SMQs. There are currently more than 100 SMQs available (CIOMS I FORM 2023). When required more SMQs are established. Small selections of the SMQs that are now available to users are as follows:

- Medication errors.
- Severe cutaneous adverse reactions.
- Hyperglycemia/new onset diabetes mellitus.
- Allergic reaction.
- Lack of efficacy/effect.
- COVID–19.
- Ischemic heart disease.
- Depression and suicide/self-injury.
- Drug abuse, addiction and withdrawal.
- Anaphylactic response.
- Central nervous system vascular disorders.
- Seizures.

In response to the MedDRA user community's recognition of the need for standardized tools to simplify the identification and retrieval of safety data SMQs were developed. Initially, similar search criteria were used to generate the MedDRA Special Search Categories (SSCs). However, after an extended period of MedDRA usage, the biopharmaceutical community (comprising supervisors and industry stakeholders) determined that there was a growing demand for expanded resources. Consequently, in early 2002, the MedDRA MSSO initiated the development of MedDRA Analytical Groupings (MAGs) in response to this need. MAGs were described as groups of terms derived from various levels of the MedDRA hierarchy (with LLTs being the general exception), spanning multiple or all MedDRA SOCs. These terms encompassed indications, symptoms, physical characteristics, lab findings, and other information from physiological tests along with associated social circumstances related to the specified medical situation or subject of interest indicated by the MAG's name (Große-Michaelis et al. 2023).

The Council for International Organisations of Medical Sciences (CIOMS) launched a separate initiative at the same time that MAGs were developed at the MSSO to address the necessity for unique inquiries or groupings using MedDRA-coded data; these groupings were known as Standardized Search Queries (SSQs). It was evident that the ideas behind MAGs and SSQs were very similar and aimed to address the perception that MedDRA needed a retrieval tool. CIOMS and the MSSO consequently concurred that combining the CIOMS Working Group's and the MSSO's efforts to produce this tool was in the best interests of the user community. The previous "MAG" and "SSQ" names were discarded to acknowledge the collaborative work and a name for these new standard groupings was decided upon. Since, May 2003 the collaborative work undertaken by the CIOMS Working Group and the MSSO has been identified as SMQs. The ICH MedDRA Management Committee approved the collaborative endeavor in November 2003 and the ICH method was used to produce SMQs. The CIOMS Working Group comprises of prominent scientists representing various drug regulatory agency, global pharmaceutical industry, the MSSO, the JMO, the WHO, and additional organizations (Standardised MedDRA Queries 2023).

4.9.4.1 Advantages

SMQs improve data analysis

1. By making it possible to aggregate safety data from many research databases or clinical trials. In order to facilitate decision-making and risk–benefit calculations, researchers and regulators can use SMQs to produce insightful summaries and comparative analyses of safety data.
2. *Saving time and money*

By offering predetermined sets of keywords and SMQs help users save time and money. Researchers and analysts can quickly apply SMQs to safety data without intensive manual coding or data mining. This simplifies the analysis procedure, lowers expenses, and enables more effective use of resources (Standardised MedDRA Queries 2023).

4.9.5 WHODRUG Global

The Uppsala Monitoring Centre maintains WHODrug Global, a global pharmaceutical information source. It offers a consistent drug vocabulary with precise wording when classifying concurrent drugs due to its distinctive drug code hierarchy and comprehensive coverage. Nearly 150 countries' pharmaceutical product information including active components, anatomical and therapeutic classifications is evaluated using the dictionary to identify medicine names (Centre UM 2023a). Both prescription drugs and herbal treatments are included in the WHODrug database. Contrast media, biotech goods, blood products, diagnostic agents, Over-the-Counter (OTC), and pharmacist-dispensed medications are all examples of conventional medicines. The US FDA and the EMA registered goods and chemicals are frequently tracked. The information is regularly updated and made available to subscribers as text and CSV files through their browsing tool. WHODrug insight, twice a year on first March and September. The WHODRUG dictionary has undergone significant growth.

4.9.5.1 Advantages

1. With the support of WHODrug Global's standardized data you may produce safer medicines by more quickly identifying drug-related issues in clinical trials and pharmacovigilance. This is because coding data with WHODrug facilitates more efficient analysis which quickens the regulatory filing procedure.

2. When understanding and assessing drug safety concerns in VigiBase, WHO's global collection of adverse event reports, WHODrug Global is crucial. WHODrug Global offers identification and data aggregation at various degrees of accuracy to provide efficient and precise safety signal analysis.
3. The US FDA has mandated WHODrug Global for studies beginning after March 15(2019) and the Pharmaceutical and Medical Devices Agency (PMDA) of Japan has endorsed it. WHODrug intends to help China's PV system grow and integrate with the global community by publishing a Chinese dictionary version.
4. WHODrug provides awareness as it is essential to have effective communication techniques in the problematic field of PV. People can keep informed about the advantages and disadvantages of medications the value of reporting adverse drug reactions (ADRs) and the significance of patient-physician communication when there is a reliable flow of pertinent information (Centre UM 2023a).

4.9.6 World Health Organization Adverse Reactions Terminology (WHO-ART)

WHO-ART is a dictionary designed to provide a foundation for the logical categorization of terminology related to adverse reactions. The WHO Collaborating Centre for International Drug Monitoring, UMC maintains the system. It has a hierarchical structure with four levels; it is presented in English and translated into French, Portuguese, Italian, German, and Spanish. It is updated quarterly.

4.9.6.1 Structure of WHO-ART

- 32 System-organ classes categorizing body organ groups
- 180 High-level terms used to group preferred terms
- 2085 Preferred terms serving as principal descriptors for adverse reactions
- 3445 Included terms acting as synonyms for preferred terms.

These are the terms that are used:

1. **Preferred terms:** PT is the main words used to describe adverse drug reactions. They are the most common terminology used on the input side and can also be used on the output side.
2. **High-level terms:** HLT are collective words for connected or related concepts that facilitate quick information retrieval. For instance, thrombophlebitis leg and thrombophlebitis arm are two distinct preferred words yet they are categorized under the high-level term thrombophlebitis. Not all Preferred words may have been given a high-level term.
3. **System-organ classes:** These are categories of adverse reactions. Preferred terminology for the same system is sometimes used on the output side. The maximum number of system-organ classes to which a preferred word can be

assigned is three. For example, respiratory depression is categorized under respiratory and central nervous system disorders. System-organ classes are given a fixed amount of a preferred word which does not fluctuate in response to particular reports. Each Preferred term's initial SOCs listed are considered the most crucial.

4. **Included terms:** These words have a solid connection to preferred terms. They help locate the appropriate preferred word for the reported adverse reaction's correct classification.
5. **Record number system:** Each preferred word is given a record number (ARECNO) assigned sequentially as it is introduced. Sequence number (SEQ) 001 is permanently assigned to preferred phrases. The record number for included terms is the same as for the corresponding preferred terms but the sequence number is more significant. Where high-level words are present all pertinent preferred terms are allocated a high-level term link (HL LINK). A record number of the preferred term which is also the high-level term is referenced by a high-level term link.

4.9.6.2 Advantages

1. Multiple language support.
2. Wide-ranging Medical Conditions, Symptoms, and Interventions are covered. WHO-ART contains comprehensive words and concepts relevant to adverse reactions. It enables accurate and exact reporting and analysis by providing extensive and specific coding of adverse occurrences.
3. Integration with PV Systems: By integrating WHO-ART with PV databases and systems adverse reaction data may be recorded and analyzed effectively and uniformly. Its integration improves data management, signal detection, and regulatory reporting processes.
4. WHO-ART has a long history and has undergone constant updating and improvement. In pharmacovigilance and drug safety its use and adoption over many years have made it a reputable and well-established word (Centre UM 2023b).

4.9.7 WHO-DDE: World Health Organization Drug Dictionary Enhanced

WHO Drug Dictionary Enhanced (WHO DDE) is the world's foremost and extensively utilized drug coding resource. Its contents guarantee the precise coding, analysis, understanding, and reporting of clinical study and safety data.

WHO DDE is accessible online through the UMC's WHO Drug Dictionary Browser. Most importantly, WHO DDE addresses the explicit need for a uniform drug dictionary and precise terminology during the coding of concurrent medications. This facilitates expedited submissions to national regulatory authorities.

The following statement from the FDA's Centre for Drug Evaluation and Research (CDER) underscores the significance it places on Clinical Research Organizations (CROs) and sponsors communicating drug data standardized. The center also emphasizes the importance of employing a standard dictionary and precise terminology throughout clinical trials and subsequent submissions including concomitant medicines, techniques, symptoms, study drug names, and medical history indications.

For instance, a sponsor or governing body receives data that deviates from dictionary conventions due to misspellings; automated data analysis processes may become unfeasible. This needs to improve the competence of the review process. It is highly recommended that a consistent drug dictionary terminology such as the WHO Drug Dictionary be employed for coding concurrent medications adapted from the CDER common data standards issues document, Version 1.1/December 2011.

4.9.7.1 Codes Serve the Purpose of Distinguishing Distinct Characteristics of a Product

Within WHO DDE, codes exist that recognize pharmaceutical names and assess details related to medicinal products, encompassing their active constituents and therapeutic applications. Each medication is identified by a drug code and an exclusive Medicinal Product ID that encapsulates essential attributes such as the country of origin, the entity holding the marketing approval, the pharmaceutical form and the potency. WHO DDE discloses information about a product's structure, therapeutic application and its chemical category as determined by the Anatomical Therapeutic Chemical (ATC) classification system.

Standardized Drug Groupings (SDGs) drug lists categorized by pharmacological class or metabolism are a featured component of WHO DDE. These lists can be employed to detect drug interactions in ICSRs, explore alternative causes of adverse events or identify medications that might impact the outcomes of a clinical study (refer to the SDG product evidence below for more information).

4.9.7.2 Improved Accuracy and Reporting of Clinical Trial and Safety Data

The hierarchical product coding and classification systems within WHO DDE, along with its array of robust analytical tools are invaluable. They facilitate the accurate and comprehensive coding, explanation and assessment of concurrent medications in clinical study and safety information. Systems like ATC and SDGs improve the consolidation of statistics during analysis and reporting.

4.9.7.3 On-Going Expansion Encompassing More Products, Countries and Services

WHO DDE continually evolves to align with the ever-changing clinical environment including new drug categories, regulatory demands and trials performed in new geographic regions. Fresh categories country-specific therapeutic practices and nomenclature are regularly incorporated.

The WHO DDE receives quarterly additions of new drug terms and substances. By December 1 (2012) it had accumulated a vast database of over two million (2,021,870) medicinal products. This comprehensive data set was compiled from information collected across more than a hundred countries globally and encompassed a total of 263,451 unique medicinal product names. Additionally, UMC provides quarterly updates for SDGs.

4.9.7.4 Related UMC Drug Dictionary Offerings

The latest expansions to the dictionary collection include the introduction of the Drug Dictionary China (DDC) and the expansion of the Cross Reference Tool (CRT) Japan, specifically designed for the Asian market. Information about these products is available below. Expect on-going development and expansion of the UMC drug dictionaries in the coming years.

4.9.7.5 Advantages

1. **Accurate Drug Identification:** WHO DDE provides precise drug coding and terminology ensuring accurate drug identification.
2. **Enhanced Safety Data:** It helps identify drug-drug interactions, adverse event causes and trial interference improving safety data analysis.
3. **Global Coverage:** With data from over 100 countries, it supports comprehensive drug information and coding worldwide.
4. **Regular Updates:** WHO DDE adapts to evolving clinical landscapes with quarterly new products and substance additions.
5. **Supports Research:** Its classification systems aid in statistical analysis and reporting facilitating research.
6. **Expanded Offerings:** Associated products like DDC and CRT Japan extend their utility for specific regions (WHO Drug Dictionary Enhanced (WHO DDE) 2023).

4.9.8 COSTART: Coding Symbols for Thesaurus of Adverse Reaction Terms

It is a standardized medical terms system used primarily to code and classify adverse reactions and events associated with drugs and other medical interventions. Developed and maintained by the US FDA, COSTART plays a crucial role in PV, medical research and healthcare data management.

4.9.8.1 Overview of COSTART

1. **Purpose and background:** COSTART was developed to provide a standardized and consistent way to code, classify adverse events and reactions related to drugs and medical interventions. Its primary purpose is to facilitate collecting, reporting, and analyzing adverse event data in PV and clinical research.
2. **Structure and organization:** COSTART has a hierarchical structure where adverse reaction terms are organized into a tree-like taxonomy. It includes a comprehensive list of AE terms; each assigned a unique alphanumeric code. The terminology is organized into various levels with broader categories at higher levels and more specific terms at lower levels. This hierarchical structure allows for detailed coding of adverse events.

3. **Utilization in PV:** COSTART is widely used by pharmaceutical companies, healthcare professionals, and regulatory agencies including the FDA, for reporting and analyzing adverse drug reactions. When reported AE are coded using COSTART terms allowing for standardized and consistent documentation. This facilitates the identification of patterns and trends in adverse events associated with specific drugs or classes of drugs.
4. **Adaptations and Changes:** Over time COSTART has undergone revisions and updates to keep pace with advancements in medicine and changing terminology. One notable update was the integration of COSTART into the MedDRA, a more comprehensive terminology system for adverse event coding. This transition aimed to improve harmonization and standardization in pharmacovigilance.

4.9.8.2 Advantages

1. COSTART provides a standardized and consistent way to document and communicate adverse event data which is crucial for patient safety and regulatory compliance.
2. It facilitates data analysis and signal detection helping to identify potential safety concerns related to specific drugs or interventions.
3. Researchers and healthcare professionals can use COSTART to conduct epidemiological studies and assess the safety profiles of medications (Coding Symbols 2023).

4.9.9 ICD-9-CM: International Classification of Disease, Ninth Revision, Clinical Modification

The International Classification of Diseases, Ninth Revision, Clinical Modification (ICD-9-CM) was a widely used coding system for classifying diseases and medical procedures. It was a critical tool for healthcare providers, insurance companies, researchers, and policymakers to document and analyze health-related data. However, it was replaced mainly by ICD-10-CM in the US with the transition completed in October 2015.

Detailed overview of ICD-9-CM concerning its historical significance given below:

4.9.9.1 Development and Purpose

ICD-9-CM was developed by the WHO and adopted in the USA to classify diseases, injuries and medical procedures for billing, statistical and epidemiological purposes. It provided a standardized way to document health-related information, ensuring consistency and accuracy in healthcare data.

4.9.9.2 Structure and Coding System

ICD-9-CM consisted of two main volumes: Volume 1 which covered diagnosis codes and Volume 2 which covered procedure codes. The diagnosis codes in Volume

1 were numeric and included three and five-digit codes. The first three digits represented the category or disease group while the additional two provided more specific details. Procedure codes in volume 2 included three-digit numeric codes that described medical procedures and interventions.

4.9.9.3 Utilization in Healthcare

Healthcare providers use ICD-9-CM codes to document patient diagnoses and procedures for billing purposes, insurance claims, and medical records. Researchers and epidemiologists relied on ICD-9-CM to analyze and study disease trends, outcomes, and healthcare utilization. It is a crucial tool for health policy and healthcare management enabling the evaluation of disease burdens and the allocation of resources.

4.9.9.4 Advantages

1. The advantages of ICD-9-CM included its wide adoption and long-standing use which allowed for consistency in healthcare coding and data exchange.
2. Transition to ICD-10-CM recognizing the need for a more comprehensive and detailed coding system. The US transitioned from ICD-9-CM to ICD-10-CM on October 1, 2015.
3. ICD-10-CM offers a broader range of codes with greater specificity, accommodating medical knowledge and technology advances.
4. Standardization: ICD-9-CM provided a standardized and consistent classification of diseases, conditions, and medical procedures. This uniformity was essential for healthcare providers, insurance companies, and government agencies to effectively communicate and exchange healthcare data.
5. Billing and Reimbursement: It was instrumental in healthcare billing and reimbursement processes. Accurate ICD-9-CM coding ensured that healthcare services were billed correctly, reducing errors, and potential disputes between providers and payers.
6. Epidemiological Research: ICD-9-CM codes facilitated epidemiological research by enabling the tracking and analysis of disease prevalence, incidence, and trends over time. Researchers could use these codes to study public health issues and identify areas that require intervention.
7. Resource Allocation: Healthcare administrators and policymakers used ICD-9-CM data to allocate resources efficiently. It helped them identify areas with high disease burdens and prioritize healthcare services and funding accordingly.
8. Clinical Decision Support: ICD-9-CM codes could be used for clinical decision support systems in clinical practice. They allowed healthcare professionals to access information about diagnoses, treatments, and associated procedures quickly.
9. Historical Data: ICD-9-CM served as a valuable historical record of healthcare data. Researchers and historians could analyze past healthcare trends and outcomes providing insights into the evolution of medical practice and public health.

10. Ease of Implementation: Due to its relatively simple coding structure, ICD-9-CM was easier to implement compared to more complex coding systems. This made it accessible to a wide range of healthcare providers and facilities.
11. Interoperability: ICD-9-CM codes were widely recognized and used internationally, fostering interoperability in healthcare data exchange. This global recognition allowed for the sharing medical information across borders (International Classification of Diseases 2023).

4.9.10 WHO Herbal Dictionary (WHO-HD)

An herbal dictionary would be a reference or resource that provides information about various medicinal herbs and plants. These dictionaries typically include details about the botanical characteristics, traditional uses, medicinal properties, preparation methods, and potential side effects or interactions of herbs. They can be valuable tools for herbalists, healthcare practitioners, researchers, and individuals interested in herbal remedies.

4.9.10.1 Advantages

1. **Standardization:** A WHO sponsored herbal dictionary could help standardize the terminology and information related to medicinal plants and their uses. This would promote consistency and accuracy in the field of herbal medicine.
2. **Global Reference:** As a product of the WHO such a dictionary would likely have international recognition and credibility making it a trusted reference for herbalists and healthcare providers worldwide.
3. **Safety and Efficacy:** The WHO-HD could provide information on the safety and efficacy of various herbal remedies helping healthcare professionals make informed decisions about their use and potential risks.
4. **Education and Research:** It could serve as an educational resource for healthcare students, traditional healers, and researchers in herbal medicine.
5. **Cross-Cultural Exchange:** A WHO-HD could facilitate the exchange of knowledge about traditional herbal practices across different cultures and regions.
6. **Regulatory Guidance:** Regulatory authorities could use the information in the dictionary to establish guidelines and regulations for using herbal products.
7. **Public Health:** By promoting the safe and effective use of herbal remedies, the WHO-HD could contribute to public health goals, particularly in regions where traditional medicine is widely practiced (WHO Herbal Dictionary (WHO HD) 2023).

4.10 Causality Assessment System

Causality assessment of ADRs plays crucial role in estimating the strength of the connection between drug exposure and the occurrence of adverse reactions. Various stakeholders undertake this assessment, including practitioner, researchers, the pharmaceutical company, and controllers. It is an essential part of all medical specialties since finding the offending substance or drugs can save lives and help to stop future damage to the body's systems (Pande 2018). Assessing causality helps to establish a link between drug exposure and adverse effects. It supports the risk–benefit analysis, signal detection, and patient safety decisions made by doctors, academics, and regulators. Diagnostic testing is frequently unavailable and adverse effects are rarely medication-specific. Therefore, establishing a causal connection is crucial for a precise diagnosis and suitable treatment with appropriate management. WHO-UMC and the Naranjo probability scale are widely used methods for causality assessment. These techniques provide a quick and efficient way to assess the possibility of a link between drug exposure and adverse effects. Due to many spontaneous ADR reports, regulatory organizations including the FDA and the EMA have emphasized the necessity for proven mechanisms and protocols for causation assessment. Recognizing the need for a systematic approach, regulatory bodies have outlined guidelines and recommendations for causality assessment. The Council for International Organizations of Medical Sciences (CIOMS) VI (2005), FDA guidance (2010), and EMA guideline (2012) provide valuable frameworks for the analysis of individual cases. These guidelines contribute to process standardization, improve the accuracy and consistency of causality determinations. Pharmaceutical businesses with a global reach have embraced organized methods for recording ADRs and doing causality analyses. These companies are aware of the value of causality analysis in assuring the security and effectiveness of their products.

However, similar structured approaches are frequently slower to be adopted in academia and general medical procedures highlighting a need for greater awareness and adoption in these contexts. Due to the complexity of adverse reactions, causality assessment is concerned with difficulties. Adverse reactions rarely fit neatly into the "certain" or "unlikely" categories. Most reactions fall within the "possible" or "probably" category falling somewhere in the middle. Rechallenges for confirmation are frequently unethically justifiable and diagnostic testing might need to be revised. These difficulties highlight the need for reliable causality assessment techniques for facilitating precise decision-making. A critical compo nent of medical practice is determining the cause(s) of ADRs which helps to identify the offending drugs and reduce patient harm. Trying-and-true techniques like the WHO-UMC system and the Naranjo probability scale offer straight forward yet efficient instruments for determining causality. Regulatory recommendations and guidelines further encourage the adoption of verified causality assessment systems. Although the pharmaceutical sector has made strides in putting organized techniques into practice, more awareness and adoption are needed in academics and ordinary medical practice. Resolving the issues with causality assessment will increase patient safety and aid in developing evidence-based risk–benefit decisions (Naidu 2013).

4.10.1 Principles of Causality Assessment

All causality evaluation techniques or instruments adhere to the following four fundamental ADR diagnosis principles: (1) The timing of the medicine administration and the drug response, (2) biological plausibility, (3) overcoming obstacles, and (4) overcoming new obstacles.

It is known as positive pre-challenge or negative pre-challenge when dechallenge or rechallenge has already happened (Pande 2018).

4.10.2 Basic Standards for Causality

- Pharmacology and prior experience with ADRs.
- The relationship between the AE and the drug (at the time and location).
- Medical and biological plausibility.
- Probability or exclusion of other explanations.
- Examine the entire report and make a note of any missing data (Nair 2013). The types of causality assessment are shown in Fig. 4.3.

4.10.3 Causality Assessment Determination Methods

4.10.3.1 Clinical Judgment/Global Introspection

When practicing global introspection, the clinician's skills and knowledge are crucial. General physicians and dermatologists have benefited from sharing information regarding suspected drug reaction cases with peers or experts via email, WhatsApp, or other modern communication platforms. This has boosted physician's clinical judgment and insight.

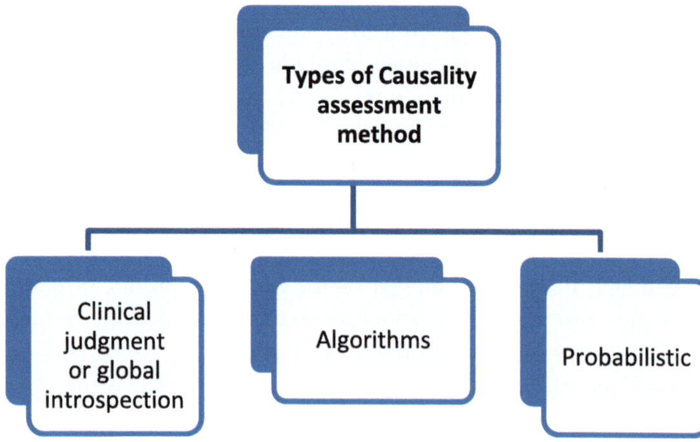

Fig. 4.3 Types of causality assessment

Two types of clinical judgment/global introspection are: WHO–UMC scale and Swedish method (Pande 2018).

4.10.3.2 WHO UPSALA Monitoring Centre (UMC) Method

WHO-UMC system is widely used approaches for assessing causality between drug usage and ADRs in admitted patients. According to a comparative study involving ten different approaches, it has been recognized as the most reliable method for establishing causal relationships. This system evaluates report quality and it is considered as a suitable and well-organized tool for individual case reports. Due to its strong performance global introspection approaches are now preferred over statistical approaches. Given the current state of the art professional judgment continues to play a crucial role in ADR causality evaluation. However, certain restrictions of global introspection techniques such as the need for reproducibility among judges have been identified. Factors like individual experience and diverse professional backgrounds may lead to discrepancies in attributing causal relationships to ADRs. To address this issue, the involvement of multi-professional teams in the assessment process becomes essential to validate the categorization of ADRs (Table 4.1).

Table 4.1 WHO-UMC Causality scale

Causality term	Assessment criteria
Certain	• Event or laboratory test abnormality with a plausible time relationship to drug intake • It cannot be explained by disease or other drugs • Response to withdrawal plausible (pharmacologically, pathologically) • Event definitive pharmacologically or phenomenologically (i.e., an objective and specific medical disorder or a recognized pharmacological phenomenon) • Rechallenge satisfactory, if necessary
Probable/Likely	• Event or laboratory test abnormality, with a reasonable time relationship to drug intake • Unlikely to be attributed to disease or other drugs • Response to withdrawal clinically reasonable • Rechallenge not required
Possible	• Event or laboratory test abnormality, with a reasonable time relationship to drug intake • It could also be explained by disease or other drugs • Information on drug withdrawal may be lacking or unclear
Unlikely	• Event or laboratory test abnormality, with a time to drug intake that makes a relationship improbable (but not impossible) • Disease or other drugs provide plausible explanations
Conditional/ Unclassified	• Event or laboratory test abnormality • More data for proper assessment is needed • Additional data under examination
Unassessable/ Unclassifiable	• A report suggesting an adverse reaction • Cannot be judged because the information is insufficient or contradictory • Data cannot be supplemented or verified (National Institutes of Health 2019)

Training session is available to these judges to standardize the application of the WHO-UMC approach for study of the causality evaluation of potential ADR. The record of ADR causality evaluation in a form created especially for this study was used in the expert adjudication procedure. According to WHO-UMC standards ADRs are divided into six classes: certain, possible, unlikely, probable, conditional, and unassessable/unclassifiable (WHO-UMC System 2023).

4.10.4 Algorithmic Methods

The given ADR is classified as certain, probable, plausible or unlikely using straightforward algorithms that are frequently questionnaire-based causality assessment tools (CATs).

These are some algorithmic methods that are commonly used: Naranjo's algorithm, Jones algorithm, Karch algorithm, Bégaud algorithm, Kramer algorithm, and adverse drug reactions advisory committee guidelines.

4.10.4.1 Naranjo Scale

The Naranjo algorithm also known as the adverse drug reaction probability scale. The ADR probability scale includes a specific form and instructions for its completion. The total scores achievable on the scale range from −4 to +13 with different point values assigned to each question. Based on the final score obtained the likelihood of the adverse drug reaction can be categorized into four levels. The reaction is come under definite if the score is 9 or more. A score ranging from 5 to 8 indicates a probable reaction. A score between 1 and 4 suggests a possible reaction, while a score of 0 or less implies a doubtful connection to the drug. The ADR Probability Scale provides a structured and standardized approach to evaluate the probability of ADRs, aiding healthcare professionals in determining the level of certainty associated with the reaction. It allows for systematically categorizing reactions into different probability levels, facilitating appropriate clinical decision-making and further evaluation.

The Naranjo algorithm, also known as the Naranjo scale, is a 10-item scale which was developed by Naranjo et al. in the year 1991 at the University of Toronto to support standardizes the causality assessment for all ADRs. Mainly the purpose of designing this scale for controlled trials and new medicine registration studies rather than routine clinical practice. However, it is simple to apply and commonly used. The Naranjo algorithm was implemented at Roche from 2001 to 2009 to assist in triaging specific cases during case processing. However, its overall effectiveness was limited resulting in its subsequent withdrawal.

The ADR probability scale comprises ten questions that require responses of "Yes," "No," or "Do not know." Each answer is assigned a specific point value, ranging from −1, 0, +1, to +2. These points help in assessing the probability of an adverse drug reaction. The scale's design enables a systematic evaluation of various factors related to the reaction. By assigning appropriate values to the responses, the scale assists in quantifying the likelihood of an adverse event being caused by a

Table 4.2 Naranjo scale

Question	Yes	No	Do Not Know	Score
1. Are there previous conclusive reports on this reaction?	+1	0	0	
2. Did the adverse event appear after the suspected drug was administered?	+2	−1	0	
3. Did the adverse event improve when the drug was discontinued or a specific antagonist was administered?	+1	0	0	
4. Did the adverse event reappear when the drug was re-administered?	+2	−1	0	
5. Are there alternative causes that could, on their own, have caused the reaction?	−1	+2	0	
6. Did the reaction reappear when a placebo was given?	−1	+1	0	
7. Was the drug detected in blood or other fluids in concentrations known to be toxic?	+1	0	0	
8. Was the reaction more severe when the dose was increased or less severe when the dose was decreased?	+1	0	0	
9. Did the patient have a similar reaction to the same or similar drugs in any previous exposure?	+1	0	0	
10. Was the adverse event confirmed by any objective evidence?	+1	0	0	
	Total score:			

drug. This structured approach aids healthcare professionals in objectively analyzing and determining the causality between a drug and an observed adverse reaction (National Institutes of Health 2019) (Table 4.2).

The scoring of the Naranjo scale shows is as follows:

- ≥9 shows definite ADR.
- 5 to 8 shows probable ADR.
- 1 to 4 shows possible ADR.
- 0 shows doubtful ADR (National Institutes of Health 2019).

4.10.5 Probabilistic Method

Bayesian probability is an interpretation of probability in which probability is understood as a reasonable expectation expressing a state of knowledge or quantifying a personal conviction rather than as frequency or tendency of some happening.

4.10.5.1 Bayesian Method

Bayesian approaches use a unique and sophisticated statistical approach to determine the reason behind ADRs. The Bayesian Adverse Reaction Diagnostic Instrument (BARDI) is a part of it (Nair 2013). It determines the "posterior probability" or "posterior odds" of a certain drug reaction being caused by the drug. The prior odds factor is defined as the ratio of the predictable drug-related risk to the inherent risk of a certain AE. The likelihood ratio is determined based on the following factors: histories, the timing of the AE in relation to the drug, the event's characteristics, dechallenge, is refers as the signs and symptoms of drug withdrawal and rechallenge. Bayesian method is a statistical technique based on Bayes' theorem, a fundamental concept in probability theory. These methods update and quantify the degree of belief (probability) in a hypothesis or model based on new evidence or data. In pharmacovigilance and medical research, Bayesian methods are crucial in analyzing ADRs, conducting clinical trials and making informed drug safety and efficacy decisions. Here is a detailed explanation of Bayesian methods:

4.10.5.2 Bayes' Theorem

Before diving into Bayesian methods, let us understand Bayes' theorem. It is a fundamental probability formula that relates the probability of a hypothesis (H) given some observed evidence (E) to the probability of the evidence given the hypothesis:

$$P(\mathrm{H}|\mathrm{E}) = \left(P(\mathrm{E}|\mathrm{H}) * P(\mathrm{H})\right) / P(\mathrm{E}).$$

where:

P (H | E) is the posterior probability of the hypothesis given the evidence (updated probability after considering the new data).

P (E | H) is the likelihood of the evidence given the hypothesis (probability of observing the evidence if the hypothesis is true).

P (H) is the prior probability of the hypothesis (initial belief in the hypothesis before observing the evidence).

P (E) is the marginal likelihood or evidence (probability of observing the evidence).

The Bayes theorem, a cornerstone of probability theory is the foundation for Bayesian procedures which are statistical approaches (Berrar 2018).

4.10.5.3 Bayesian Methods in PV

Bayesian methods have several applications in pharmacovigilance and medical research:

1. **Signal Detection and ADR Analysis:** Bayesian methods are used to analyze safety data and detect potential signals of adverse drug reactions. By incorporating prior knowledge about drug safety and using observed ADR data, Bayesian approaches can provide more robust estimates of the risk associated with medication than traditional methods.
2. **Bayesian Network Analysis:** Bayesian networks are graphical models representing the relationships between variables and their conditional dependencies. In PV, Bayesian networks are employed to model complex interactions between drugs, diseases, and adverse events facilitating a better understanding of causality and contributing factors.
3. **Bayesian Meta-Analysis:** Bayesian meta-analysis combines data from multiple studies or clinical trials allowing for a more flexible and coherent analysis of

safety and efficacy data. This approach considers both within-study and between-study variability providing more precise estimates of treatment effects.

4. **Bayesian Adaptive Clinical Trials:** Bayesian methods are increasingly used in adaptive clinical trials where trial designs can be modified based on accumulating data. This approach allows for more efficient and informative trials as the sample size and design can be adjusted during the trial to optimize the decision-making process.
5. **Bayesian Hierarchical Models:** Bayesian hierarchical models account for heterogeneity in safety data, especially when dealing with data from different sources or populations. These models enable the borrowing of strength from related data subsets leading to improved estimates of ADR probabilities (Berry 2006).

4.11 Conclusion

The processing ADRs start from identification of ADRs, assessing, collecting, and reporting. Known ADR should be also mentioned in medical dictionary so that public will aware of the ADR. Every step plays a significant role and they have team member from different specialization overall, this is the most important PV guideline. However, underreporting is one of the major challenges which need to overcome in future.

References

18.i. Listedness/Expectedness Assessment—Introduction I Pharmacovigilance (2019). https://allaboutpharmacovigilance.org/18-i-listedness-expectedness-assessment-introduction/. Accessed 20 Sept 2023

Allen EN, Chandler CI, Mandimika N, Leisegang C, Barnes K (2018) Eliciting adverse effects data from participants in clinical trials. Cochrane Database Syst Rev 1:MR000039. https://doi.org/10.1002/14651858.MR000039.pub2

Argus. https://www.oracle.com/in/life-sciences/pharmacovigilance/argus-safety-case-management/. Accessed 20 September 2023

Asiamah M, Akuffo KO, Nortey P, Donkor N, Danso-Appiah A (2022) Spontaneous reporting of adverse drug reaction among health professionals in Ghana. Arch Publ Health 80(1):1–1. https://doi.org/10.1186/s13690-021-00783-1

Assessing Labelling, Listedness, Expectedness in Pharmacovigilance: Differences & Methodology used in assessment. https://www.linkedin.com/pulse/assessing-labelling-listedness-expectedness-used-and-vigilance/?trackingId=Kjertg2oT8aD0EmiNJ3aug%3D%3D. Accessed 20 Sept 2023

Babre D (2010) Medical coding in clinical trials. Perspect Clin Res 1(1):29. PMID: 21829779

Berrar D (2018) Bayes' theorem and naive Bayes classifier. In: Encyclopedia of bioinformatics and computational biology: ABC of bioinformatics, pp 403–412. https://www.researchgate.net/publication/324933572_Bayes'_Theorem_and_Naive_Bayes_Classifier

Berry DA (2006) Bayesian clinical trials. Nat Rev Drug Discov 5(1):27–36. https://doi.org/10.1038/nrd1927

Bhangale R, Vaity S, Kulkarni N (2017) A day in the life of a pharmacovigilance case processor. Perspect Clin Res 8(4):192. https://doi.org/10.4103/picr.PICR_120_17

Centre UM (2023a) WHODrug Global. https://who-umc.org/whodrug/whodrug-global/. Accessed 20 Sept 2023
Centre UM (2023b) WHO-ART legacy service. https://who-umc.org/vigibase/vigibase-services/who-art/. Accessed 20 Sept 2023
Chen RT, Rastogi SC, Mullen JR, Hayes SW, Cochi SL, Donlon JA, Wassilak SG (1994) The vaccine adverse event reporting system (VAERS). Vaccine 12(6):542–550. https://doi.org/10.1016/0264-410X(94)90315-8
CIOMS I FORM. https://cioms.ch/wp-content/uploads/2019/11/Fillable-Form_CIOMS-to-E2B.pdf. Accessed 20 Sept 2023
Coding Symbols for a Thesaurus of Adverse Reaction Terms—Classes. https://bioportal.bioontology.org/ontologies/COSTART. Accessed 20 Sept 2023
Coleman JJ, Pontefract SK (2016) Adverse drug reactions. Clin Med 16(5):481. https://doi.org/10.7861/clinmedicine.16-5-481
EMA. European Medicines Agency. Serious adverse reaction. https://www.ema.europa.eu/en/glossary/serious-adverse-reaction. Accessed 20 Sept 2023
European Medicines Agency (EMA). https://www.ema.europa.eu/en. Accessed 20 Sept 2023
FDA Adverse Event Reporting System. https://www.fda.gov/drugs/questions-and-answers-fdas-adverse-event-reporting-system-faers/fda-adverse-event-reporting-system-faers-public-dashboard. Accessed 20 Sept 2023
Feng C, Le D, McCoy AB (2019) Using electronic health records to identify adverse drug events in ambulatory care: a systematic review. Appl Clin Inform 10(01):123–128. https://doi.org/10.1055/s-0039-1677738
Große-Michaelis I, Proestel S, Rao RM, Dillman BS, Bader-Weder S, Macdonald L, Gregory W (2023) MedDRA labeling groupings to improve safety communication in product labels. Ther Innov Regul Sci 57(1):1–6. https://doi.org/10.1007/s43441-022-00393-1
Huang YL, Moon J, Segal JB (2014) A comparison of active adverse event surveillance systems worldwide. Drug Saf 37:581–596. https://doi.org/10.1007/s40264-014-0194-3
Inácio P, Cavaco A, Airaksinen M (2017) The value of patient reporting to the pharmacovigilance system: a systematic review. Br J Clin Pharmacol 83(2):227–246. https://doi.org/10.1111/bcp.13098
Indian Pharmacopoeia Commission (IPC). https://www.ipc.gov.in/. Accessed 20 Sept 2023
International Classification of Diseases, Ninth Revision, Clinical Modification (ICD-9-CM). https://www.cdc.gov/nchs/icd/icd9cm.htm. Accessed 20 Sept 2023
Katusiime B, Semakula D, Lubinga SJ (2015) Adverse drug reaction reporting among health care workers at Mulago National Referral and Teaching Hospital in Uganda. Afr Health Sci 15(4):1308–1317. https://doi.org/10.4314/ahs.v15i4.34
MedDRA. Welcome to MedDRA | MedDRA. https://www.meddra.org/. Accessed 20 Sept 2023
MedWatch: The FDA Safety Information and Adverse Event Reporting Program. https://www.fda.gov/safety/medwatch-fda-safety-information-and-adverse-event-reporting-program. Accessed 20 Sept 2023
MedWatch Forms for FDA Safety Reporting. https://www.fda.gov/safety/medical-product-safety-information/medwatch-forms-fda-safety-reporting. Accessed 20 Sept 2023
Montané E, Santesmases J (2020) Adverse drug reactions. Med Clin (Barc) 154(5):178–184. https://doi.org/10.1016/j.medcli.2019.08.007
Naidu RP (2013) Causality assessment: a brief insight into practices in pharmaceutical industry. Perspect Clin Res 4(4):233. https://doi.org/10.4103/2229-3485.120173
Nair GJ (2013) Ensuring quality in the coding process: a key differentiator for the accurate interpretation of safety data. Perspect Clin Res 4(3):181. https://doi.org/10.4103/2229-3485.115383
National Institutes of Health (2019) Adverse drug reaction probability scale (Naranjo) in drug induced liver injury. Clinical and Research Information on Drug-Induced Liver Injury, LiverTox. https://www.ncbi.nlm.nih.gov/books/NBK548069/
Omar I, Harris E (2016) The use of social media in ADR monitoring and reporting. J Pharmacovigil 4(223):2. https://doi.org/10.4172/2329-6887.1000223

Pande S (2018) Causality or relatedness assessment in adverse drug reaction and its relevance in dermatology. Indian J Dermatol 63(1):18. https://doi.org/10.4103/ijd.IJD_579_17

Standardised MedDRA Queries | MedDRA [Internet]. https://www.meddra.org/standardised-meddra-queries. Accessed 20 Sept 2023

VigiFlow|UMC. https://who-umc.org/pv-products/vigiflow/. Accessed 20 Sept 2023

WHO Drug Dictionary Enhanced (WHO DDE)—Pharmaceutical Business review. https://www.pharmaceutical-business-review.com/products/who-drug-dictionary-enhanced-who-dde/. Accessed 20 Sept 2023

WHO Herbal Dictionary (WHO HD)—Pharmaceutical Business review. https://www.pharmaceutical-business-review.com/products/who-herbal-dictionary-who-hd/. Accessed 20 Sept 2023

WHO-UMC System. The use of the WHO-UMC System for standardised case causality assessment. https://www.who.int/publications/m/item/WHO-causality-assessment. Accessed 20 Sept 2023

Aggregate Reporting

5

Rima Singh, Mukesh Nandave, Anoop Kumar, and Deepti Pandita

5.1 Introduction

From the development of a new drug to post-market surveillance, it is necessary to keep track of the entire information on a benefit–risk ratio before it reaches the market and is used in a larger, much wider population (Han 2022). Therefore, a systemic approach, i.e., aggregate report (AR) has been included to look at the safety profile.

An aggregate report is a cumulative report that examines the combined safety data from various sources systematically and gives conclusions to regulators worldwide with the gathered information on the safety profile for medicine over a longer time duration, it can be months or years, as opposed to solitary event reporting which involves only individual adverse event (AE) reports (Hendrickson et al. 2021). The International Council for Harmonization (ICH) first harmonized AR with regulatory authorities in 1996, with the ICH guideline E2C, clinical safety data management (Ojha and Bhargava 2022). These reports focus not on individual cases, but preferably on the outline of adverse drug reaction (ADR) and the serious adverse event (SAE) and pregnancy reports (Wang et al. 2021).

Marketing authorization holders (MAH) cannot evaluate the benefit–risk ratio profile and recognize a medicinal product's detailed safety characteristics at individual case safety levels (Karale and Patil 2022). In addition to presenting individual case safety reports, MAH also examines regular estimation of collective safety

R. Singh (✉) · M. Nandave · A. Kumar · D. Pandita
Department of Pharmacology, Delhi Pharmaceutical Sciences and Research University, New Delhi, India
e-mail: mukeshnandave@gmail.com; anoopdpsru@dpsru.edu.in

M. Nandave, A. Kumar (eds.), *Pharmacovigilance Essentials*,
https://doi.org/10.1007/978-981-99-8949-2_5

information obtained from different sources and presents the conclusions of ARs to drug regulators (Amiri et al. 2021).

5.2 Importance

Aggregate report has a vital role in ensuring patient safety profile, regulatory compliance, and the ongoing monitoring of the benefit–risk profile of drugs and medical products, such as:

5.2.1 Patient Safety

It allows for the identification and analysis of potential safety signals. By collecting AE data from various sources, patterns, and trends can emerge that might not be evident in individual case reports. This helps in detecting safety concerns early and taking appropriate actions to mitigate risks to patients.

5.2.2 Signal Detection

By analyzing aggregated safety data, potential safety signals can be detected. These signals might indicate previously unrecognized AE or patterns of ADR, which can then be investigated further to determine their significance and potential impact.

5.2.3 Risk Management

Aggregate report contributes to the overall risk management strategy for a drug or medical product. Identifying and understanding risks associated with a product allows regulatory agencies and manufacturers to implement risk minimization strategies, update product labeling, or even consider regulatory actions if necessary.

5.2.4 Regulatory Compliance

Regulatory authorities such as the Food and Drug Administration (FDA), European Medicines Agency (EMA), and others require pharmaceutical firms to submit AR at specific intervals as part of their post-marketing surveillance obligations. Compliance with these reporting requirements is essential to maintain regulatory approval and continue marketing the product.

5.2.5 Decision-Making

Healthcare professionals, regulatory authorities, and pharmaceutical companies rely on aggregate safety reports to make informed decisions. These reports provide a comprehensive overview of the safety profile of a product, enabling informed decisions about patient care, regulatory actions, labeling updates, and more.

5.2.6 Public Health Monitoring

Aggregated safety data contribute to the broader understanding of public health by providing insights into AE and their prevalence. This information can be used to monitor public health trends, allocate resources, and improve patient care.

5.2.7 Long-Term Safety Assessment

As products continue to be used in real-world settings, their safety profiles can evolve. AR facilitates the assessment of long-term safety, helping to identify any changes in the safety profile that might emerge over time.

5.2.8 Communication with Healthcare Professionals

Healthcare professionals rely on accurate and timely safety information to make informed treatment decisions. AR provide them with comprehensive insights into potential risks associated with specific drugs or medical products.

5.2.9 Research and Development

It contribute valuable data to research and development efforts. Analyzing safety data from multiple products can inform the development of safer and more effective drugs in the future.

5.2.10 Global Monitoring

For products marketed internationally, AR helps maintain consistency in safety monitoring across different regions and regulatory bodies.

5.3 Types of Aggregate Reporting

The AR scrutinizes and precises all prevailing safety measures with a new drug or marketed pharmaceutical products. These AR includes the information on benefit–risk evaluation of various ADR and the SAE followed by pregnancy reports. Investigational New Drug (IND) report in United States (US) and yearly safety report in European Union (EU) are specified as the pre-approval AR. Specifically, there are various types of post-marketing AR such as development safety update report (DSUR) which is required for a molecule in development whereas for marketing approval products or drugs, periodic adverse drug experience report (PADER), periodic safety update report (PSUR), and periodic benefit–risk evaluation report (PBRER) are need to be submitted (Nandhini et al. 2019) (Fig. 5.1). Periodic examination is necessity to optimize safe use of a pharmaceuticals of worldwide safety data (Sardella et al. 2021).

5.3.1 Periodic Safety Update Report (PSUR)

Periodic safety update report is a documented AR that consents a regular and complete evaluation of the wide-reaching safety data of a marketed drug or biologicals. PSUR plays a significant role as a pharmacovigilance tool for the detection of novel safety signals (Klepper 2004). The conception for the PSUR originated from the Council for International Organizations of Medical Sciences (CIOMS, 1992)

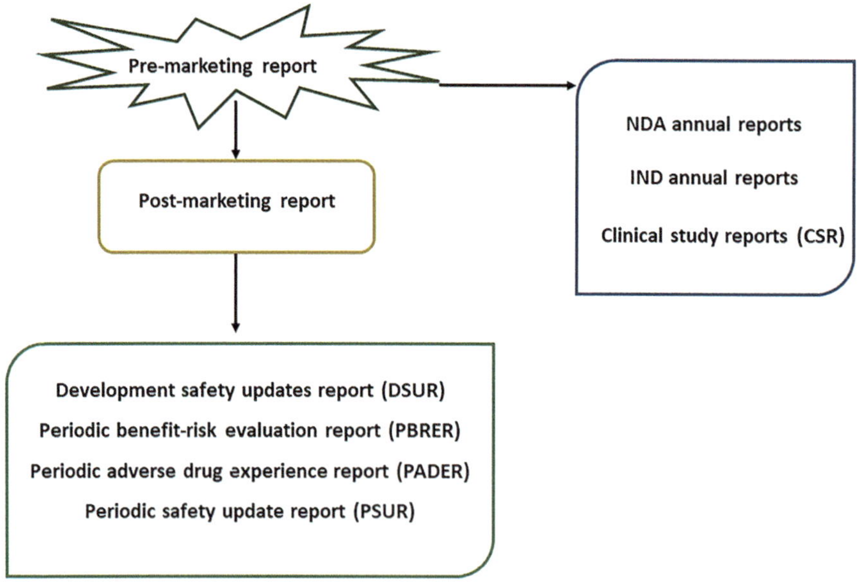

Fig. 5.1 Types of AR on the basis of pre- and post-marketing surveillance

Working Group II report and the ICH guidance for Industry, "E2C Clinical Safety Data Management: PSUR for marketed drugs" (Bahri 2014). It is an essential source of significant variations in the benefit–risk profile and an effectual mode of risk communication to monitoring authorities. In India, PSURs of pharmaceuticals are needed to be submitted to the Drugs Controller General of India (DCGI) in consonance with the guidelines of section 4 of Schedule "Y" Drugs and Cosmetics Rules now New Drugs and Clinical Trials Rule (NDCT).

Periodic safety update report provides an upgraded data which comprises and bring up-to-date on emerging or crucial safety-related matters. Numerous stages are concerned in the PSUR method that includes the intake of ADR data, case processing, data recovery, data examination, therapeutic assessment and risk assessment (Santoro et al. 2017). These progressions are profoundly dependent on the accessibility of adequate resources. Normally, PSUR also contains the information of dosage forms and preparations along with signals for a recognized pharmacologically active substance for medicinal products which are authorized to MAH (Arlett et al. 2014). Within the single PSUR, distinct arrangements of data for various dosage forms, signs, or inhabitants such as adults with children are appropriated possibly (Agrawal 2014). It is necessary to submit PSUR to the regulatory authorities for monitoring of benefit–risk profile of marketed drugs (Figs. 5.2, 5.3 and Table 5.1). The format and sections of the PSUR are mentioned in Table 5.2.

5.3.2 Periodic Adverse Drug Experience Report (PADER)

PADER is another collective safety description that summarizes the AE and reactions for the approved medicinal product within a specific period of time. PADERs required to be presented to the FDA for products or drugs approved for marketing

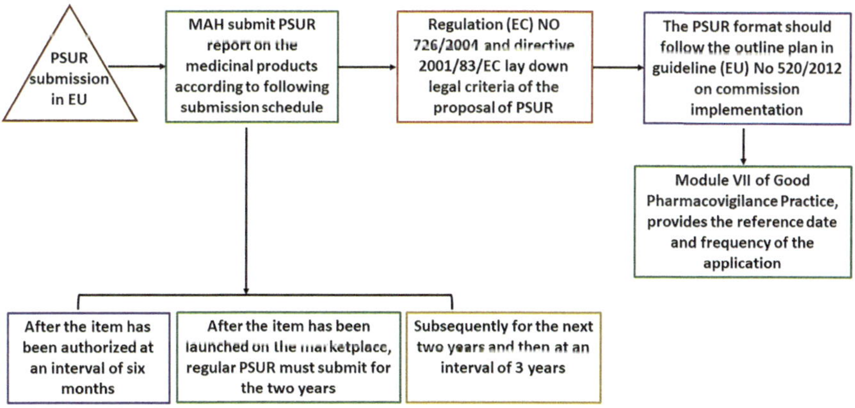

Fig. 5.2 Submission of PSUR in EU

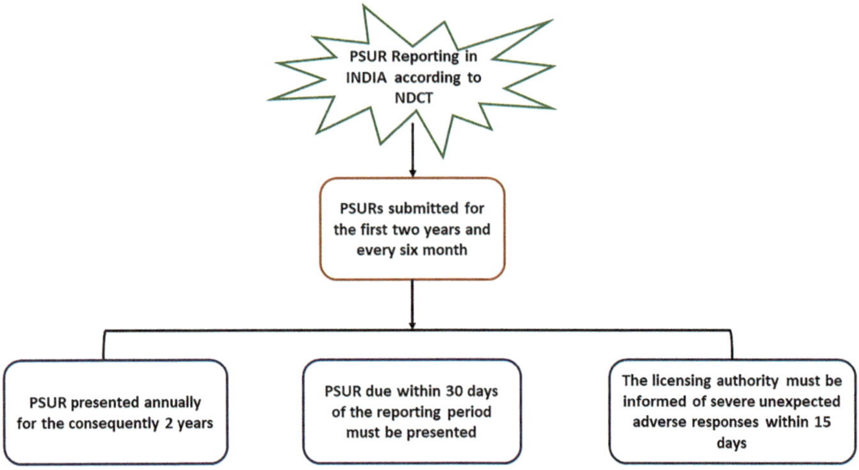

Fig. 5.3 Submission of PSUR in India

Table 5.1 Submission of PSUR in different countries

Requirement for PSUR	EU	India	Japan	Singapore
	Regulation EC 726/2004; Directive 2010/84/EU; Regulation (EU) 1235/2010; EU Vol. 9A	Drugs and Cosmetics Act 1940; Drugs and Cosmetics Rules 1945 (Schedule Y), *the New Drugs and Clinical Trials (NDCT)*	Pharmaceutical Affairs Law; MHLW Ordinance No.135 of 2004; GVP and Good Post-Marketing Study Practice (GPSP)	Medicine Act Chapter 176, 1977
	In EU it is submitted in every 6 months for the first 2 years	Every 6 months for the first 2 years and then annually thereafter	Every 6 months for the first 2 years	Every 6 months for the first 2 years

in the US and EU (Kulkarni and Kulkarni 2019). On a global scale, countries outside of the EU and US typically use the PSUR such as in India (Furlan et al. 2016).

For drafting a PADER, source documents are needed such as 1. line listings: It includes all the serious unlisted national and external cases in a 15 days alert and non-15 days alert which are serious listed, nonserious unlisted, and nonserious listed national cases are described all through the reporting period. It also includes evaluation table for all the AE and submitted to FDA for the NDA number. PADER also covers all the reports where the medicinal product is reported as a co-suspect medication, 2. regulatory input: It covers the whole evident data on actions taken for safety reasons, safety-related labeling changes, and bring up-to-date on

Table 5.2 Sections of PSUR by NDCT

1	Introduction: This section of PSUR should capture the reporting interval; drugs intended use, mode of action, therapeutic class, dose, route of administration, formulation and a brief description of the approved indication and population
2	Current worldwide marketing authorization status: This section of periodic safety update reports should capture the brief narrative over view including details of countries where the drug is currently approved along with date of first approval etc.
3	Actions taken in reporting interval for safety reasons: This section of PSUR should include a description of significant actions related to safety that have been taken during the reporting interval, related to either investigational uses or marketing experience by the licence holder, sponsor of a clinical trial, regulatory authorities, data monitoring committees, or ethics committees
4	Changes to reference safety information: This section should capture any significant changes to the reference safety information within the reporting interval
5	Estimated patient exposure: It contains a brief description of the methods used to estimate the subject or patient exposure should be provided, —(i) Cumulative and interval subject exposure in clinical trial. (ii) Cumulative and interval patient exposure from Marketing Experience from India. (iii) Cumulative and interval patient exposure from Marketing Experience from rest of the world
6	Presentation of individual case histories: Provide following information: (i) Reference prescribing information (ii) Individual cases received from India (iii) Individual cases received from rest of the world (iv) Cumulative and interval summary tabulations of SAE from clinical investigations. (v) Cumulative and interval summary tabulations from post-marketing data sources
7	Studies: PSUR should capture the brief summary of clinically important emerging efficacy or effectiveness and safety findings obtained from the licence holder, sponsored clinical trials and published safety studies that became available during the reporting interval of the report which has potential impact on product safety information
8	Other information: This section of periodic safety update reports should include the details about signals and Risk Management Plan in place by licence holder (if any). (a) Signal and risk evaluation: In this section licence holder will provide the details of signal and risk identified during the reporting period and evaluation of signals identified during the reporting period. (b) Risk management plan: In this section licence holder will provide the brief details of safety concern and necessary action taken by him to mitigate these safety concerns
9	Overall safety evaluation: This section of PSUR should capture the overall safety evaluation of the drug based upon its risk benefit evaluation for approved indication. (i) Summary of safety concerns (ii) Benefit evaluation (iii) Benefit risk analysis evaluation
10	Conclusion: This section should provide the details on the safety profile of drug and necessary action taken by the licence holder in this regard

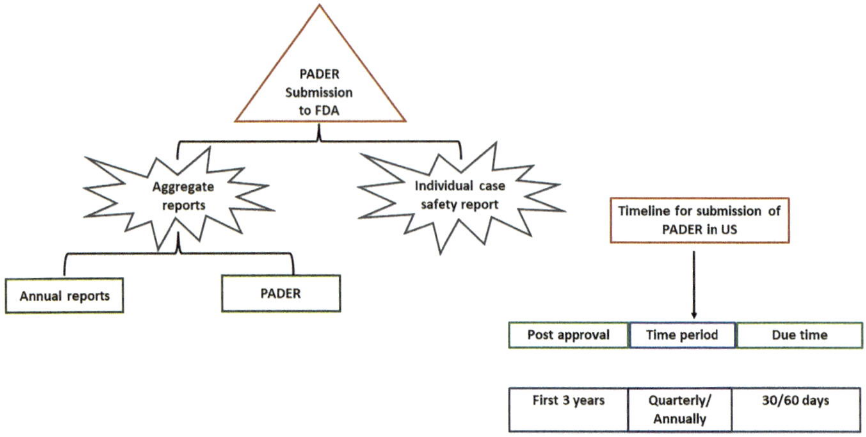

Fig. 5.4 Submission of PADER to USFDA

clinical trials started, ongoing, or accomplished throughout the reporting interval (Samara et al. 2023; Westergren et al. 2022). PADER is obligatory to be submitted by a sponsor or MAH to the USFDA after the authorization of the medicinal product is approved as in the US, the existing periodic report is the PADER (Johnson and Barash 1991). It summarizes altering post-approval AE profiles, safety information of an approved drug, and the benefit–risk profile assessment. The approved/authorized companies must submit the report quarterly within 30 days of the quarter's close. It is also required to submit annually within 60 days of the US approval date for initial 3 years (Kishore et al. 2021) (Fig. 5.4). It is necessary to report all the novel data from existing sources in consistent with the guideline of PADER, such data should be related to the patient safety interaction with the medicinal product or any major safety associated variations should be described (Khurana et al. 2015). The collective information which gathered from marketable sources, post-marketing clinical investigation, the under review scientific article, and already published literature should be reviewed by the MAH (Dollen 2014). From PSUR to PBRER if there is a alter in the data lock point (DLP) reporting rate, the marketing authorization holder can continue without changing the novel waiver submission and if there are any variations to the DLP, MAH must submit a new waiver appeal and a 1 time PADER application (Jalali 2018). The format and sections of the PSUR are mentioned in Table 5.3.

5.3.3 Periodic Benefit Risk Evaluation Report (PBRER)

ICH issued the revised ICH E2C (R2) in 2012, PBRER. The PBRER comprises all the appropriate assessment of benefit–risk ratio (Sharma et al. 2020). PBRER is essential to provide as a norm for periodic benefit–risk assessment report on

Table 5.3 Sections of PADER

1	Title page: This section includes the name of the pharmacovigilance report author, reviewer, and person and the molecule name, strength, formulation, etc.
2	Cover letter: This includes a number of serious expected, nonserious unexpected, and nonserious expected cases
3	Introduction: Includes an overview of the product, reporting interval, authorization information
4	Summary and evaluation of the data: Details of safety problem recognized and evaluation of the reporting period of 15 days finding
5	Discussion and action taken for safety reasons: Information about the labeling changes, studies initiated and submitted, drug safety recommendations from FDA
6	Appendices: Table of the frequency of AE occurrence from the reporting period

marketed pharmaceuticals and as the PBRER highlights "risk–benefit ratio" it should consequently comprise facts on benefits and safety along with the reference facts for report (Arora 2012; Klepper and Cobert 2010). Furthermore, the PBRER should thus include details on benefits and safety other than the reference information. In overall, having 1 reference data is not feasible for the MAH. Altogether new safety and efficacy signal should be presented in the proper unit of PBRER. The effectiveness on efficiency accessible from the International Birth Date (IBD), the date of the first world marketing approval or the Developmental International Birth Date (DIBD), the date of the first authorization for initiating the clinical trial from which the novel safety evidence is obtainable. Development of a drug clinically continues after marketing consent, data from post-marketing research or clinical trials should be comprised in PBRER format. The format and sections of the PSUR are mentioned in Table 5.4.

5.3.4 Development Safety Updates Report (DSUR)

In the ICH region DSUR is prevalent for the reporting of drugs or products being marketed under research (Samara et al. 2023). Regulatory body monitors the DSUR and states that the report need to be submitted yearly, on the basis of fulfillment of the regional and countrywide necessities (Pernice and Colley 2020). It is a collective information intensive process which provides the required efficient communication between the different effectual stakeholders (Pianka et al. 2021). Regulatory authorities determine the ongoing detailed examination, alteration in production, and comprehensive development position and approaches should be acquiesced in the form of the periodic report (Parkinson 2021). DSUR also delivers data on sponsored medications under additional examination. Whatsoever the data found at the period of reporting should be in correspondence with the earlier investigational drug

Table 5.4 Sections of PBRER

1	Introduction
2	Worldwide marketing authorization status
3	Actions taken in the reporting interval for safety reasons
4	Changes to reference safety information
5	Estimated exposure and use patterns: 5.1. Cumulative subject exposure in clinical trials 5.2. Cumulative and interval patient exposure from marketing experience
6.	Data in summary tabulations 6.1. Reference information 6.2. Cumulative summary tabulations of serious AE from clinical trials 6.3. Cumulative and interval summary tabulations from post-marketing data sources
7.	Summaries of significant findings from clinical trials during the reporting interval 7.1. Completed clinical trials 7.2. Ongoing clinical trials 7.3. Long-term follow-up 7.4. Other therapeutic use of medicinal product 7.5. New safety data related to fixed combination therapies
8.	Findings from noninterventional studies
9.	Information from other clinical trials and sources 9.1. Other clinical trials 9.2. Medication errors
10.	Nonclinical data
11.	Literature
12.	Other periodic reports
13.	Lack of efficacy in controlled clinical trials
14.	Late-breaking information
15.	Overview of signals: New, ongoing or closed
16.	Signal and risk evaluation 16.1. Summaries of safety concerns 16.2. Signal evaluation 16.3. Evaluation of risks and new information 16.4. Characterization of risks 16.5. Effectiveness of risk minimization (if applicable)
17.	Benefit evaluation 17.1. Important baseline efficacy and effectiveness information 17.2. Newly identified information on efficacy and effectiveness 17.3. Characterization of benefits
18.	Integrated benefit–risk analysis for authorized indications 18.1. Benefit–risk context—Medical need and important alternatives 18.2. Benefit–risk analysis evaluation
19.	Conclusions and actions
20.	Appendices

safety reports (Phillips et al. 2019). It is also mandatory that the clinical examination and evaluation result should be rationalized. If any issues identified in the reporting disclosures it should be specified in the DSUR in a proper order (Lee et al. 2021). Also, it is required to summarize all the mandatory data of DSUR to the authorities and sponsor that the risk frameworks of new drug is satisfactorily monitored (Makhene et al. 2023).

It should also provide the safety evidence from all enduring clinical trials or has completed during the assessment time. It includes clinical trials of a new drug, i.e., (from Phase 1 trial to phase 3 trial) Clinical trials initiated by means of promoted medications in approved indications (Phase 4 trial), Therapeutic use of an novel drug (e.g., sympathetic use programs, particular patient use, single patient INDs, and treatment INDs, and clinical trials conducted to provision changes in the manufacturing development of pharmaceuticals (Rechtsteiner and von Bruchhausen 2022). The format and sections of the PSUR are mentioned in Table 5.5.

Table 5.5 Sections of DSUR

1.	Introduction
2.	Worldwide Marketing Approval Status
3.	Actions Taken in the Reporting Period for Safety Reasons
4.	Changes to Reference Safety Information
5.	Inventory of Clinical Trials Ongoing and Completed during the Reporting Period
6.	Estimated Cumulative Exposure: 6.1 Cumulative Subject Exposure in the Development Program 6.2 Patient Exposure from Marketing Experience
7.	Data in Line Listings and Summary Tabulations: 7.1 Reference Information 7.2 Line Listings of SAE during the reporting period 7.3 Cumulative Summary Tabulations of SAE
8.	Significant Findings from Clinical Trials during the Reporting Period: 8.1 Completed Clinical Trials 8.2 Ongoing Clinical Trials 8.3 Long-term Follow-up 8.4 Other Therapeutic Use of Investigational Drug 8.5 New Safety Data Related to Combination Therapies
9.	Safety Findings from Noninterventional Studies
10.	Other Clinical Trial/Study Safety Information
11.	Safety Findings from Marketing Experience
12.	Nonclinical Data
13.	Literature
14.	Other DSURs
15.	Lack of Efficacy
16.	Region-Specific Information
17.	Late-Breaking Information
18.	Overall Safety Assessment: 18.1. Evaluation of the Risks 18.2 Benefit-risk Considerations
19.	Summary of Important Risks
20.	Conclusions

5.4 Significance

The opportunities in the pharmacovigilance has grown over time for the identification, evaluation, understanding, and prevention of ADRs and it is mandatory to check the safety profile of a drug (Nyagah et al. 2020). Recognition of the significance of an efficient approach for examine and developing the safe use of medications reporting of ADR is necessary. For individual case safety reports, it is difficult for MAH to monitor on benefit–risk profile and recognize the comprehensive safety parameters of a pharmaceuticals (Jeetu and Anusha 2010). Along with submission of individual case safety data, MAH also analyze occasionally, collective safety information accomplished from numerous sources and acquiesce the results as AR to drug regulators. AR gives broader viewpoint of the drug's safety profile that benefits the worldwide population. From the development of a new drug to the post-market observation it is essential to keep track of the complete information on a benefit–risk ratio before it reached the market. Therefore, regular examination of safety reports received cumulatively globally becomes extremely significant (Wadhwa et al. 2021). These reports need exceptional diligence and attention to detail, including an overview and a sense of what is essential, on the other hand (Almenoff 2007).

5.5 Challenges

AR provide a brief summary of safety data connected to a specific drug or medical product. Despite its benefits, AR has some challenges also:

5.5.1 Data Quality

The precision of safety data is decisive for AR. Incomplete or inaccurate data can lead to misleading conclusions and compromise patient safety.

5.5.2 Appropriateness

Regulatory bodies have firm timelines for submitting AR. Ensuring that data is gathered, monitored, and reported within a deadline can be demanding, especially for products with extensive safety profiles.

5.5.3 Signal Detection and Evaluation

Identifying potential safety signals within the collected data requires sophisticated arithmetical and analytical approaches. Distinguishing between actual safety concerns and random variations can be complex.

5.5.4 Regulatory Acquiescence

Different regulatory bodies, such as the FDA, EMA, and others, have their own specific requirements for a AR. Compliance with these varying regulations can be challenging, particularly for corporations or companies operating in multiple regions.

5.5.5 Risk Minimization and Management

Based on AR, regulatory actions may be required, such as updating safety labeling, adding cautions, or implementing risk evaluation and mitigation Strategies (REMS). Managing these regulatory actions efficiently can be challenging.

5.5.6 Resource Allocation

Generating AR involves significant resources, including personnel, time, and financial investments. Allocating these resources efficiently while meeting reporting requirements can be a challenge.

5.5.7 Communication and Collaboration

AR often requires collaboration between different departments within a pharmaceutical company, as well as communication with regulatory agencies. Ensuring effective communication and coordination among these stakeholders is essential.

5.5.8 Updating Safety Databases

As new data is collected and safety signals are identified, it's important to update safety databases and reports accordingly. Ensuring that the most current information is available while maintaining consistency can be difficult.

5.6 Conclusion

Aggregate reports should be submitted to regulatory authorities' time to time such as pre-marketing, DSUR and post-marketing, PSUR report need to be submitted. The sections and time period of AR varies across the different countries. Overall, AR plays a significant role in benefit–risk evaluation of medicinal products at regular interval.

References

Agrawal P (2014) Drug discovery and development: an insight into pharmacovigilance. J Pharmacovigil 2(3):120

Almenoff JS (2007) Innovations for the future of pharmacovigilance. Drug Saf 30:631–633

Amiri A, Okai J, Bahri P, Sarinić VM (2021) The fundamental value of exposure data for pharmacovigilance: review of different aggregation levels of exposure data in pharmaceutical companies' PSURs. Drug Saf 44:1402–1402

Arlett P, Portier G, De Lisa R, Blake K, Wathion N, Dogne JM, Spooner A, Raine J, Rasi G (2014) Proactively managing the risk of marketed drugs: experience with the EMA pharmacovigilance risk assessment committee. Nat Rev Drug Discov 13(5):395–397

Arora D (2012) Pharmacovigilance—an industry perspective. Pharmapublisher, Navi Mumbai

Bahri P (2014) Pharmacovigilance-related topics at the level of the international conference on harmonization. In: Mann's pharmacovigilance, pp 47–62

Dollen MZ (2014) Pharmacovigilance legislation: the impact of what is happening in Europe. Ther Innov Regul Sci 48:190–199

Furlan G, Edwards B, Mastroianni A, Koski G (2016) The future of pharmacovigilance: proposals for more efficient and effective systems-based approaches. Pharmaceut Med 30(3):137–142

Han M (2022) The application of Big Data in pharmacovigilance: a systematic review. In: 2021 International conference on public art and human development (ICPAHD 2021). Atlantis Press, Amsterdam, pp 533–537

Hendrickson BA, Wang W, Ball G, Bennett D, Bhattacharyya A, Fries M et al (2021) Aggregate safety assessment planning for the drug development life-cycle. Ther Innov Regul Sci 55:717–732

Jalali RK (2018) Pharmacovigilance and drug safety. In: Pharmaceutical medicine and translational clinical research, pp 403–406

Jeetu G, Anusha G (2010) Pharmacovigilance: a worldwide master key for drug safety monitoring. J Young Pharm 2:315–320

Johnson JM, Barash D (1991) A review of postmarketing adverse drug experience reporting requirements. Food Drug Cosm LJ 46:665

Karale AB, Patil V (2022) The role of periodic/regular safety update reports in biopharmaceutical. Saf Manag 12(1):1023–1039

Khurana A, Rastogi R, Gamperl H-J (2015) Ready for pharmacovigilance inspection—USFDA. Int J Pharm Sci Rev Res 35:210–217

Kishore TS, Aswani V, Nikhitha SSL, Bonthagarala B, Sindhu YR, Ramakrishna G et al (2021) Current scenario of pharmacovigilance in India and its comparision with USA and EU. World J Pharmaceut Res 10(11):826–837

Klepper MJ (2004) The periodic safety update report as a pharmacovigilance tool. Drug Saf 27:569–578

Klepper MJ, Cobert B (2010) Drug safety data: how to analyze, summarize and interpret to determine risk. Jones & Bartlett Publishers, Burlington, MA

Kulkarni TN, Kulkarni NG (2019) Authoring a periodic adverse drug experience report... here's what you need to know! Perspect Clin Res 10:95

Lee BM, Park S-J, Shim D-Y, Rhee HE, Lee J-E, Kim SH et al (2021) A survey for management of drug safety evaluation system for investigational product. Korean J Clin Pharm 31:53–60

Makhene NL, Steyn H, Vorster M, Lubbe MS, Burger JR (2023) Development of a checklist for the assessment of pharmacovigilance guidelines in southern Africa: a document review. Therapeut Adv Drug Saf 14:20420986221143272

Nandhini B, Venkatesh MP, Balamuralidhara V, Kumar TP (2019) Aggregate reporting and regulatory requirements. J Pharm Sci Res 11:2504–2514

Nyagah DM, Mokaya D, Karanja SM (2020) The reporting of adverse drug reactions by healthcare providers in Kenya. South Sudan Med J 13(4):141–145

Ojha A, Bhargava S (2022) International council for harmonisation (ICH) guidelines. Regulatory affairs in the pharmaceutical industry. Elsevier, Amsterdam, pp 47–74

Parkinson C (2021) Regulatory affairs. In: Drug discovery and development E-book: technology in transition, p 290

Pernice M, Colley A (2020) Principles and practice of clinical trials: regulatory requirements in clinical trials. In: Principles and practice of clinical trials. Springer, Cham, pp 1–20

Phillips R, Hazell L, Sauzet O, Cornelius V (2019) Analysis and reporting of adverse events in randomised controlled trials: a review. BMJ Open 9:e024537

Pianka K, Cichone J, Vashist A, Parikh N, Rahman M (2021) Increasing efficiency and cost-effectiveness by automating the authoring of the development safety update report. Pharmaceut Med 35:297–305

Rechtsteiner S, von Bruchhausen T (2022) Pharmacovigilance. Med Writing 31:116–119

Samara C, Garcia A, Henry C, Vallotton L, Cariolato L, Desmeules J et al (2023) Safety surveillance during drug development: comparative evaluation of existing regulations. Adv Ther 40:2147–2185

Santoro A, Genov G, Spooner A, Raine J, Arlett P (2017) Promoting and protecting public health: how the European Union pharmacovigilance system works. Drug Saf 40:855–869

Sardella M, Belcher G, Lungu C, Ignoni T, Camisa M, Stenver DI et al (2021) Monitoring the manufacturing and quality of medicines: a fundamental task of pharmacovigilance. Therapeut Adv Drug Saf 12:20420986211038436

Sharma R, Kant K, Kumar A (2020) Overview of periodic safety update reports: where have we reached? Appl Clin Res Clin Trial Regul Affairs 7:4–11

Wadhwa D, Kumar K, Batra S, Sharma S (2021) Automation in signal management in pharmacovigilance—an insight. Brief Bioinform 22:bbaa363

Wang W, Munsaka M, Buchanan J, Li J (2021) Quantitative drug safety and benefit risk evaluation: practical and cross-disciplinary approaches. CRC, Boca Raton, FL, pp 1–381

Westergren T, Narum S, Klemp M (2022) Biases in reporting of adverse effects in clinical trials, and potential impact on safety assessments in systematic reviews and therapy guidelines. Basic Clin Pharmacol Toxicol 131:465–473

Reporting of ADRs Across the Globe: India, USA, EU, and Non-EU

6

Priyanka Sharma, Mukesh Nandave, and Anoop Kumar

6.1 Introduction

Reporting adverse drug reactions (ADRs) is crucial in ensuring the safety and efficacy of pharmaceutical products worldwide. ADRs are the undesirable and unwanted effects that are produced by using medications. Therefore, monitoring and reporting are crucial for identifying and mitigating risks to reduce drug-related hazards and improving patient safety and overall healthcare quality.

The comparative study of this chapter for the ADR reporting system in India, the United States of America, the European Union, and the European Union is intended to examine similarities, differences, and the best practices in ADR reporting, which could improve the international efforts toward the pharmacovigilance. The Pharmacovigilance Programme of India (PvPI), a national program started by the Indian Pharmacopoeia Commission (IPC), is mainly responsible for regulating the reporting of ADRs in India. The PvPI obtains, tracks, and examines ADR data from patients, healthcare providers, and pharmaceutical corporations.

In this chapter, we have examine the PvPI's functioning, composition, and challenges with a specific emphasis on their impact on drug safety in India. The all-over charge of ADR reporting in the USA lies with the Food and Drug Administration (FDA), where the Adverse Event Reporting System (FAERS), a sizable database that compiles and evaluates reports of Adverse Drug Reactions (ADRs) provided by medical professionals, patients, and pharmaceutical corporations, is under the FDA's supervision. Moreover, the regulatory framework for ADR reporting in the

P. Sharma (✉) · M. Nandave · A. Kumar
Department of Pharmacology, Delhi Pharmaceutical Sciences and Research University, New Delhi, India
e-mail: mukeshnandave@gmail.com; anoopdpsru@dpsru.edu.in

M. Nandave, A. Kumar (eds.), *Pharmacovigilance Essentials*,
https://doi.org/10.1007/978-981-99-8949-2_6

USA and their related procedures regulating through FDAs to improve pharmacovigilance practices. The European Medicines Agency (EMA) and its member states have established a robust pharmacovigilance system in the European Union. EudraVigilance is a European repository for suspected ADRs where healthcare experts, patients, and owners of marketing authorizations submit information. Through this chapter, we have investigated the cooperative efforts between EMA and its member states. We have also highlighted EudraVigilance's crucial role in facilitating the exchange of ADR data among the EU.

This chapter's primary concern is recognizing shared challenges, regulatory variance, and efficient approaches in ADR reporting by comparing and constructing ADR reporting systems among India, the USA, the EU, and the non-EU regions. Exploring the harmonization of reporting standards, the value of international cooperation, and the involvement of technological advancement for pharmacovigilance on a global scale. The advantages and disadvantages of ADR reporting protocols in India, the USA, the EU, and non-EU regions have also discussed.

6.2 Overview of ADR Reporting

The crucial aspect of pharmacovigilance and drug safety monitoring is reporting ADRs. The harmful and unwanted drug reactions and their responses are essential for ensuring patient safety. ADRs are unanticipated to medications and can occur even when medications are taken as prescribed. ADR reporting identifies, evaluates, comprehends, and ensures patient safety by preventing adverse reactions and other drug-related issues. This chapter provides a comparative overview of the ADR reporting systems in four major regions: India, the USA, the EU, and non-EU.

6.2.1 Definition and Importance of ADR Reporting

ADR reporting, also known as adverse drug reaction reporting, is collecting, documenting, and evaluating information about adverse events or side effects in patients taking medications or pharmaceutical products. It involves systematically reporting any unexpected, harmful, or unintended reactions resulting from using drugs, vaccines, herbal medicines, or medical devices (Walker et al. 2023). The importance of ADRs is listed in Table 6.1.

6.2.2 Objectives and Benefits of ADR Reporting

The schematic representation in Fig. 6.1 outlines the key objectives of ADR reporting, which collectively aim to improve patient safety and enhance drug safety practices (Kim et al. 2015). At the core of this framework lies the objective of "Patient Safety," emphasizing the paramount importance of safeguarding patients from potential medication-related harm.

Table 6.1 The significance of ADR reporting

Importance of ADR Reporting	Description
Patient safety	Ensures patient safety by identifying and addressing potential medication risks
Early detection of safety issues	Helps in the early detection of safety issues by monitoring and analyzing adverse events beyond clinical trials
Post-marketing surveillance	Extends drug safety surveillance beyond clinical trials to monitor the real-world safety of medications in a larger patient population
Signal detection	Aids in signal detection and identifying potential safety concerns related to specific drugs based on reported adverse events
Regulatory decision-making	Data collected from ADR reports influence regulatory decisions such as updating safety labels, issuing warnings, or withdrawing drugs if necessary
Pharmacovigilance and risk management	Integral to pharmacovigilance, ensuring better risk management and patient safety in the context of drug use
Improving drug development	Insights from ADR reports contribute to drug development, creating safer medications with reduced side effects
Public health and epidemiology	Aggregated ADR data aids public health and epidemiological research, helping to identify trends and patterns in adverse events on a broader scale
Enhancing healthcare practices	Healthcare professionals use ADR reports to make informed decisions about drug choices, dosages, and patient management, thus enhancing healthcare practices

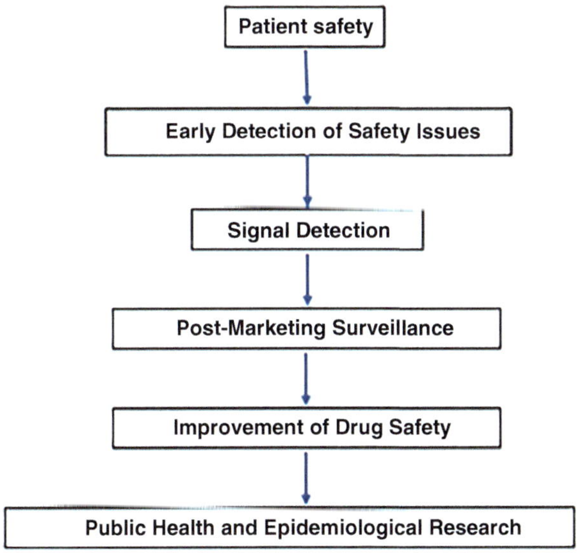

Fig. 6.1 Objectives of ADR reporting

The quick recognition of ADR and resolving any pharmaceutical concern provides many advantages to patient care and drug safety. The personnel and regulatory bodies can recognize early safety risks and take preventive actions to safeguard patients from harm through ADR reporting (Singh et al. 2023). Moreover, the Reporting of ADR also plays an essential role in risk management and facilitating better monitoring of the safety of medications outside the clinical study. It intends to create an alarming system that enables the detection of safety signals and the patterns of unfavorable events that might invite further research. Additionally, the regulatory implementation promotes scholarly investigation, medical education, and research.

Overall, ADR reporting empowers patients, enhances global health initiatives, and supports informed decision-making by regulatory bodies, ultimately culminating in improved drug safety standards and patient outcomes (Singh et al. 2020).

6.3 ADR Reporting in India

ADR reporting in India is an essential component of pharmacovigilance, overseen by the Indian Pharmacopoeia Commission (IPC) and the National Coordination Centre (NCC) for pharmacovigilance. Healthcare professionals and consumers can submit reports of suspected ADRs to ensure patient safety (Suke et al. 2015). Regulatory requirements mandate pharmaceutical companies to report ADRs, contributing to post-marketing surveillance and continuous improvement of drug safety practices in the country.

6.3.1 Regulatory Framework and Authorities

The Central Drugs Standard Control Organization (CDSCO) under the Ministry of Health and Family Welfare governs the regulatory framework for ADR reporting in India. The primary authority overseeing pharmacovigilance activities, including ADR reporting, is the Indian Pharmacopoeia Commission (IPC) (Joshi et al. 2022). The IPC acts as NCC for Pharmacovigilance and is central in coordinating and monitoring ADR reports from various stakeholders.

Healthcare professionals, consumers, and pharmaceutical companies must report suspected Adverse Drug Reactions to the IPC through the PvPI. The PvPI operates a web-based reporting system, VigiFlow, for the submission of Individual Case Safety Reports (ICSRs) containing relevant information on ADRs (Thota et al. 2018). The data collected through ADR reporting contributes to post-marketing surveillance and signal detection and enhances drug safety measures in India.

6.3.2 Structure of ADR Reporting System

The ADR reporting system in India follows a structured approach to ensure comprehensive collection, evaluation, and monitoring of adverse drug reactions (Mulchandani and Kakkar 2019). The main components of the ADR reporting system in India are as follows in Fig. 6.2:

India's organized ADR reporting system supports regulatory authorities in ensuring patient safety and improving drug safety standards by continuously monitoring drug safety and detecting safety issues early.

6.3.3 Challenges and Improvements

Several challenges hinder the effectiveness of the ADR system in India, and it faces difficulties in ensuring comprehensive drug safety surveillance. The primary challenge is the underreporting of ADRs by healthcare professionals and consumers (Li et al. 2022), which might be due to a lack of knowledge regarding pharmacovigilance and ADR reporting concerning possible repercussions or time restraints. The quality and completeness of ADR data are affected by insufficient awareness campaigns and training programs. The inadequate resources and infrastructure of

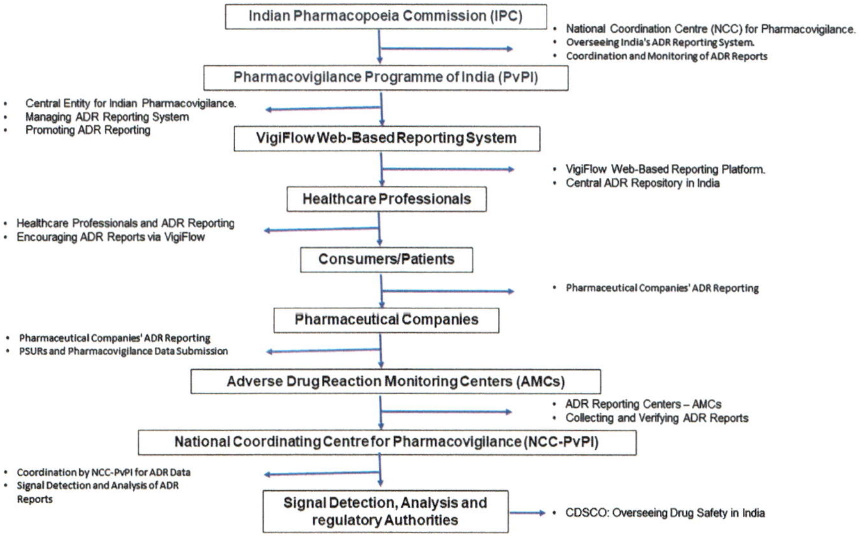

Fig. 6.2 Structured workflow of ADR Reporting in India

certain regions facilitate low reporting rates, particularly in rural areas. The accuracy and reliability of reported data pose another challenge in identifying potential safety signals and overall analysis of ADR reports (Simera et al. 2010). The challenge of getting patients to report their symptoms often resulting in a failure to consistently connect their symptoms to the use of prescribed medications. Addressing these challenges will be simplified reporting mechanisms, feedback systems, and capacity building that can strengthen India's ADR reporting system, resulting in better patient safety and more effective drug safety monitoring practices.

Many efforts have been made to enhance ADR reporting in India through various initiatives. To emphasize the importance of ADR reporting many awareness campaigns targeting healthcare professionals, consumers, and pharmaceutical companies. To educate and encourage the active participation of healthcare workers regarding reporting procedures, various training programs have been designed to inform ADR recognition. User-friendly and simplified mechanisms of reporting ADRs, including online portals and mobile applications, have been launched to streamline the reporting process and facilitate more convenient submission. Feedback mechanisms have also been established to inform reporters about the action taken based on their ADR reports, promoting continued reporting and related transparency. Encouragement for participation in the ADR reporting program by engaging patients through patient support groups and consumer reporting programs (Dylan Fernandes et al. 2019). The motive of the ADR reporting system in India is to strengthen drug safety through digital integration of the ADR reporting system with electronic health records for effective ADR monitoring and enhance patient safety by improved data collection efficiency.

6.4 ADR Reporting in the United States

ADR reporting in the United States is managed by the FDA. The FDA operates FAERS, where healthcare professionals, consumers, and pharmaceutical companies submit reports of suspected adverse drug reactions (Ahmad et al. 2013). ADR reporting helps monitor drug safety, signal detection, and risk assessment for medications in the US market. The structured Workflow of ADR Reporting in US is shown in Fig. 6.3.

6.4.1 Regulatory Framework and Authorities

In the United States, the regulatory framework and authorities for ADR reporting are overseen by the FDA. The FDA plays a central role in drug safety and pharmacovigilance, ensuring the post-marketing surveillance of medications in the US market. Healthcare professionals, consumers, and pharmaceutical companies must report suspected adverse drug reactions through the FDA's Adverse Event Reporting System (FAERS) (Stergiopoulos et al. 2016; Patel et al. 2022). The FDA evaluates these reports, conducts signal detection, and takes regulatory actions, such as

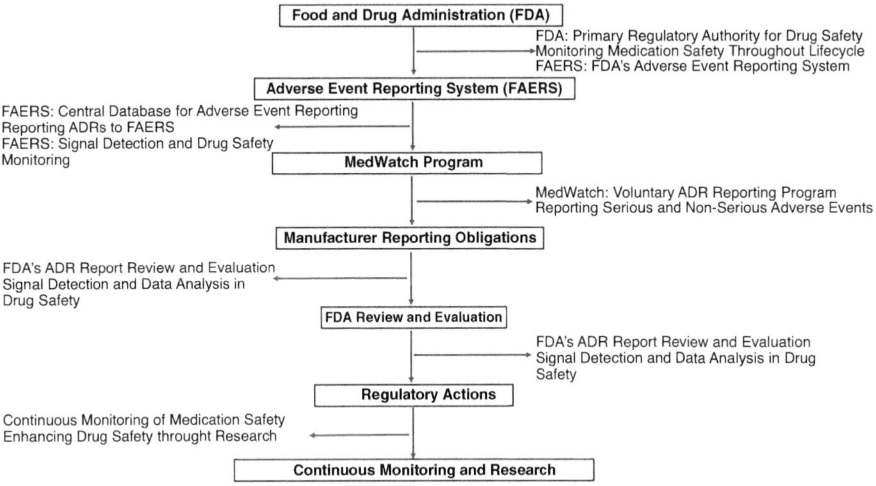

Fig. 6.3 Structured workflow of ADR reporting in US

updating drug labels or issuing warnings, to ensure patient safety and enhance drug safety practices in the country.

6.4.2 Structure of ADR Reporting System

The US's FDA-led structured ADR reporting system, backed by FAERS and the MedWatch program (Nguyen et al. 2012), is essential for keeping track of medication safety, spotting warning signs, and guaranteeing patient safety.

6.4.3 Challenges and Improvements

There are some obstacles that the ADR reporting system in the US must overcome to monitor drug safety effectively. Healthcare personnel and patients must disclose adverse drug responses, which results in insufficient data and prevents the detection of possible safety signals. Inconsistencies in ADR reports are also a result of varying report criteria, which makes it challenging to compare and analyze data from various sources. Having high-quality data is essential for accurate signal recognition and analysis. However, completeness and accuracy problems might jeopardize the correctness of medication safety evaluations (Daller 2016). Timeliness is critical since ADR reporting delays could prevent prompt regulatory steps to reduce risks. Another challenge is encouraging patients to report adverse events directly to regulatory authorities since they might not be aware of reporting options or might not always link their discomfort to pharmaceutical use. To overcome these obstacles, increasing public and medical professional knowledge is imperative, expediting reporting procedures, establishing uniform standards, and encouraging patient involvement in reporting is imperative. The ADR reporting mechanism may be strengthened by utilizing digital integration, data mining, and stakeholder participation, improving medication oversight and patient healthcare.

6.5 ADR Reporting in the European Union

The EMA oversees ADR reporting in the EU. The EudraVigilance system, run by the EMA, allows consumers and pharmaceutical companies to report alleged adverse medication reactions (Brucker and King 2017). ADR reporting supports drug safety surveillance, signal detection, and drug risk assessment in all EU member states.

6.5.1 Regulatory Framework and Authorities

The EMA and the European Commission are in charge of the legal framework for ADR reporting in the EU (Felix et al. 2019). To coordinate pharmacovigilance efforts among EU member states, the EMA is a key player. The EudraVigilance system, which acts as the central database for ADR reporting, is under the control of the EMA. The EMA works with National Competent Authorities (NCAs) in each member state to monitor drug safety, assess ADR reports, and implement regulatory measures to guarantee patient safety. The regulatory framework of the EU strives to improve drug safety surveillance across the area and harmonize ADR reporting.

6.5.2 Structure of ADR Reporting System

To ensure the prompt and thorough collection, analysis (Ferrajolo et al. 2014), and evaluation of ADR reports, contributing to improved drug safety and patient care throughout the European Union, the structure of the ADR reporting system in the EU places a focus on collaboration between the EMA, NCAs, and other stakeholders, as shown in Fig. 6.4.

6.5.3 Challenges and Improvements

Numerous obstacles could hinder the EU's ADR reporting system's ability to monitor medication safety and guarantee patient care. One of the main issues is the underreporting of adverse drug reactions (ADRs), which results in inadequate data because ADRs may not consistently be recognized or reported by consumers, healthcare professionals, or pharmaceutical corporations. Additionally, there are

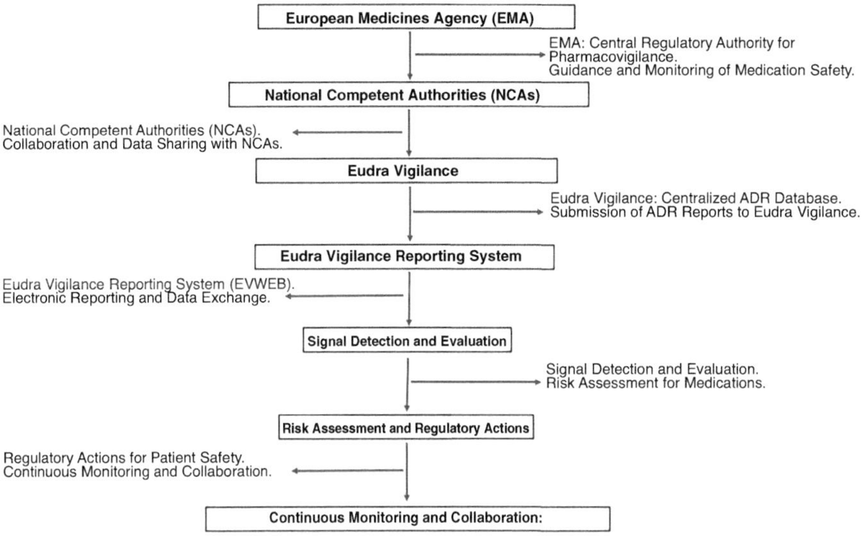

Fig. 6.4 Structured workflow of ADR reporting in the European Union

differences and challenges in comparing and analyzing. ADR data can arise from differences in reporting standards among EU member states (Blake et al. 2014; Schrama 2022). As consistent and complete data can make it easier to make correct risk assessments, ensuring data quality and completeness is essential for reliable signal identification and analysis. Language constraints brought on by the EU's many official languages can make it challenging to gather and analyze data effectively. Timely ADR reporting is essential for the prompt identification of safety risks and the implementation of regulatory procedures. Harmonizing reporting criteria, improved training and awareness, digital integration, centralized data analysis, multilingual support, and cooperation between member states and stakeholders can all help overcome these issues. By implementing these changes, the EU's ADR reporting system can be reinforced, which will enhance patient care and allow for better drug safety monitoring.

6.6 ADR Reporting in the Non-European Union

A key component of pharmacovigilance is the reporting of adverse drug reactions (ADRs), which helps to identify and reduce medication-related hazards and ensure patient safety. Pharmacovigilance is well-established in the European Union (EU), but ADR reporting procedures vary in non-EU regions because to different legal frameworks, reporting protocols, and challenges.

6.6.1 Regulatory Framework and Authorities

To maintain adequate pharmacovigilance procedures, the Health Regulatory Agency in non-EU regions (aside from the US, India, and EU) creates thorough rules for reporting Adverse Drug Reactions (ADRs). These regulations cover the criteria for submitting reports, the range of adverse events, and the precise deadlines for reporting given in Table 6.2.

6.6.2 Structure of ADR Reporting System

In non-EU regions, the ADR reporting system is governed by a Health Regulatory Authority (HRA) which establishes comprehensive guidelines. Healthcare professionals, consumers, and pharmaceutical companies play crucial roles as reporters. Adverse events linked to pharmaceutical products are identified, prompting the reporting process. Healthcare professionals must report within 7 days of the event, while consumers and companies have a 15-day window. An electronic reporting platform named "PharmaSafe" facilitates secure submissions. Reporters access PharmaSafe, complete the provided ADR reporting form, and attach necessary documents. The data is swiftly transferred to a central database within 24 h, where advanced pharmacovigilance tools are employed for analysis. Techniques like signal detection and data mining are used to identify potential safety concerns. Expert committees evaluate signals, resulting in regulatory actions such as updates to drug labeling or product withdrawals. Collaboration with international bodies ensures global data sharing and signal assessment, contributing to robust pharmacovigilance. Regular feedback and

Table 6.2 Authorities and regulatory framework in European Union

Aspect	Instructions for ADR Reporting in non-EU regions
Regulatory Authority and Oversight	Health Regulatory Agency establishes guidelines for ADR reporting
Who Can Report	Healthcare professionals, consumers, and pharmaceutical companies
What Should Be Reported	Any unexpected adverse event, serious or non-serious, linked to a pharmaceutical product
Reporting Timeframes	As soon as possible after becoming aware, typically within 15 days
Mechanism of Reporting	Electronic reporting systems are established for streamlined submission
Electronic Reporting System	Named Electronic ADR Reporting System (E-ADR)
How to Report ADRs	The regulatory authority provides an online portal or mobile application
Data Transfer or Registration	Data is transferred to a central database or regulatory authority within 30 days
Data Analysis Techniques for Signal Detection	Automated data analysis, statistical methods, and data mining tools are employed

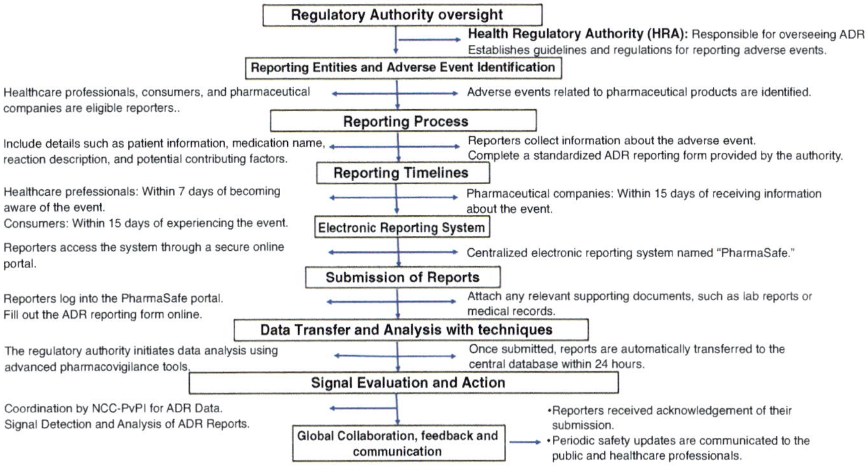

Fig. 6.5 Structured workflow of ADR Reporting in non-European Union

updates keep reporters and the public informed about ongoing efforts to ensure drug safety, as shown in Fig. 6.5.

6.6.3 Challenges and Improvements

In non-EU regions, reporting ADRs faces significant challenges while striving for improvements. One major obstacle is the underreporting of ADRs due to limited awareness among healthcare professionals, consumers, and pharmaceutical companies. This lack of awareness can stem from concerns about potential consequences or a general need for more understanding of the importance of reporting. Furthermore, resource constraints and inefficient reporting mechanisms contribute to incomplete data and hinder the detection of potential safety signals. Another challenge arises from inconsistent data quality and incomplete reports, which affect the reliability of the information gathered, making it difficult to identify patterns and trends that could indicate emerging safety concerns. Due to the process's increased complexity and regional differences in reporting requirements, comparing and analyzing data effectively is more complicated. Non-EU regions are actively working on improvements to address these issues. Healthcare professionals and the general public are educated about the importance of ADR reporting through public awareness campaigns and training initiatives. The goal of simplified reporting procedures and the incorporation of multilingual support is to increase the usability and accessibility of reporting. Standardized criteria are used to ensure that reports contain all pertinent information, enhancing the data's quality and completeness. The reporting procedure can be significantly streamlined with the use of digital integration. Healthcare workers and patients may now report incidents more quickly and conveniently because of the introduction of user-friendly web platforms and mobile applications that make it easier to submit ADR reports.

Additionally, by automating some steps in the reporting process, these digital technologies lower the possibility of error and speed up data delivery. Collaboration is another critical aspect of improvement. Non-EU regions collaborate with international organizations and neighboring countries to share knowledge and best practices. This exchange of information helps adopt successful strategies from other regions and implement them effectively. Enhancing data quality is a priority, and this is being achieved through validation checks and automated analysis tools. These tools assist in detecting patterns and trends in large datasets, making it easier to identify potential safety signals promptly. This proactive approach ensures that any emerging safety concerns are addressed on time (Table 6.3).

Table 6.3 Challenges and corresponding improvements in Adverse Drug Reaction (ADR) Reporting within non-EU regions

Challenges in ADR Reporting	Improvements and solutions
Underreporting: Limited awareness among healthcare professionals, consumers, and pharmaceutical companies leads to underreported ADRs	*Public awareness campaigns*: Conducting educational campaigns to raise awareness about the importance of reporting ADRs
	Healthcare training: Providing training to healthcare professionals on recognizing and reporting ADRs to encourage active participation
Resource constraints: Limited resources and infrastructure hinder efficient reporting and data collection	*Simplified reporting processes*: Streamlining the reporting process through user-friendly digital platforms and applications
	Digital integration: Introducing online reporting systems and mobile apps to make reporting quicker and more convenient
Incomplete data: Consistent data quality and complete reports impede the identification of patterns and trends	*Standardized reporting criteria*: Implementing standardized criteria to ensure comprehensive and accurate reporting
	Multilingual support: Providing support in multiple languages to facilitate reporting from diverse regions
Language barriers: Different languages used across regions challenge the comparison and analysis of data	*Collaboration and knowledge sharing*: Collaborate with international organizations and neighboring countries to adopt best practices and share strategies
	Data validation and analysis tools: Implementing automated analysis tools to enhance data quality and detect emerging safety signals
Lack of digitalization: Manual reporting processes lead to errors and delays in data transfer	*Automated data transfer*: Introducing digital systems to automate data transfer and reduce the chances of errors

(continued)

Table 6.3 (continued)

Challenges in ADR Reporting	Improvements and solutions
	Efficient oversight: Establishing dedicated authorities to oversee ADR reporting and ensure compliance with guidelines
Insufficient data analysis: Inadequate tools for analyzing large datasets prevent timely detection of safety concerns	*Advanced data analysis*: Utilize advanced analytics tools to identify potential safety signals from extensive datasets proactively
	Timely intervention: Promptly addressing emerging safety concerns to prevent adverse effects on public health

6.7 Comparative Analysis and Lessons Learned

In Table 6.4, the key aspects (Regulatory Framework and Authorities, ADR Reporting System Structure, Challenges, Best Practices, and Lessons Learned) are compared for ADR reporting practices in India, the US, and the EU (Kramer et al. 2013). The table highlights the similarities and differences in their practices, their everyday challenges, the best practices they implement, and the valuable lessons they have learned from their experiences. Collaboration, data quality improvement, and standardized reporting criteria are important themes across all regions.

6.8 Case Studies or Examples of ADR Reporting in India, US, EU, and Non-EU

Table 6.5 describes the ADR reporting process for the pharmaceutical product Thalidomide and Vioxx (Rofecoxib) in different countries: India, the United States, the European Union, and Non-European Union countries (excluding India, the US, and EU).

6.9 Future Perspectives and Recommendations

6.9.1 Advancements in ADR Reporting Technology

The advancements in ADR reporting technology have revolutionized pharmacovigilance practices, making the process more efficient, data-driven, and patient-centered. Implementing these technological advancements continues to be crucial in enhancing drug safety surveillance and ultimately improving patient outcomes (Tandon et al. 2015; Kharkar and Bowalekar 2012).

Digital Reporting Platforms: A significant advancement is the widespread adoption of digital reporting platforms. These platforms, like EudraVigilance in the EU,

Table 6.4 ADR Reporting Practices Comparison: India, US, and EU (Vashisth et al. 2012)

Aspect	Similarities	Differences	Challenges faced by all regions	Best practices	Lessons learned
Regulatory Framework and Authorities	Central regulatory authorities (CDSCO, FDA, EMA)	Differences in specific regulatory bodies and their roles in ADR reporting	Underreporting of ADRs	Standardization of reporting criteria and guidelines	Patient engagement is crucial for complete reporting
ADR Reporting System Structure	Centralized databases (VigiFlow, FAERS, EudraVigilance)	Differences in reporting platforms and structures	Data quality and completeness	Digital integration for streamlined reporting	Collaboration among stakeholders is essential
Challenges	Underreporting, data quality, language barriers (EU)	Each region faces unique challenges in its ADR reporting practices	Timeliness in reporting	Awareness campaigns for improved reporting	Data sharing and exchange for signal detection
Best practices	Standardization, digital integration, patient engagement	Best practices vary, but sharing expertise and lessons can lead to improvement	Harmonization of reporting criteria	Electronic reporting systems for efficiency	Continuous monitoring of drug safety
Lessons learned	Collaboration, timely regulatory actions, patient safety	Lessons from each region can inform and improve ADR reporting practices globally	Language diversity and multilingual support	Patient reporting to enhance data completeness	Harmonization of reporting criteria

FAERS in the US, and VigiFlow in India, enable the electronic submission of ADR reports. Digital reporting streamlines the process, reduces paperwork, and allows faster data transmission and analysis.

Automated data analysis: Its capabilities have been integrated into ADR reporting technology as it has developed. These techniques aid in the rapid identification of potential safety risks by identifying patterns and trends in massive datasets. ADR reporting systems are more effective and accurate when automated signal detection is used.

Table 6.5 ADR Reporting for Thalidomide and Vioxx (Rofecoxib) in different countries

Country	Regulatory authority	Reporting structure	Timelines for reporting	Outcome and actions
Vioxx (Rofecoxib)				
India	Health Regulatory Agency India	Healthcare professionals, consumers, and pharmaceutical companies report to the Health Regulatory Agency	Within 15 days of awareness	Cases of cardiovascular risks reported, regulatory action taken, product withdrawal
United States	Food and Drug Administration (FDA)	Healthcare professionals, consumers, and pharmaceutical companies report to the FDA's Adverse Event Reporting System (FAERS)	Within 15 days of awareness	Significant cardiovascular risks observed, FDA strengthens warnings, eventual market withdrawal
European Union	European Medicines Agency (EMA)	Healthcare professionals, consumers, and pharmaceutical companies report to EudraVigilance	Within 15 days of awareness	Cardiovascular issues identified, EMA advises updated warnings, product suspension
Non-EU (Excluding India, US)	Respective Health Regulatory Authority	Healthcare professionals, consumers, and pharmaceutical companies report to the Health Regulatory Authority	Within 30 days of awareness	Emerging cardiovascular concerns, regulatory intervention, safety label change
Thalidomide				
India	Health Regulatory Agency India	Healthcare professionals, consumers, and pharmaceutical companies report to the Health Regulatory Agency	Within 15 days of awareness	Birth deformities were reported immediately banned, and stringent regulations were enforced
United States	Food and Drug Administration (FDA)	Healthcare professionals, consumers, and pharmaceutical companies report to the FDA's Adverse Event Reporting System (FAERS)	Within 15 days of awareness	Congenital disability cases documented, FDA introduces rigorous drug approval process

(continued)

Table 6.5 (continued)

Country	Regulatory authority	Reporting structure	Timelines for reporting	Outcome and actions
European Union	European Medicines Agency (EMA)	Healthcare professionals, consumers, and pharmaceutical companies report to EudraVigilance	Within 15 days of awareness	With widespread birth abnormalities, EMA strengthens drug evaluation procedures
Non-EU (Excluding India, US)	Respective Health Regulatory Authority	Healthcare professionals, consumers, and pharmaceutical companies report to the Health Regulatory Authority	Within 30 days of awareness	Instances of congenital disabilities trigger regulatory responses, and products are banned or restricted

Mobile Applications: In some areas, mobile applications that allow consumers and healthcare professionals to report ADRs straight from their cellphones or tablets have been released. Mobile reporting improves accessibility and convenience, promoting more frequent and widespread reporting.

Artificial *intelligence (AI):* ADR reporting systems incorporate AI technologies like machine learning and natural language processing. AI makes Advanced data analytics possible, which also helps improve data quality and extract pertinent information from unstructured data.

Integration and Interoperability: Better data integration and interoperability between various ADR reporting databases and systems have been made possible by technological advancements. Harmonized data interchange fosters regional cooperation and improves worldwide pharmacovigilance initiatives.

Real-Time Monitoring: A few systems now allow users to keep track of reported ADRs in real-time. This capability can quickly identify and address emergent safety signals, resulting in more prompt regulatory measures.

Social Media Monitoring: Technology has expanded ADR reporting beyond conventional means. Using social media monitoring techniques, prospective ADR reports users to share on sites like Twitter and Facebook are collected and analyzed.

Data Visualization: Advancements in technology have allowed better data integration and interoperability between different ADR reporting databases and systems. Harmonized data exchange supports collaboration among regions and enhances global pharmacovigilance efforts.

Real-Time Monitoring: Some systems now offer real-time monitoring of reported ADRs. This capability enables rapid identification and response to emerging safety signals, leading to more timely regulatory actions.

Social Media Monitoring: Technology has extended ADR reporting beyond traditional channels. Social media monitoring tools are being used to capture and analyze potential ADR reports users share on platforms like Twitter and Facebook.

Data Visualization: Improved data visualization tools aid in presenting ADR data in a user-friendly and informative manner. Visualizations like heatmaps and interactive dashboards enable a more straightforward interpretation of ADR trends and patterns.

Blockchain Technology: Blockchain technology is being investigated to improve data security and integrity in ADR reporting. It can offer a decentralized, impenetrable system that guarantees data trust and transparency.

6.10 Collaboration and Information Sharing Among Regions

Regional cooperation and information sharing are crucial to improve global pharmacovigilance efforts and ensure patient safety. Countries and regulatory bodies work together in ADR reporting to exchange safety data, best practices, and lessons learned. Sharing information on reported adverse drug reactions, signal detection outcomes, and regulatory actions helps identify potential safety concerns associated with specific medications (Collaboration and Information Sharing Among India, US and EU—Google Scholar n.d.; Stojčić 2021). Collaborative efforts allow for a broader perspective on drug safety profiles, especially for rare or delayed adverse events that may not be evident within individual regions. Through shared knowledge and experiences, regions can collectively address common challenges, harmonize reporting standards, and implement more effective risk management strategies. This collaborative approach fosters a more proactive and responsive pharmacovigilance system, benefiting patients worldwide and promoting a safer and more reliable pharmaceutical landscape (Sachdeva 2008).

6.11 Recommendations for Enhancing ADR Reporting Globally

Enhancing ADR reporting requires a concerted effort to strengthen drug safety monitoring and promote patient well-being. First and foremost, awareness and education campaigns should be implemented to raise understanding among healthcare professionals, consumers, and pharmaceutical companies about the significance of ADR reporting. Standardizing reporting criteria and guidelines across regions is essential for streamlined data collection and improved data exchange between countries. Embracing digital reporting platforms and automated data analysis tools will accelerate reporting processes and enhance signal detection capabilities (Kharkar and Bowalekar 2012). Empowering patients to actively report adverse events through user-friendly channels, such as mobile applications, will contribute to more comprehensive safety data. Creating a secure and standardized platform for global data exchange will facilitate international collaboration and research efforts. Leveraging AI technologies and social media monitoring will strengthen data analysis and complement traditional reporting systems. All regions can actively participate in ADR reporting thanks to international collaboration and capacity building activities, resulting in a more effective global pharmacovigilance system. The continual improvement that results from regular input and evaluation of regulatory activities will strengthen a patient-centered approach to medication safety (Chatterjee et al. 2006). The global pharmacovigilance community can collaborate to create a safer and more dependable pharmaceutical environment to help patients all around the world by putting these ideas into practice, eventually helping patients all around the world.

6.12 Conclusion

This chapter provided a comparative analysis of ADR reporting practices in India, The United States of America, the European Union, and the non-European Union concerning each region's strengths, difficulties, and best practices. ADR is a crucial component of pharmacovigilance, ensuring patient safety and advancing drug safety procedures globally. Case studies demonstrating the influence of ADR reporting on medication safety were examined, along with the regulatory frameworks, reporting procedures, and difficulties experienced by these regions. While there were some commonalities in ADR reporting practices among the regions, such as the use of centralized databases and central regulatory agencies, some variances reflected the distinct approaches and laws of each jurisdiction. Recommendations were made to improve ADR reporting globally with a focus on patient participation, standardization, digital integration, awareness campaigns, artificial intelligence (AI) use, data sharing, and international cooperation. The global pharmacovigilance community may strive toward a more secure and dependable pharmaceutical landscape, assuring better patient safety and better healthcare practices globally, by implementing these guidelines and learning from one another's experiences.

References

Ahmad A, Patel I, Balkrishnan R, Mohanta GP, Manna PK (2013) An evaluation of knowledge, attitude and practice of Indian pharmacists towards adverse drug reaction reporting: a pilot study. Perspect Clin Res 4:204–210. https://www.ncbi.nlm.nih.gov/pmc/articles/PMC3835963/. Accessed 18 Jul 2023

Blake KV, Zaccaria C, Domergue F, La Mache E, Saint-Raymond A, Hidalgo-Simon A (2014) Comparison between paediatric and adult suspected adverse drug reactions reported to the European Medicines Agency: implications for pharmacovigilance. Pediatr Drugs 16(4):309–319. https://doi.org/10.1007/S40272-014-0076-2

Brucker MC, King TL (2017) The 2015 US Food and Drug Administration pregnancy and lactation labeling rule. J Midwifery Womens Health 62(3):308–316. https://doi.org/10.1111/JMWH.12611

Chatterjee S, Lyle N, Ghosh S (2006) A survey of the knowledge, attitude and practice of adverse drug reaction reporting by clinicians in eastern India. Drug Saf 29(7):641–642. https://doi.org/10.2165/00002018-200629070-00009

Collaboration and Information Sharing Among India, US and EU—Google Scholar (n.d.). Available from https://scholar.google.com/scholar?hl=en&as_sdt=0%2C5&q=Collaboration+and+Information+Sharing+Among+India%2C+US+and+EU&btnG=. Accessed 18 July 2023
Daller J (2016) Biosimilars: a consideration of the regulations in the United States and European Union. Regul Toxicol Pharmacol 76:199–208. https://www.sciencedirect.com/science/article/pii/S0273230015301483. Accessed 18 Jul 2023
Dylan Fernandes S, Anoop NV, Castelino LJ, Narayana Charyulu R (2019) A national approach to pharmacovigilance: the case of India as a growing hub of global clinical trials. Res Social Adm Pharm 15(1):109–113. https://doi.org/10.1016/j.sapharm.2018.03.061
Felix T, Jordan JB, Akers C, Patel B, Drago D (2019) Current state of biologic pharmacovigilance in the European Union: improvements are needed. Expert Opin Drug Saf 18(3):231–240. https://doi.org/10.1080/14740338.2019.1577818
Ferrajolo C, Capuano A, Trifirò G, Moretti U, Rossi F, Santuccio C (2014) Pediatric drug safety surveillance in Italian pharmacovigilance network: an overview of adverse drug reactions in the years 2001-2012. Expert Opin Drug Saf 13 Suppl 1:S9–S20. https://doi.org/10.1517/14740338.2014.939581
Joshi D, Gupta S, Singh TG, Parashar A, Singh SK (2022) A qualitative evaluation of ADR reporting in India: non-regulatory confronts and their possible solutions. ECS Trans 107(1):6763–6780. https://doi.org/10.1149/10701.6763ECST/META
Kharkar M, Bowalekar S (2012) Knowledge, attitude and perception/practices (KAP) of medical practitioners in India towards adverse drug reaction (ADR) reporting. Perspect Clin Res 3:90–94. https://www.ncbi.nlm.nih.gov/pmc/articles/PMC3487231/. Accessed 18 Jul 2023
Kim FJ, da Silva RD, Gustafson D, Nogueira L, Harlin T, Paul DL (2015) Current issues in patient safety in surgery: a review. Patient Saf Surg 9(1):26. https://doi.org/10.1186/S13037-015-0067-4
Kramer DB, Tan YT, Sato C, Kesselheim AS (2013) Postmarket surveillance of medical devices: a comparison of strategies in the US, EU, Japan, and China. PLoS Med 10(9):e1001519. https://doi.org/10.1371/journal.pmed.1001519
Li R, Curtis K, Zaidi ST, Van C, Castelino R (2022) A new paradigm in adverse drug reaction reporting: consolidating the evidence for an intervention to improve reporting. Expert Opin Drug Saf 21(9):1193–1204. https://doi.org/10.1080/14740338.2022.2118712
Mulchandani R, Kakkar AK (2019) Reporting of adverse drug reactions in India: a review of the current scenario, obstacles and possible solutions. Int J Risk Saf Med 30(1):33–44
Nguyen M, Ball R, Midthun K, Lieu TA (2012) The Food and Drug Administration's post-licensure rapid immunization Safety monitoring program: strengthening the federal vaccine safety enterprise. Pharmacoepidemiol Drug Saf 21(SUPPL. 1):291–297. https://doi.org/10.1002/PDS.2323
Patel NM, Stottlemyer BA, Gray MP, Boyce RD, Kane-Gill SL (2022) A pharmacovigilance study of adverse drug reactions reported for cardiovascular disease medications approved between 2012 and 2017 in the United States Food and Drug Administration adverse event reporting system (FAERS) database. Cardiovasc Drugs Ther 36(2):309–322. https://doi.org/10.1007/S10557-021-07157-3
Sachdeva G (2008) India and the European Union: broadening strategic partnership beyond economic linkages. Int Stud 45(4):341–367. https://doi.org/10.1177/002088170904500403
Schrama R (2022) Expert network interaction in the European Medicines Agency. Regul Governance 17(2):491–511. https://doi.org/10.1111/rego.12466
Simera I, Moher D, Hoey J, Schulz KF, Altman DG (2010) A catalogue of reporting guidelines for health research. Eur J Clin Invest 40(1):35–53. https://doi.org/10.1111/j.1365-2362.2009.02234.x
Singh A, Kalaivani M, Srivastava S, Goyal RK, Gupta SK (2020) Post-marketing safety of biosimilars: current status, challenges, and opportunities in the spontaneous reporting system. Therapeut Innov Regul Sci 54(3):667–680. https://doi.org/10.1007/S43441-019-00101-6
Singh P, Vaishnav Y, Verma S (2023) Development of pharmacovigilance system in India and paradigm of pharmacovigilance research: an overview. Curr Drug Saf 18(4):448–464. https://doi.org/10.2174/1574886317666220930145603

Stergiopoulos S, Brown C, Felix T, Safety GG-D (2016) A survey of adverse event reporting practices among US healthcare professionals. Drug Saf 39:1117–1127. https://doi.org/10.1007/s40264-016-0455-4

Stojčić N (2021) Collaborative innovation in emerging innovation systems: evidence from central and Eastern Europe. J Technol Transfer 46(2):531–562. Accessed 18 Jul 2023. https://doi.org/10.1007/s10961-020-09792-8

Suke SG, Kosta P, Negi H (2015) Role of pharmacovigilance in India: an overview. Online J Public Health Inform 7:e223. https://www.ncbi.nlm.nih.gov/pmc/articles/PMC4576445/. Accessed 18 Jul 2023

Tandon VR, Mahajan V, Khajuria V, Gillani Z (2015) Under-reporting of adverse drug reactions: a challenge for pharmacovigilance in India. Indian J Pharm 47:65–71. https://www.ncbi.nlm.nih.gov/pmc/articles/PMC4375822/. Accessed 18 Jul 2023

Thota P, Thota A, Medhi B, Sidhu S, Kumar P, Selvan VK, Singh GN (2018) Drug safety alerts of pharmacovigilance programme of India: a scope for targeted spontaneous reporting in India. Perspect Clin Res 9(1):51–55. https://doi.org/10.4103/picr.PICR_29_17

Vashisth S, Singh G, Generic AN-J (2012) A comparative study of regulatory trends of pharmaceuticals in Brazil, Russia, India and China (BRIC) countries. J Gene Med 9(3):128–143. https://doi.org/10.1177/1741134312459187

Walker KEW, Bankay R, Jankie S, Dhingra S (2023) Pharmacovigilance in the Caribbean countries: an overview. Curr Pharmacol Rep:1–11. https://doi.org/10.1007/s40495-023-00320-4

Pharmacovigilance System in India

7

Megha Sahu, Mukesh Nandave, and Anoop Kumar

Abstract

This chapter provides an overview of the pharmacovigilance system in India, concentrating on history, development, functions, different pharmacovigilance programs, framework, and current scenario. This chapter aims to offer insights to readers seeking a deeper understanding of the pharmacovigilance system in India. In 2010, the Pharmacovigilance Programme of India (PvPI) was launched by the Ministry of Health and Family Welfare, Government of India, after recognizing the need to improve ADRs reporting system in India. PvPI plays a significant role in collecting drug safety-related data and submitting it to World Health Organization (WHO) database. IPC, Ghaziabad is the national coordination centre (NCC) under the PvPI responsible for collecting, analyzing, and suggesting regulatory actions to Central Drugs Standard Control Organization (CDSCO). There are 760 Adverse Drug Monitoring Centres (AMCs) in India. Globally, India is now considered as a hub of clinical trials and research studies. Furthermore, there is a thrust need to a robust pharmacovigilance system in India to ensure patient safety.

Keywords

ADR reporting · Adverse reactions · Pharmcovigilance Program · Suspected drugs · VigiBase · Vigiflow

---

M. Sahu (✉) · M. Nandave · A. Kumar
Department of Pharmacology, Delhi Pharmaceutical Sciences and Research University, New Delhi, India
e-mail: mukeshnandave@gmail.com; anoopdpsru@dpsru.edu.in

M. Nandave, A. Kumar (eds.), *Pharmacovigilance Essentials*,
https://doi.org/10.1007/978-981-99-8949-2_7

7.1 Introduction

Before establishing a formal pharmacovigilance system in India, Adverse Drug Reactions (ADR) and safety concerns associated with drug are underreported and or poorly monitored. However, in 1986, pharmacovigilance activities took a step forward with the proposal of ADR monitoring system in India. The establishment of 12 centers in India for drug monitoring was planned. Some were set up in New Delhi, Mumbai, Kolkata, Lucknow, Chandigarh, and Pondicherry and monitored ADRs. This step strengthens the pharmacovigilance efforts and ensures the drug safety in Indian population. In 1997, India also joined the World Health Organization (WHO) Programme for International Drug Monitoring (PIDM), which has six centers for drug monitoring. All India Institute of Medical Sciences (AIIMS), New Delhi, was chosen as the national center, while King Edward Memorial (KEM) hospital in Mumbai was identified as WHO special center (Gupta 2010; Olsson 1998).

7.1.1 History of Pharmacovigilance System in India

In 1983, Dr. Molly Thomas, Clinical Pharmacologist at Christian Medical College, Vellore, initiated the ADR monitoring program in India at her hospital. Dr. Thomas took the initiative to educate about 1650 doctors and implemented a voluntary ADR reporting system within her hospital. At that time, she received around 600–900 ADR reports yearly and published newsletters quarterly. She was the first to identify low rates of ADR reporting and found that clinicians reported only significant reactions while ignoring minor ones. Most of the developed countries had initiated their pharmacovigilance program in early 1960. However, the Drug Controller General of India established the country's pharmacovigilance system in 1986 with 12 regional centers. District hospitals and primary health centers were affiliated with these main centers that are spread all over the country. Each center serves around 50 million people across the country.

In 1997, program was modified in India as it joined the PIDM, which was managed by the Uppsala Monitoring Centre (UMC), Sweden. This collaboration of India with PIDM further strengthened its commitment to ensuring drug safety and promoting world efforts in ADR reporting. Additionally, India had six centers running a pharmacovigilance program spread all over the country: New Delhi, Mumbai, Lucknow, Pondicherry, Kolkata, and Chandigarh. However, efforts made in the 1980s and 1990s failed to propel the growth of the pharmacovigilance program in India (CDSCO 2004). Indian Council of Medical Research (ICMR), New Delhi, initiated its independent ADR monitoring system having a total 12 centers across the country. A special task force was assigned to regulate this independent program, which started in 1992. This ICMR task force project is the evolved version of the previous program initiated in 1989. During this program a total number of 4490 ADRs in 82,761 patients were observed at different centers

(Thatte et al. 2018). Unfortunately, this program faced some challenges and was discontinued. Still, the assigned task force observed some improvement points that could be made if this program needed to be resumed. Improvement points include identifying centers, training in data analysis and interpretation, dedicated staff for data entry and its management, and identification of coordinating centers. In 2004, the pharmacovigilance program in India started to get successful with funding support from the World Bank, and the WHO continued to support India in the pharmacovigilance discipline. The pharmacovigilance program in India is officially termed the "National Pharmacovigilance Programme of India." India got funding of 0.1 million USD per year by the World Bank for 5 years (Adithan 2005). Figure 7.1 summarizes the pharmacovigilance system's history in India for easy understanding.

7.2 Advantages of Pharmacovigilance System in India

- It develops a nationwide strategy to enhance patient safety by ensuring the safety of medications.
- Evaluate the benefit–risk ratio of marketed medication, thus assuring the safety of patients.
- Identify and evaluate emerging signals from already reported cases.
- Assist competent regulatory authorities in decision-making process associated with medication usage.
- Disseminate information to various stakeholders to reduce or prevent the risk related to medication usage.
- It allows us to collaborate with other national centers to exchange and manage information and data.

7.3 National Pharmacovigilance Programme

In November 2004, the Government of India launched a pharmacovigilance program in the country and named the National Programme of Pharmacovigilance with funding support from the World Bank, and this program became operational on first January 2005. This pharmacovigilance program was managed by the National Pharmacovigilance Advisory Committee (NPAC), located at the office of Central Drugs Standard Control Organization (CDSCO). The ADRs report was received and processed by the South-West Zonal Center at KEM Hospital in Mumbai and North East Zonal center at AIIMS, New Delhi. The South West and North East Zonal Centers have 3 and 2 regional centers, respectively. There was a total of 26 peripheral centers across the country. The three main objectives of this program were to create a culture for ADR reporting, especially among healthcare professionals and to disseminate information on drug safety among the healthcare professionals and the public. The long-term objective was to set India as a critical player in

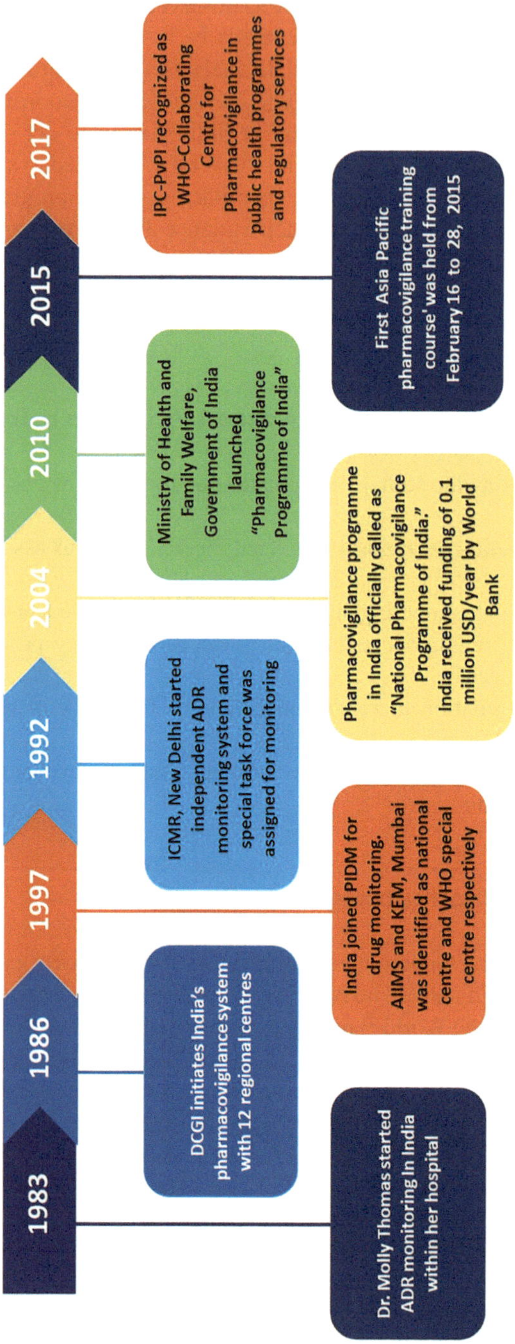

Fig. 7.1 Evolution of Pharmacovigilance System in India

pharmacovigilance globally (Biswas and Biswas 2007). However, the funding from the World Bank stopped, and this program faced some challenges and did not meet expectations. Therefore, it was suspended for the time being (Gupta 2010).

7.3.1 Peripheral Pharmacovigilance Centers

Primary or peripheral pharmacovigilance centers played a significant role in ADR reporting. They were smaller medical facilities such as private hospitals, medical practitioner's clinics, pharmacies, and nursing homes than Regional and Zonal Pharmacovigilance Centers. The identification and management of these types of centers were regulated by the Regional or Zonal Pharmacovigilance centers in collaboration with CDSCO. Including smaller hospitals and private practices in the National Pharmacovigilance Programme ensures the fulfillment of the aim to receive a wide range of ADR data from all over the country. There was a total of 28 Peripheral Pharmacovigilance Centers spread throughout the country that were attached to their nearest Regional or Zonal Centers (Adithan 2005).

7.3.2 Regional Pharmacovigilance Centers

Secondary or Regional Pharmacovigilance were more extensive healthcare facilities affiliated with medical college. They used to handle a broad range of ADRs as they serve a larger number of populations. They were identified and regulated by Zonal Pharmacovigilance Centers in collaboration with CDSCO. There were five Regional Pharmacovigilance Centers in the nation situated at TN Medical College and BYL Nair Charitable Hospital, Mumbai; IGPMR-SSKM hospital, Kolkata; Lady Hardinge Medical College, New Delhi; JIPMER, Pondicherry; Indira Gandhi Medical College, Nagpur (Adithan 2005).

7.3.3 Zonal Pharmacovigilance Centers

Tertiary or Zonal Pharmacovigilance Centers were more extensive healthcare facilities affiliated with medical colleges, identified and coordinated by CDSCO. Zonal Pharmacovigilance Centers analyze and forward the received ADRs report to CDSCO. There were two Zonal Pharmacovigilance Centers in the country at AIIMS, New Delhi, and Seth GS Medical College, Mumbai (Adithan 2005).

7.4 Pharmacovigilance Programme of India (PvPI)

In 2010, PvPI was launched by the Ministry of Health and Family Welfare, Government of India after recognizing the need for improving the ADRs reporting system in India. AIIMS, New Delhi, was recognized as the National Coordination

Center (NCC) with 22 Adverse Drug Reaction Monitoring Centers (AMC) nationwide. In 2011, the Ministry of Health and Family Welfare, Government of India, reforge this program, and NCC was shifted to the Indian Pharmacopoeia Commission (IPC), Ghaziabad (Thota et al. 2018). There are about 760 AMCs in India up to date, which is increasing every year, and India has the highest number of AMCs around the globe (Indian Pharmacopoeia Commission 2022). India is one of the top ten countries under WHO PIDM and one of the most significant contributors of ADR reporting. Individual Case Safety Reports (ICSRs) are gathered in the standard ADR report form, and these ICSRs are forwarded to NCC through VigiFlow software. All the AMCs have access to WHO PIDM world's ICSRs database via VigiBase (Thota et al. 2018). VigiBase is the database of ICSRs from membered countries enrolled in WHO PIDM. Figure 7.2 depicts how the data of ADR is reported and transferred in PvPI.

Spontaneous Reporting (SR): This method is widely used and termed "voluntary" reporting. SR depends on community and healthcare professionals volunteering to report ADRs. Therefore, it is necessary for the reporters to be educated and should be motivated to submit their observations. Training should be provided to healthcare professionals to disseminate information in relation to what, whom, where how, and whom to report ADRs. Underreporting is the major challenge of SR; therefore, it is crucial to conduct subsequent training (Hazell and Shakir 2006). This system has the advantage of getting ADRs reports from actual clinical practice, unlike clinical trials, which are for limited time and excludes a liable population (Olsson et al. 2010). However, this also has disadvantages like underreporting and

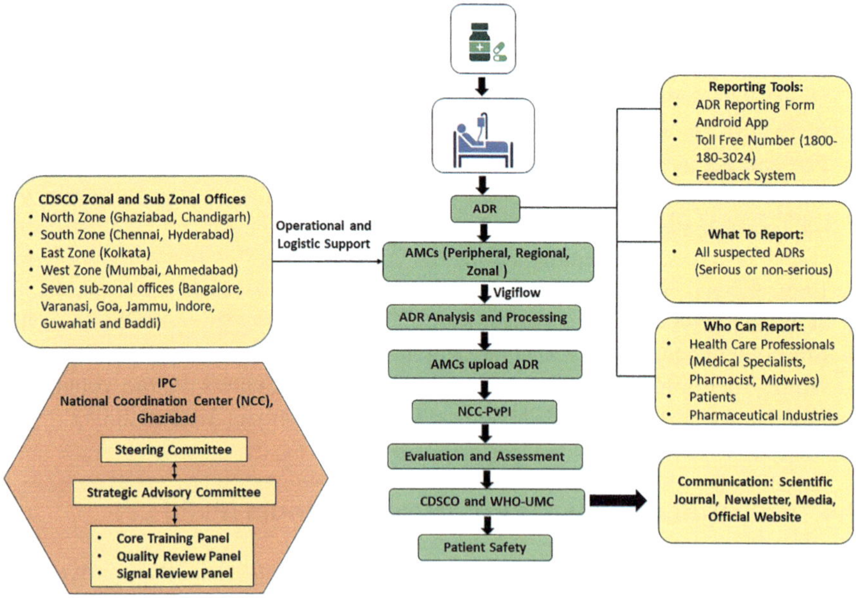

Fig. 7.2 Framework of Pharmacovigilance Programme of India (PvPI)

insufficient information on the exposed population. Therefore, measuring risk associated with suspected drugs becomes challenging, and bias reporting is possible. Despite these demerits, SR remains the foundation of PvPI as it ensures the early detection of potential ADRs linked with suspected drug (Team WHO 2006).

Targeted Spontaneous Reporting (TSR): In 2010, TSR was launched by WHO, which was built on the principles of the system but implemented within a specific context (WHO 2012). In this method of reporting, specific patients are selected to report particular safety issues associated with suspected drugs. TSR is undergoing pilot phase in three countries (Uganda, Vietnam, and Kenya) within HIV treatment programs. TSR method may be applied in specific populations to document suspected ADRs of particular interest. Patients undergoing therapy under the TSR method are closely monitored as part of their medical care. Healthcare providers' vigilance toward ADRs and their immediate reporting contributes to the success of these efforts (Clarkson 2001).

7.4.1 Achievements of PvPI

- A total of 760 AMCs have been established, along with framework of pharmacovigilance and a reporting culture across the country (Indian Pharmacopoeia Commission 2022).
- The PvPI made remarkable contributions to several health programs, including tuberculosis, HIV-AIDS, immunization, vector-borne disease, and neglected tropical disease. The drug safety concerns for particular drugs received have been shared with national health programs to ensure patient safety.
- PvPI has started a skill development program "Basic & Regulatory Aspects of Pharmacovigilance" to educate healthcare professionals. To community outreach, AMCs have conducted awareness program to reinforce the ADR reporting system across the country. As a result, this culture has improved throughout the nation (Anon 2016). As antimicrobial resistance is reaching an alarming rate in the country, PvPI is vigorously working and taking every measure to combat this danger. The pharmacovigilance endeavors are being improved at national, regional and district level to assure public health. National Health Policy 2017, initiated by Ministry of Health and Family Welfare, Government of India, explicitly addresses pharmacovigilance and antimicrobial resistance. This policy aims to ensure ADRs reporting and prevent ADRs wherever possible.
- Under regulations of IPC and Ministry of Health and Family Welfare, Govt of India. PvPI successfully underwent the assessment by National Regulatory Authority (WHO-NRA) 2017 Global Benchmarking Tool. Therefore, vigilance reached a maturity level of 4 (PvPI. 2017).
- NCC-PvPI accomplished quality and quantitative work toward WHO-PIDM over the years. This noteworthy contribution made the IPC recognized as the "WHO Collaborating Center for Pharmacovigilance in Public Health Programmes and Regulatory Science."

- PvPI has submitted 88,360 ICSRs to VigiBase, making it the ninth largest reporter of ICSRS in Vigibase on a global scale.
- PvPI has organized 5926 workshops, training courses, Continuing Medical Education (CME) and Advance Level Training (ALT) programs with approximately 3,16,912 participants trained during these initiatives. PvPI has celebrated its first national pharmacovigilance week from 17th-23rd September 2021 nationwide (Indian Pharmacopoeia Commission 2022).

7.4.2 Committee of NCC-PvPI

Steering Committee: The principal administrative body and monitoring body in NCC-PvPI, offers guidance and supervision to the program.

Working Group: This is directed by Secretary-cum-Scientific Director, IPC, and handles all the technical aspects related to the establishment and implementation of the pharmacovigilance program as well as it is responsible for providing technical guidance.

Quality Review Panel: It evaluates quality, completeness score, causality assessment, and other parts of ICSRs. This panel recommends PvPI working group after data analysis and develops the format and instructional materials for subsequent actions.

Signal Review Panel: This panel includes clinical experts and scientists from government and non-governmental hospitals and academic institutions. According to the recruitment, experts from the pharmaceutical industry are invited to analyze ICSRs, collate and give their valuable suggestions. This panel is responsible for confirming and validating the computerized results of ICSRs after appropriate evaluation. It established biostatistical methods for assessment and developed post-analytical reports to facilitate the smooth interpretation of information from ICSRs.

Core Training Panel: This panel helps conduct training programs for healthcare professionals and other stakeholders and guides in designing training modules. They also communicate with national and international organizations to facilitate participation and the successful execution of training programs. Moreover, the Core Training Panel receives support from the PvPI internal training team (Indian Pharmacopoeia Commission 2022).

7.5 Overview of CDSCO

CDSCO is the regulatory authority overseeing drugs and medical devices in India. CDSCO operates in collaboration with IPC, and NCC-PvPI to monitor the safety of medicines usage and takes appropriate regulatory action as required. CDSCO also communicates decisions associated with drug safety to PvPI stakeholders. CDSCO and NCC-PvPI conduct regular training sessions for the personnel involved in pharmacovigilance to make them aware of pharmacovigilance terminology, standards, concepts, and processes for ADR reporting and causality evaluation. Zonal and sub-zonal CDSCO offices offer technical and logistical support to AMCs in their respective zones. Additionally, respective zonal and sub-zonal CDSCO offices are responsible for monitoring the functionality of AMCs (Kumar 2015). There are six zonal offices (Ghaziabad, North zone; Kolkata, East zone; Mumbai, West zone; Chennai, South zone; Ahmedabad and Hyderabad, zonal offices) and seven sub-zonal offices (Bangalore, Varanasi, Goa, Jammu, Indore, Guwahati and Baddi) (CDSCO n.d.).

7.6 Introduction to AMCs

In India, Medical colleges and hospitals play a pivotal role in education and providing specialized services to patients. AMCs under PvPI working in these institutions also play a crucial role in ADR monitoring. Letter of Intent is attached in Annexure-1.

Who can enroll for AMC: government, district, private hospitals, autonomous bodies, medical or pharmacy colleges, and primary, or community health centers.

7.6.1 Terms and Conditions for AMCs Enrollment

- Availability of infrastructure and logistics support for pharmacovigilance at the proposed center.
- The Dean or Head of the Institution or Head of Department is responsible for establishing and executing pharmacovigilance activities at the proposed center.
- Prominent track record of the proposed center demonstrated through both quality and quantity of reported ADR and frequency of ADR reporting.
- The proposed center's AMC coordinator or deputy coordinator should have appropriate experience.
- State or Union Territories with limited or no existing AMC will be preferred.
- AMCs will be selected based on demographic considerations.

Standard procedure is followed during the enrollment of new AMCs as shown in Fig 7.3. After recognition, NCC-PvPI provides consistent training, skill development, and technical training to the individuals engaged in PvPI-associated activities.

7.6.2 Criteria for Disenrollment of AMC

- Lack of reporting or activity.
- Non-adherence to the quality management system (Indian Pharmacopoeia Commission 2022).

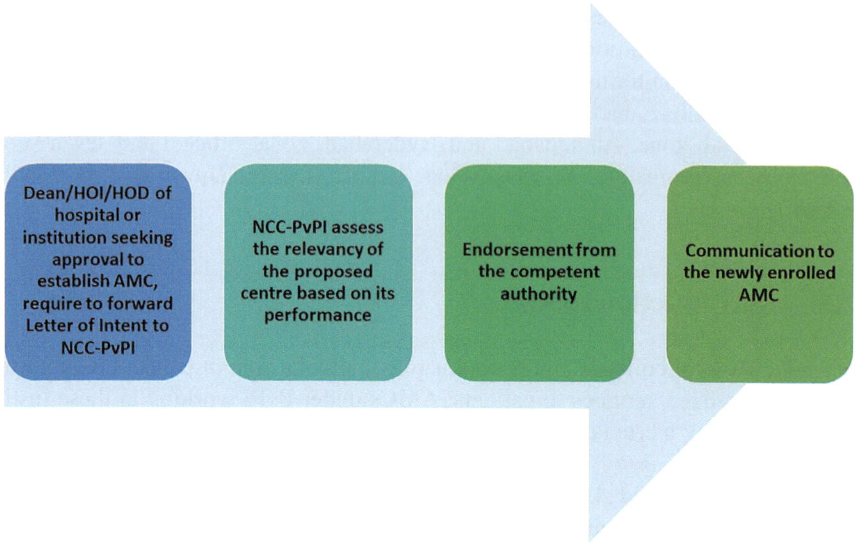

Fig. 7.3 Figure Depicting Procedure for ADR Monitoring Centre (AMC) Enrollment

7.7 The UMC, Sweden

After the thalidomide disaster, WHO initiated an international drug monitoring program, which was executed at UMC, Sweden, UMC provides technical assistance to several countries, including India for drug safety. The primary role of the UMC is to manage all the ADRs related databases submitted by national centers. NCC-PvPI has been providing drug safety data of the Indian population to the safety database Vigibase after collaboration with UMC. NCC has access to most of the web tools developed by UMC. The UMC identifies and evaluates new ADR signals from participating countries (Kumar 2015).

7.8 Pharmacovigilance Regulations in India

A vigorous regulatory system forms the foundation of a national approach toward drug safety and fosters public trust in drug therapy. The pharmacovigilance program needs to maintain a strong association with regulatory authority to inform the latter about safety issues in routine clinical practice. This association is essential to address any potential future regulatory action or concerns that may arise in public.

7.8.1 Schedule Y

In India, Legislative obligations for pharmacovigilance are driven by the provisions mentioned in Drugs and Cosmetics Act 1940 and Rules 1945. Schedule Y encompasses regulations for preclinical and clinical research studies for new drugs and deals with clinical requirements for importing, manufacturing, and getting approval to introduce a new drug in the Indian market. In January 2005, Schedule Y underwent changes and was amended as the continued dedication of the Drug Controller General of India (DCGI) to ensure that pharmaceutical companies stick to their pharmacovigilance duties. Amendment of Schedule Y included a better explanation of the roles and responsibilities of pharmaceutical companies related to their products and reporting of ADRs from clinical trials (Bhave and Menon 2017).

7.8.2 Spontaneous ADR

Schedule Y depicts that unexpected serious adverse reactions received should be forwarded to licensing authorities within 15 days of receiving the applicant's primary data, followed by follow-up data provided (Pant 2021). Individual adverse event reports should be submitted in successive safety update reports without requiring immediate urgency. However, Schedule Y does not include additional information on recording, evaluation, and subsequent monitoring of adverse events. Therefore, pharma companies follow the guidelines provided by ICH E28 to manage spontaneous reaction reports associated with marketed products (Biswas 2013).

7.8.3 Safety Reporting During Clinical Trial

According to amended Schedule Y, investigators and sponsors need to report severe adverse reactions as follows:

Suppose an unexpected serious adverse reaction is observed. In that case, the investigator must report it promptly to the sponsor within 24 h of first occurrence and to the ethical committee that endorsed the study within 7 days.

Consequently, the sponsor must report serious adverse events during the clinical trial to the licensing agency and other investigators involved in the clinical trial on an urgent basis (Appendix XI).

Schedule Y states that during the clinical trial or follow-up, it is the investigator's responsibility to ensure that adequate medical care is available to subjects experiencing adverse reactions.

Schedule Y does not outline the guidelines for reporting adverse reactions observed in multinational trials. Additionally, it lacks information on the process for unblinding, data monitoring committee, coding, and managing ADRs related to comparator drug or placebo (Arora 2008; Don 2006).

7.9 Procedure for the Release of Drug Safety Alert in India

All received ICSRs are processed according to the standard operating procedure of PvPI. Subsequently, the collected safety data will be submitted to VigiBase to identify the global drug safety signal. The grading completeness score of ICSRs is based on the WHO-UMC VigiGrade algorithm. Received ICSRs at NCC undergo filtration through vigiflow that identifies unlisted ICSRs. Unlisted ICSRs are segregated as drug-ADR combinations followed by further validation to confirm them as unlisted ICSRs or potential drug alerts. PvPI reviews diverse drug information, including primary, secondary, tertiary, production information leaflets, and authorized government websites. In addition, PvPI also compares the drug-ADR combination data with the VigilyZe database and publications by national centers of other countries. The drug safety alerts will be distributed among the NCC-PvPI stakeholders or partners by NCC-PvPI. NCC-PvPI published drug safety alerts in newsletters for better patient safety. These newsletters help patients, hospital staff, pharmacists, and clinicians to prevent medication usage that could have potential ADR. Furthermore, AMCs will monitor closely all the patients who are receiving drug which is indicated to cause ADR (Thota et al. 2018).

7.10 Current Scenario

Globally, India is one of the largest producers of pharmaceuticals and is establishing itself as a hub for clinical trials. Many novel drugs are being launched into the market, so it is necessary to strengthen the pharmacovigilance system in India to prevent potential risks associated with novel drugs. In India, pharmacovigilance is constantly evolving, growing, and improving with time. The ADR reporting tools, including the PvPI helpline number, ADR reporting form, and PvPI mobile application, is now not only confined to AMCs, but these tools are also available at pharmacies, corporate and private hospitals to their broaden access to patients and caregivers (Prakash et al. 2021). On 11th October 2013 and 15th September 2014, the Revised National Tuberculosis Control Program (RNTCP) and National AIDS Control Organization (NACO) collaborated with PvPI, respectively. The aim of this collaboration was to ensure patient safety with the usage of the anti-tubercular drug and anti-retroviral drug.

Additionally, CDSCO and NCC websites were upgraded so that it could be used to communicate with stakeholders and make it feasible for public to search for specific information. Aforementioned websites provide pharmacovigilance-related guidance documents, including AMCs list, the procedure for ADR reporting, training modules, and newsletters. The newsletter is a recent initiative by PvPI, which is published every 4 months in a year, it includes ADR-associated information. It is available online and hard copies are supplied to the institutions associated with pharmacovigilance (Kalaiselvan et al. 2016).

NCC-PvPI accomplished quality and quantitative work toward WHO-PIDM over the years. This noteworthy contribution led the IPC to be recognized as the "WHO Collaborating Center for Pharmacovigilance in Public Health Programmes and Regulatory Science" on 18th July 2017. In 2021, NCC-PvPI started to celebrate first National Pharmacovigilance Week Pan India from 17th—23rd September with the theme "Pharmacovigilance: A step toward patient safety" (Anon 2021).

PvPI has identified 39 new AMCs altogether now there are a total of 760 AMCs across the nation (Indian Pharmacopoeia Commission 2022). In 2022, NCC-PvPI has suggested 12 signals and 56 modifications in the Prescribing Information Leaflet (PIL) to CDSCO to take appropriate regulatory measures. PvPI has released 150 drug safety alerts to promote awareness among healthcare professionals and the general public. Table 7.1 illustrates the recently released drug safety alerts by PvPI-NCC, IPC. Currently, there is a pressing need to foster the growth of skilled human resource therefore PvPI has conducted 5926 training programs, including Induction-cum training programs, ALT programs, etc. (Indian Pharmacopoeia Commission 2022). Recently, CDSCO approved PIL modification recommended by NCC-PvPI for cephalosporins, haloperidol, remdesivir, hyponatremia, Minoxidil, and Tigecycline. India holds eighth position among WHO PIDM member countries in relation to ICSRs submitted on VigiBase around the globe (Anon 2023a).

7.11 Conclusions

In India, the pharmacovigilance concept was in a very early stage, although its concept was existed since the 1980s. Accessibility of pharmacovigilance was confined to some institutions thus it was not accessible to everyone. However, this field started to emerge and develop from 2009 with exponential growth, specifically from 2012. PvPI is raising awareness of ADR reporting among the public. The issue of low reporting rates is being resolved due to the facilities that are easily accessible such as toll-free messages, helpline numbers, email, and ADR forms in regional languages. Although the pharmacovigilance system has made progress in India, but it has a considerable journey to go ahead to achieve its full potential so that it can align with international standards. Furthermore, progress and development are required in the Indian pharmacovigilance system to match global benchmarks.

Table 7.1 Drug safety alerts identified and issued by PvPI from January 2022 to March 2023 (Anon 2022a,b, c; 2023b)

S.No.	Issue Date	Suspected Drugs	Indications	Adverse drug reactions
1	29th March 2023	Sulfasalazine	• In the treatment of rheumatoid arthritis, Crohn's disease, ulcerative colitis	Visual impairment
2	29th March 2023	Olmesartan	• Used in the hypertension	Muscle spasm and taste disorder
3	29th March 2023	Nebivolol	• In the treatment of hypertension	Hyperkalemia
4	29th March 2023	Metoprolol	• Hypertension, migraine prophylaxis, heart disorders, cardiac arrythmia, stable symptomatic CHF	Hyponatremia
5	20th February 2023	Amikacin	• In infections with amikacin sensitive organism	Vision blurred
6	20th February 2023	Cephalosporins	• Beta-lactam antimicrobials used to deal with broad range of gram positive and negative bacteria	Purpura
7	31st Jan 2023	Amphotericin B (liposomal)	• For invasive fungal infection patients who are intolerant to conventional treatment of amphotericin B • Febrile neutropenia in cancer patients	Hearing disorder and tachycardia
8	26th Sep 2022	Piroxicam	• In the treatment of osteoarthritis, cervical spondylitis, rheumatoid arthritis, ankylosing spondylitis, and others	Fixed drug eruption
9	23rd August 2022	Cefoperazone	• To treat respiratory infections, UTI, skin tissue infections, meningitis, biliary infections, septicemia, salmonella typhi., fragilis infections, pseudomonas	Coagulopathy
10	15th July 2022	Tacrolimus	• As prophylaxis in kidney transplant or liver or heart allograft rejection • In the treatment of moderate to severe atopic dermatitis	Gingival hypertrophy

(continued)

Table 7.1 (continued)

S.No.	Issue Date	Suspected Drugs	Indications	Adverse drug reactions
11	17th June 2022	Trimetazidine	• Used in angina pectoris, ischemic heart disease, infarction, intermittent claudication	Drug reaction with eosinophilia and systemic symptoms (DRESS)
12	30th May 2022	Itraconazole	• Used in cryptococcosis, sporotrichosis, blastomycosis, systemic aspergillosis, and candidiasis. • Therapy of febrile neutropenic patients with fungal infections	Symmetrical drug related intertriginous and flexural exanthema (SDRIFE)
13	28th April 2022	Cefuroxime	• Antibiotic prescribed for lower and upper respiratory tract infection, gynecological infection, urinary tract infection skin or soft tissue infection, etc.	Drug reaction with eosinophilia and systemic symptoms (DRESS)
14	17th March 2022	Cephalosporin class	• Beta-lactam antimicrobials used to deal with a broad range of gram positive and negative bacteria	Fixed drug eruption
15	28th February 2022	Losartan	• Used in the treatment of hypertension	Muscle spasm
16	18th January 2022	Ibuprofen	• To treat arthritic disorder and musculoskeletal painful condition	Fixed drug eruption

References

Adithan C (2005) National pharmacovigilance programme. Indian J Pharmacol 37(6):347

Anon (2016) PvPI. Newsletter Pharmacovigilance Programme of India. 6(16). https://www.ipc.gov.in/PvPI/newsletter/Newsletter%20Vol%206%20Issue%2016%202016%20PDF.pdf

Anon (2021) Pharmacovigilance Programme of India. PvPI Newsletter 11(37). https://www.ipc.gov.in/images/PvPI_Newsletter_37_1.pdf

Anon (2022a) Pharmacovigilance Programme of India. PvPI Newsletter 12(3). https://www.ipc.gov.in/images/PvPI_Newsletter_Vol._12_Issue_3_2022_compressed.pdf

Anon (2022b) Pharmacovigilance Programme of India. PvPI Newsletter. 12(1). https://www.ipc.gov.in/images/PvPI_Newsletter_-_Vol._12_Issue_1_2022-.pdf

Anon (2022c) Pharmacovigilance Programme of India. PvPI Newsletter 12(2). https://www.ipc.gov.in/images/PvPI_Newsletter_Issue_2.pdf

Anon (2023a) Pharmacovigilance Programme of India. PvPI Newsletter 13(2). https://www.ipc.gov.in/images/PvPI_Newsletter_-_Vol._13_Issue-2_Comp.pdf

Anon (2023b) Pharmacovigilance Programme of India. PvPI N\ewsletter 13(1). https://www.ipc.gov.in/images/PvPI_Newsletter_-_Vol._13_Issue_1_16.6.2023_compressed.pdf

Arora D (2008) Pharmacovigilance obligations of the pharmaceutical companies in India. Indian J Pharmacol 40(Suppl 1):S13–S16
Bhave A, Menon S (2017) Regulatory environment for clinical research: recent past and expected future. Perspect Clin Res 8(1):11
Biswas P (2013) Pharmacovigilance in Asia. J Pharmacol Pharmacother 4(1_suppl):S7
Biswas P, Biswas A (2007) Setting standards for proactive pharmacovigilance in India: the way forward. Indian J Pharmacol. 39(3):124
CDSCO 2004 Protocol for National Pharmacovigilance Program
CDSCO (n.d.) Introduction. https://cdsco.gov.in/opencms/opencms/en/About-us/Introduction/
Clarkson A (2001) A novel scheme for the reporting of adverse drug reactions. Arch Dis Child 84(4):337–339
Don M (2006) Safety reporting during clinical trials: the new amended regulations in India. Pipeline 9:4–7
Gupta Y (2010) Ensuring patient safety—launching the new pharmacovigilance programme of India. Pharma Times 42:21–26
Hazell L, Shakir SAW (2006) Under-reporting of adverse drug reactions. Drug Saf 29(5):385–396
Indian Pharmacopoeia Commission (2022) Annual Report-2022. https://www.ipc.gov.in/images/Annual_Report_2022_.pdf
Kalaiselvan V, Thota P, Singh G (2016) Pharmacovigilance Programme of India: recent developments and future perspectives. Indian J Pharmacol. 48(6):624
Kumar RKV (2015) Indian pharmacopoeia Commission's partners for promoting public health. Adv Pharmacoepidemiol Drug Saf 04(03):1000181
Olsson S (1998) The role of the WHO Programme on international drug monitoring in coordinating worldwide drug safety efforts. Drug Saf 19(1):1–10
Olsson S, Pal SN, Stergachis A, Couper M (2010) Pharmacovigilance activities in 55 low- and middle-income countries. Drug Saf 33(8):689–703
Pant JSR (2021) Drug safety monitoring (pharmacovigilance) in India and different tools for detection and monitoring of adverse effects. SPAST Abs 1(1)
Prakash J, Sachdeva R, Shrivastava T, Jayachandran C, Sahu A (2021) Adverse event reporting tools and regulatory measures in India through outcome of pharmacovigilance Programme of India. Indian J Pharmacol. 53(2):143
PvPI (2017) Newsletter Pharmacovigilance Programme of India (PvPI) striving for excellence: a professional "skill development programme" for healthcare stakeholders 7(18) https://www.ipc.gov.in/PvPI/newsletter/Newsletter%20Vol%207%20Issue%2018%202017%20PDF-min.pdf
Team WHO (2006) The safety of medicines in public health programmes: pharmacovigilance, an essential tool. World Health Organization, Geneva. https://apps.who.int/iris/handle/10665/43384
Thatte UM, Chaudhari NL, Gogtay NJ (2018) Pharmacovigilance program of India: history, evolution and current status. Adverse Drug React Bull 312(1):1207–1210
Thota P, Thota A, Medhi B, Sidhu S, Kumar P, Selvan V et al (2018) Drug safety alerts of pharmacovigilance programme of India: a scope for targeted spontaneous reporting in India. Perspect Clin Res 9(1):51
WHO (2012) A practical handbook on the pharmacovigilance of medicines used in the treatment of tuberculosis enhancing the safety of the TB patient. WHO, Geneva

Pharmacovigilance System in EU

8

Deepali Siwan, Mukesh Nandave, and Anoop Kumar

Abstract

The primary goal of the pharmacovigilance system is to assess every element of risk management in reporting an adverse drug reaction via the pharmacovigilance risk assessment committee. The primary goal of a system is to stimulate the availability of medicine, particularly those that address traditionally unmet therapeutic needs, and lessen the incidence of adverse drug reactions to endorse and protect public health. These are accomplished by using a proactive, risk-proportionate, patient-centered approach, involving civil society, and maintaining significant transparency. Preparation and execution of pharmacovigilance actions before medicine is put on the market in the European Union, which encourages the start of an early development process for high innovation outcomes. The European Union (EU) is a multi-level organization. The role of pharmacovigilance and several institutional relationships at the European and national levels represent the system's condensed visual depiction. This chapter outlines the system workflow, applications, components, significant challenges, and drivers for future change.

Keywords

Pharmacovigilance system · European Union · Modules

D. Siwan (✉) · M. Nandave · A. Kumar
Department of Pharmacology, Delhi Pharmaceutical Sciences and Research University, New Delhi, India
e-mail: mukeshnandave@gmail.com; anoopdpsru@dpsru.edu.in

M. Nandave, A. Kumar (eds.), *Pharmacovigilance Essentials*,
https://doi.org/10.1007/978-981-99-8949-2_8

8.1 Introduction

All approved drugs inside the European Union (EU) have been evaluated for their effectiveness, safety, and quality and a favorable benefit–risk profile at the moment of permission. However, due to the acknowledged limitations of clinical research, not all safety concerns may be considered at the point of authorization. It is possible to discover more about a safety prescription post-authorization (Vandenbroucke 2008).

Therefore, to detect and reduce risk, it is crucial to continuously and meticulously evaluate the safety profile of all medications throughout their lifespan. Important pharmacovigilance tasks include risk management strategies, marketing authorization holder (MAH) studies, and recurring safety update reports. Effective post-marketing monitoring, particularly the spontaneous disclosure of suspected adverse drug reactions (ADRs), continues to be a crucial component of pharmacovigilance and the primary method for finding relatively uncommon and unexpected ADRs (Anon 2022).

A total of >eight million individual cases were referenced by 14.6 million particular case safety reports (ICSRs) in EudraVigilance (EV) as of the end of 2018. Pharmacovigilance is essential for promoting and safeguarding public health by reducing risk ADRs and maximizing the benefit–risk ratio for individual investor patients (Anon 2022).

The Pharmacovigilance Risk Assessment Committee (PRAC), developed in 2012 by the EU Pharmacovigilance Legislation, is at the center of the EU signal management process and plays a crucial role in the safety monitoring and evaluation of pharmaceutical products for human use (Santoro et al. 2017; Bilia et al. 2021).

Along with assistance for product research, authorization, manufacturing monitoring, inspection, and compliance, pharmacovigilance is a crucial tenet of medication regulation. The EC is responsible for medications covered by Regulation (EC) No. 726/2004, often known as Centrally Approved Products (CAP). Marketing authorization for CAPs is granted following a scientific assessment by the European Medicines Agency (EMA), acting through its committees, and is valid in all EU Member states (MS). The National Competent Authorities (NCA) are the agencies responsible for managing National Authorised Products (NAP) or medications covered by Directive 2001/83/EC (Edwards and Gandhi n.d.). The EMA coordinates some operations, including pharmacovigilance, for nationally approved medicines, which are given marketing authorizations by NCAs that are valid in their area (Fig. 8.1).

In this chapter, we provide a summary of the EU's pharmacovigilance system. First, we provide an overview of the EU's significant legislative and executive bodies, including the European Commission (Commission), the EU Council of Ministers (Council), the EP, and the key players in the pharmacovigilance policy implementation process. Then, we provide a brief overview of recent developments in pharmacovigilance legislation, including Directive 2001/83/EC and its reform through Directive 2010/84/EU. Finally, we present the most significant modifications generated by the update to the Directive and review its ADR provisions.

8.2 The EU Pharmacovigilance System

The center of the EU pharmacovigilance system is the EMA Pharmacovigilance Risk Assessment Committee (PRAC), in which the EU chooses member states, independent specialists are selected by the European Committee (EC), representatives of Healthcare Providers (HCP), and patients (Bilia et al. 2021). In the national system of EU residents, over 500 million may have access to new medicines, which approves nearly all innovative goods and results in authorization by Member States (MS).

The EU pharmacovigilance system experienced a significant rationalization and reinforcement in July 2012 due to the introduction and operationalization of the updated pharmacovigilance law, with the primary goal being to lessen the health impact of ADRs. A legally binding document that gives information on operational elements, the Commission Implementation Regulation (EU) No. 520/2012, was included with the law.

Researchers from the EMA and NCAs have created a set of GVPs for pharmacovigilance in the EU as advice to promote implementation and adherence to the legal requirements outlined in the law (Edwards and Gandhi n.d.). The legislation's enactment intends to create a more robust EU pharmacovigilance system, as illustrated in (Fig. 8.1).

Pharmacovigilance has undergone a paradigm shift in the past 10 years, moving from a reactive approach to responding to new hazards to a planned, proactive, and risk-appropriate strategy. The planning of pharmacovigilance operations occurs before the product is approved for the EU market, integrating pharmacovigilance into the life cycle of a product. The EU pharmacovigilance system provides the premarketing planning of risk management operations, inspections, and capacity building.

8.2.1 Good Pharmacovigilance Practice

Based on the guidelines of GVP, it can be divided into two groups. The first group covers the significant process of the pharmacovigilance system, and the second group covers the product or population-specific reflections. Major pharmacovigilance procedures are covered in the GVP modules I through XVI. Most modules are accessible in their most recent iteration. However, several have already changed. As shown in Fig. 8.2, further modules are still being developed. All subjects initially scheduled to be covered in GVP Module XIII are now incorporated into Module XII. Hence, this module is no longer being produced.

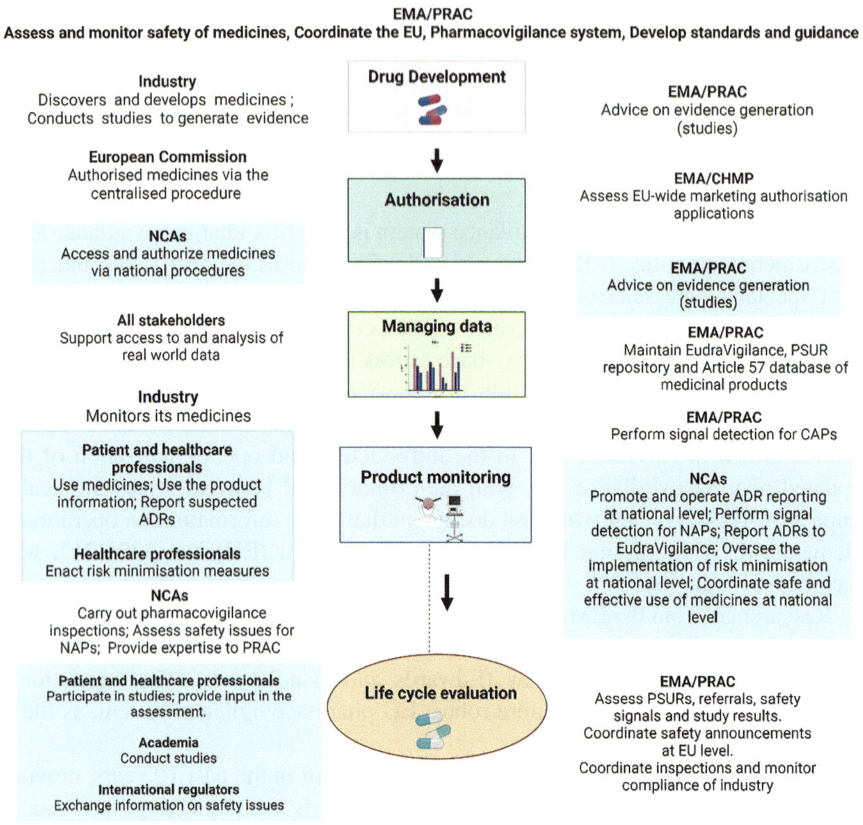

Fig. 8.1 Pharmacovigilance system at the European Union: function and responsibilities of drug life cycle

8.3 Role of Pharmacovigilance Systems in the EU

When a medication is suspected of having caused an adverse event, an unexpected report alerts the drug surveillance system (Fig. 8.3). The EMA defines a spontaneous report as a voluntary, unsolicited notice to medicine regulators by a patient, a healthcare provider, or anyone else to inform them of a potential adverse drug reaction (Durand et al. 2023). The regulatory authorities will next conduct a process known as a causality evaluation to evaluate whether the observed response is caused by the medicine or not. A database of possible adverse reactions to drugs approved for sale or being investigated in European clinical studies is available through EudraVigilance (Guideline 2003). The pharmaceutical business, which is the marketing authorization holder (MAH), receives spontaneous reports from EudraVigilance so that it may look into the issue. Signal detection and signal validation were reported under the EMA and MAHs (Durand et al. 2023).

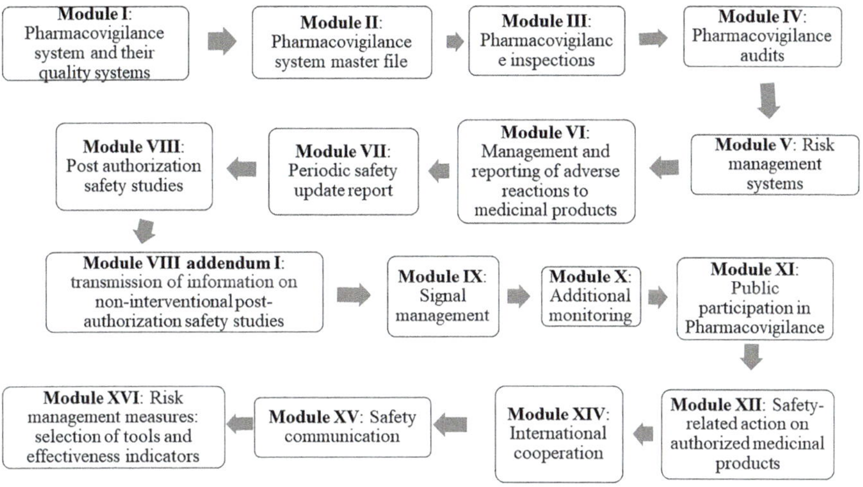

Fig. 8.2 Representation of modules in GVP

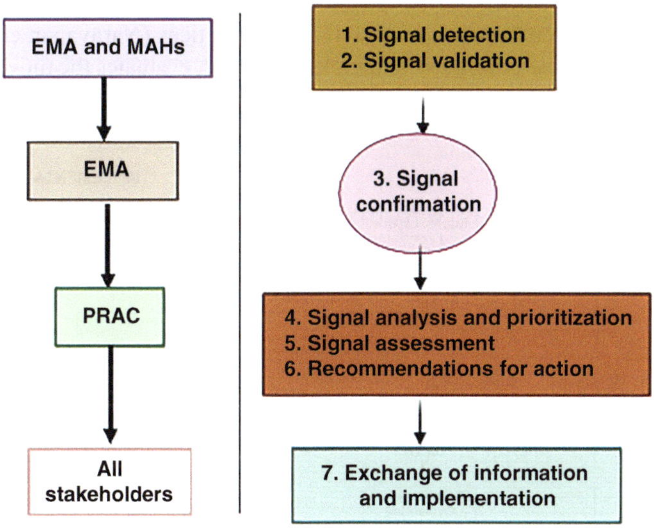

Fig. 8.3 Pharmacovigilance workflow in the EU

Additionally, MAHs communicate to EudraVigilance anything that they receive from patients. It is known as "re-routing" when EudraVigilance delivers the reports to AIFA. Lastly, EudraVigilance shares spontaneous reports with the WHO-Uppsala Monitoring Centre.

Spontaneous reports are not required, unlike solicited messages, which originate through organized data-collecting methods (such as clinical trials, non-interventional research, registries, and healthcare organizations). A causality evaluation is conducted when an ADR is suspected in these situations. A requested report is made only when a robust causal relationship between the adverse response and the medicine is proven (Baldo and De Paoli 2014; Council for International Organizations of Medical Sciences 2010). ADR reports, both spontaneous and requested, are crucial since they point to the need for more research to validate the drug's relationship and may raise alarms.

According to the EMA, a signal is "Information from one or more sources (including reports and experiments), which suggests a new probably causal association in or an entirely novel component of a known association in among a measure and a particular incident or sequence of related occurrences, either negative or positive, that is evaluated to be enough potential to justify verificatory action" (Esslinger et al. 2022).

Signal analysis and prioritization are crucially significant. ADR only sometimes occurs just because a signal was detected. The Overview of Products Characteristics (SmPC) is a legal document accepted throughout the marketing authorization procedure. It is intended for healthcare professionals and provides instructions on using a medicine based on data from clinical trials (Sultana et al. 2019).

The phases of the information management procedure include identification, confirmation, and verification by EMA with the MAHs (Fig. 8.4), as stated in Module IX of EMA's Good Pharmacovigilance Practices (Narayanan et al. 2020). The EMA's PRAC then examines and ranks the signal, evaluates the movement, and suggests taking regulatory action if necessary. People working in medical services

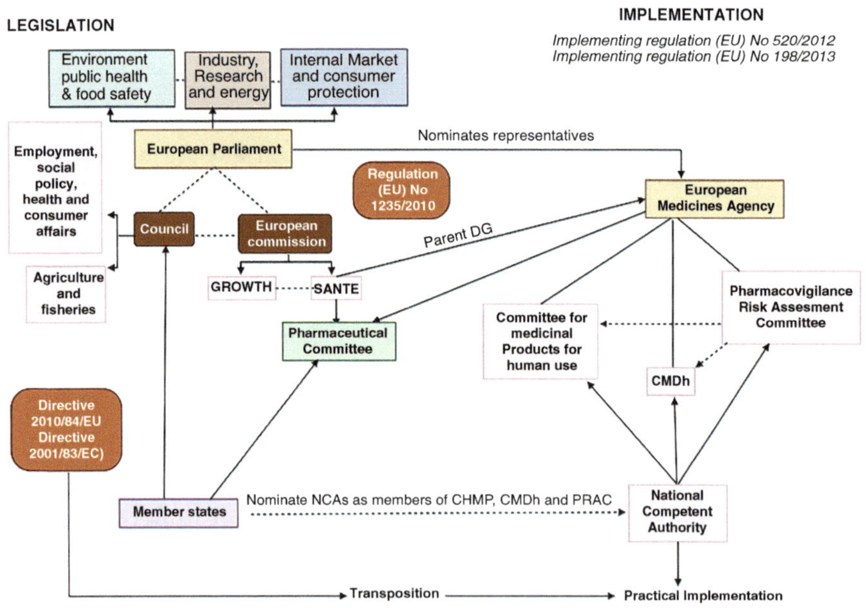

Fig. 8.4 The European Pharmacovigilance networks

are informed of the recommended steps to provide them with additional information about medications and their safety. MAHs amend the risk management plans (RMPs) and other records needed by EMA during the process of applying for drug marketing, using the fresh information produced by signal detection. RMPs include planned actions to learn more about the efficacy and safety update reports (PSUR) and post-authorization safety studies (PASS). PASS is performed to detect, characterize, and quantify ADRs after a medication hits the market. PSUR, on the other hand, are reports created by MAHs to evaluate the risk–benefit ratio of a drug. EMA uses this data to provide suggestions, warnings, and actions to reduce the possible impact of ADRs.

8.3.1 Application of Pharmacovigilance Systems

The pharmacovigilance regulation is now being implemented differently in each Member State of the European Union, ranging from simple absorption into domestic law to full implementation, reflected in modifications to pertinent national systems. Fundamental disparities between Member States regarding the proper designation of biological medications as drugs and not small-molecule pharmaceuticals inside their national pharmacovigilance databases are an example of such variances. The categorization of several physical medications, such as somatropin, epoetins, filgrastim, and monoclonal antibodies (MA), has been the subject of substantial disagreement, according to Klein et al.'s analysis of pharmacovigilance data from five Member States. According to the nation of origin and the analyzed biologic, the percentage of correctly classified biologics varied between 0% and 100% (Vermeer et al. 2019).

In ADR reports sent to EudraVigilance, more restrictions have been found. Vermeer et al. examined information from the EudraVigilance database between 2004 and 2010 to investigate the transparency of drugs and bio-identical drugs in this repository (Borg et al. 2015). The research covered medicinal products for which a biosimilar had obtained European Union approval (at the time, only a handful of biosimilars, including epoetin, filgrastim, and somatropin, had achieved acceptance) (Borg et al. 2015). In 96% of the cases reported for the three brand classes, the suspected drug's recognizable product name (such as a brand name, INN, or name of the marketing authorization holder) was supplied (Klein et al. 2015). Comparatively, only 5.3% of the filings for the three drug classes with authorized biosimilars included the batch number, as opposed to 21.1% of reports for all medications (Vermeer et al. 2019). Epoetin reports comprised 70.7% of all suspected ADR complaints, indicating that the information disproportionately weighted epoetins. This is probably because of increased public knowledge of safety issues with epoetins related to the PRCA pandemic. Compared to reports for the other pharmacological classes, reports for epoetins showed superior name attribution (i.e., recognizable brand names in 98.9% of records for epoetins), inflating the general precision of product identification (Vermeer et al. 2019). Except for data for epoetins, 89.7% of ADRs submitted to EudraVigilance had a product name that could be easily identified (Vermeer et al. 2019). It should be noted that this study examined data at a time when reporting on brand awareness and batch identification was required. The 2010 EU drug surveillance regulation on ADR reporting was implemented during this time. ExclVermeer et al. subsequently released a comparable study of ADR data from EudraVigilance between January 2011 and June 2016 (Borg et al. 2015). The study included ten classes of biologics for which biosimilars or related products, such as human normal immunoglobulin, interferon β-1a, and octocog α, have received European regulatory approval (Felix et al. 2019). These classes of biologics included etanercept, infliximab, glargine insulin, filgrastim, epoetin α, somatropin, and follitropin α. 86.3% of biologics were classified as concurrent or interacting medicines, and 96.7% of suspected biologics had appropriate IDs in ADR reports. The identifiability of putative biologics rose to 97.2% when narration and reporter remarks were considered. However, data submitted to the Amgen health database indicate that additional work needs to be done to increase identification accuracy (Vermeer et al. 2016). Between 89.5% for filgrastim to over 100% for interferon β-1a, being identifiable varied by class (Felix et al. 2019). Etanercept accounted for 37.5% of all reports as the most often reported suspected biologic (Felix et al. 2019). From the initial evaluation (2004 to 2010) and the most recent one (2011–2016) (Arora et al. 2017), there were appreciable improvements in the percentage of ADR reports with recognized products, with states via identifiable products increasing for filgrastim from 85.0% to 85.9% and somatropin from 91.3% to 96.2%. For epoetins, reports with distinguishable products dropped somewhat from 98.9% to 96.4% (Felix et al. 2019). Batch traceability fluctuated between 1.8% for follitropin α products to 69.3% for things that used normal human immunoglobulins between 2011 and 2016 for the 10 classes of drugs analyzed (Klein et al. 2016), which is identical to the 21.1% reported for all medicinal products between 2004 and 2010 (Klein et al. 2016). The authors contend that the lack of a trend toward enhanced batch traceability in their most recent analysis and the relatively low level of batch traceability indicate that European Union pharmacovigilance legislation has yet to have an impact on the requirement to include batches when reporting suspected ADR for biologics (Klein et al. 2016). The 2010 EU drug surveillance legislation's effects on ADR reporting have been studied. Using April 2012 to December 2014, health authorities and Amgen received ADR reports on filgrastim throughout the EU. From these reports, brand names were checked to ensure that the right manufacturer could be identified (Felix et al. 2019). This corresponds to the period when identical filgrastims were offered and the time after adopting the EU's pharmacovigilance law in 2010, which compelled Member States to promote brand names in health data and report adverse reactions (Felix et al. 2019). The finding that 21% of filgrastim reports obtained by Amgen's safety department after 2011 were unattributed and the passage of the EU pharmacovigilance legislation in 2010 coincides with the 85% rate of responsibility reported, especially for filgrastims before 2011, indicating insufficient enforcement of this aspect of the Directive. The inability to identify a drug identity in pharmacovigilance databases has several effects, including a delay in detecting the safety signal. For instance, Vermeer et al. 2016 report simulation research to investigate the impact of ADR misattribution more recently (Siu et al. 2019). The authors discovered that incorrect attribution can cause a delay in the detection of ADRs related to medicine. A significant impact of misinterpretation was shown for infliximab-induced hypersensitivity responses; in the event of a 34% misclassification, the number of cases doubled, and the time to identify the risk increased from 6 months to 1 year (Cohen et al. 2018). The marketplace's share of the medicine had a major impact on the misclassification's outcome. For instance, a 50% rate of misattribution for drugs with a low market share would nearly double the number of cases and time to detect new safety information. In contrast, a 5% rate of misattribution for drugs with a high market share would only be twice the number of cases and time to detect (Jørgensen et al. 2017). This model's application to infliximab ADR data from 27 European nations obtained from VigiBase revealed that unclear ADR reports would cause a delay in the discovery of product-specific safety signals (Moots et al. 2017). Approximately, 22% of infliximab ADR reports were submitted using the international nonproprietary name before introducing the biosimilar infliximab in late 2013. Additionally, pilot research in the Netherlands found that biosimilars lacked distinguishable product names (McKinnon et al. 2018). Between January 1, 2009, and December 31, 2014, the Netherlands Pharmacovigilance Centre Lareb collected 1523 natural ADR reports for recombinant biologics. Only 5% of the findings had a batch number, but 76% included a distinguishable brand name (Lunddahl 2016). The MHRA's experience in the UK has shown how pharmacovigilance regulations may be implemented. For instance, the MHRA employs the Yellow Card Scheme to "monitor the safety of all medicinal products in the UK" and gathers data on ADRs, medications with subpar quality, and fake or counterfeit drugs (Johal et al. 2022). ADRs recorded on Yellow Cards are examined, coupled with extra sources for details including clinical trial data, scientific journals, or data from overseas pharmaceuticals authorities, to detect previously unknown safety problems (World Health Organization n.d.). The MHRA has aggressively pushed medical professionals to provide the drug's name and batch number to remove doubt when reporting ADRs according to the 2010 EU law. As a result, the Yellow Cards are now altered to contain a place for the brand's name and batch identification and a notice stating where this information is crucial (Vermeer et al. 2016).

8.4 Pharmacovigilance Risk Assessment Committee

The PRAC is crucial in creating and managing the European Union's framework. The PRAC is a group in charge of evaluating all facets of risk management for medications intended for human use while considering the medicinal product's therapeutic impact (de Langen et al. 2008). Considering the drug's therapeutic effect involves the detection, assessment, minimization, and communication relative to the risk of adverse events. Additionally, it is in charge of planning and assessing pharmacovigilance audits and post-authorization safety studies (PASSs). Directly binding judgments made by PRAC regarding enforced non-interventional PASS. The PRAC meets once a month to review RMPs, signals, in-depth analyses of safety concerns, and benefit–risk studies of pharmaceuticals and to formulate recommendations on any issues about pharmacovigilance activities and risk management systems involving the evaluation of their efficacy. PRAC recommendations are considered when the Committee for Medical Products for Human Use adopts opinions for medications that include a CAP. The Coordination Group for Mutually Recognition and Decentralized Procedures—Human also considers PRAC recommendations when it recommends drugs only authorized in the MSs. After working with PRAC over the past 5 years, it has become clear that the Committee is essential for advancing strategic pharmacovigilance concerns, advancing in the science field, and bolstering its operational procedures (Kaeding et al. 2017a).

8.4.1 European Pharmacovigilance Bodies

It is crucial to distinguish between two groups of participants to comprehend the EU's pharmacovigilance system. The EU institutions were the first to pass pharmaceutical rules and establish the basis for pharmacovigilance. The EU institutions with legislative and executive responsibilities are the Commission, the Council, and the EP. In combination, they might be seen as a legislative triangle (Haycock-Stuart et al. 2014).

The European Commission is the body tasked with representing the interests of Europe, and it performs several duties. The so-called Directorate Generals (DGs) address various policy concerns. Since DG SANTE serves as EMA's "parent" DG, its representatives are crucial resources for the organization's daily operation. However, membership within the EMA Management Board, the organization's primary governing body, includes representatives from both DGs.

Initiating legislation is one of the Commission's numerous responsibilities. Additionally, the Commission's recommendations are the only ones that may be used to pass EU legislation. The Pharmaceutical Committee, a professional body of Member States and EMA members, was founded in 1975 and supported the Commission in its executive tasks (Haycock-Stuart et al. 2014). DG SANTE controls it and is primarily responsible for implementing Directive 2001/83/EC and other pharmaceutical regulations. The entity representing the nations that are members of the Council of Ministers mainly has legislative responsibilities. The Council meets in various formats and negotiates with national ministers participating according to the policy issue. The Council met in two groups to discuss the amendment of Directive 2001/83/EC: the EPSCO and the AGRIFISH groups. The Council, along with the EP, enacts laws like the pharmacovigilance mentioned above legislation (Haycock-Stuart et al. 2014).

The European Union's legislative body is comprised of the Council and the European Parliament (EP), representing the continent's citizens. Some parliamentary committees handle legislative recommendations brought forward by the Commission. For instance, the ENVI committee managed Directive 2001/83/EC with input from two other committees on the proposed legislation (Kaeding et al. 2017b). Two representatives from the EP may attend meetings of the EMA

Management Board. Scientific specialists often represent the EP. The EP, a legislature component, is crucial to EMA's fiscal monitoring and management. However, the EP has a limited impact on implementing pharmacovigilance rules (Kaeding et al. 2017b). Based on the laws enacted by the EU institutions, the second group of actors is responsible for carrying out pharmacovigilance policy at the national and EU levels. Additionally, the EU passes implementing legislation at the EU level. The EMA, federal competent authorities, pharmaceutical firms, and other stakeholders are also included in this group (Kaeding et al. 2017b).

The EMA's primary duties include coordinating the assessment of pharmaceutical products and providing guidance on regulating medicines to EU institutions and Member States. Since it started working in 1995, the Commission has emerged as a critical player in many facets of pharmaceutical Regulation. It is crucial in setting up the framework for EU pharmacovigilance (Haycock-Stuart et al. 2014; Kaeding et al. 2017b). The Committee for Medicinal Products for Human Use (CMPH), which makes recommendations to the Commission on the centralized authorization procedure, is one of the bodies the agency uses for its scientific evaluations. Additionally, the PRAC has been evaluating and monitoring the safety of pharmaceuticals since 2012. PRAC offers comments and suggestions regarding centralized and decentralized authorization processes (Kaeding et al. 2017b).

The EMA collects complaints of alleged adverse reactions using its EudraVigilance database, an internet-based information system. ADRs in the EU must be officially recorded in a central repository by the Member States and those possessing the marketing authorization. Furthermore, the Member States and the national competent bodies play a significant role in the EU's pharmacovigilance system (Kaeding et al. 2017b). Members of Member State actors participate in practically all pharmacovigilance activities, as shown in (Fig. 8.4).

The national responsible authorities implement and enforce pharmacovigilance, drawing on local knowledge and resources. These agencies not only play a vital role in the national level's actual implementation, but also they additionally have representation at the EU level in the numerous EMA committees that deal with pharmacovigilance and authorization. When pharmaceutical goods are marketed via a decentralized system, decisions are made at the EU level by the CMDh. Additionally, the EU pharmacovigilance is supported by the Strengthening Collaboration for Operating Pharmacovigilance in Europe (SCOPE) Joint Action program, which provides training, resources, and templates to promote best practices (Kaeding et al. 2017b). Additionally, the science and application of pharmacovigilance are also goals for the ENCePP. The significant organizations regulating the gathering of data on suspected ADRs reported by medical personnel, owners of marketing authorizations, and patients are the national competent authorities. These authorities, therefore, supply the tools, information, and skills necessary for causality analysis and signal identification (Kaeding et al. 2017b).

Pharmacovigilance, which includes risk management plans and post-authorization safety investigations, is based on the EMA's close ties to the pharmaceutical sector. These are crucial components of the authorization procedure and product surveillance after commercialization. Marketing authorization holders are required to adhere to a variety of requirements outlined in EU law on pharmacovigilance. For instance, they must designate a responsible individual to oversee pharmacovigilance and act as regulatory authorities' primary point of contact (Kaeding et al. 2017b). Furthermore, marketing authorization holders are required by law to disclose ADRs. Finally, several other parties are crucial in practically applying EU pharmacovigilance regulations.

The involvement of interest groups in EU healthcare regulations is mentioned explicitly in law (EC) No. 726/2004. A working party for patients and consumers has been formed within the EMA and a network of European medical and consumer associations. Patients can now immediately report potential adverse effects to either the appropriate national agencies or the marketing authorization holders as part of the drug surveillance reform by Directive 2010/84/EU (Kaeding et al. 2017b).

8.4.2 Legislative Developments

Although the EU started regulating medicines in the 1960s, pharmacovigilance was given little attention in the 1990s, when the EU began to pass several laws addressing it (Kaeding et al. 2017b). Member States are already required to set up pharmacovigilance systems and urge medical staff to report adverse drug reactions (ADRs) under Directive 93/39/EEC. Holders of marketing authorizations were likewise asked to choose a capable pharmacovigilance representative. At the time, the EU's regulatory framework for medicines was comprised of several intricately interrelated laws. To simplify things, the various parts were codified into a single document, giving rise to Directive 2001/83/EC (Kaeding et al. 2017b).

The EU's pharmacovigilance law is based on this Directive, which has undergone ten amendments. The obligations of governments and marketing permit holders to establish and maintain systems for pharmacovigilance remained relatively the same from Directive 93/39/EEC. Thus, Title IX of Directive 2001/83/EC, which was devoted to pharmacovigilance, only served to solidify the pertinent requirements established in principle in the early 1990s (de Langen et al. 2008). The Commission began a public consultation in 2006 to reform the pharmacovigilance system. Clarifying stakeholder duties, guaranteeing the engagement of various stakeholders (which includes healthcare professionals and consumers), and recognizing overlaps and obligations were among the objectives listed by the Commission (Borg et al. 2011). A report that evaluated the public consultation discovered "differences and inconsistencies due to a non-optimal conformity between national law and practice with the EC regulations" (Borg et al. 2011).

The Commission released a proposal for legislation in December 2008 in response to the consultation. The Commission stated in this proposal that it attempted to achieve the following goals: improved public health protection, appropriate internal market functioning, and simplifying present laws and processes (Borg et al. 2011). The next year, the idea was addressed by member nations in the relevant council working group. To ensure the swift approval of the Directive, the Council of Europe and the EP held several informal meetings (referred to as trialogues) after starting preliminary discussions in late 2009 (Council of the European

Union 2010). The legislative process was completed in September 2010 when Directive 2010/84/EU was approved by the EP with a majority vote (Borg et al. 2011). The EU drug surveillance system has to be maintained by further laws.

Directive 2010/84/EU covers pharmacovigilance for decentralized approval, whereas centralized authorization is covered by Regulation (EU) No 1235/2010. The Commission Implementing Regulation No. 520/2012 was established to address the operational issues of these laws. The rule, for instance, mandates that batch numbers be included in specific safety reports for biologicals. The "black triangle" (▲) is a new concept introduced by Implementing Regulation No. 198/2013.

8.4.3 The Pharmacovigilance Reform: Directive 2010/84/EU and Article 102

The recently adopted Pharmacovigilance Directive 2010/84/EU seeks, in the words of Recital 3, "to enhance the functioning of European Union legislation on the pharmacovigilance of pharmaceutical products." In conclusion, the new legislation altered the EU pharmacovigilance system in the ways listed below:

ADRs are expanded to include medications, and the reason for additional monitoring is broadened to include biologicals. The appropriate authorities might call for further tracking of items subject to research after marketing. Medicinal products liable to other observations must be identified by the black triangle (▲) and be included in a publicly available list (European Commission 2007). With a focus on recognizing biologicals, the EU pharmacovigilance system reform aims to make ADR reporting easier (European Commission 2007).

The latter part is primarily extended due to the revisions made by Directive 2010/84/EU, whereas the first two elements were left alone. With the Member States, the expansion of these measures turned out to be a contentious issue. Article 102 of the Commission report drew 14 responses based on its initial language, with nine nations asking for revisions (de Langen et al. 2008). The precise wording of these rules was the topic of much debate among Member States throughout the legislative process. Over 70 changes were submitted to the Commission proposal by the various legislative committees. During the informal trialogue discussions with the Council, an agreement on language was created that included some of the changes made to the original phrasing but left out other significant clauses added by the EP (de Langen et al. 2008).

8.5 Role of Signal Detection and Management in EU

A signal is described as "information that comes from a few sources, such as experiments and observations, which indicate a new possibly causal organization, or an additional component of a known connection between a measure and a particular incident or collection of associated occurrences, either negative or positive, that is assessed to be enough probability to justify verificatory action" (Postigo et al. 2018). Signal management in the European Union focuses on unfavorable outcomes. It entails a series of actions to ascertain whether new risks are related to an active substance or medication or whether bets have changed based on an analysis of ICSRs, collected data from dynamic surveillance networks or studies, literature data, or other data sources (Kaeding et al. 2017b).

Regulators and MAHs continuously monitor and review the safety data to ensure that any safety signals are quickly identified, thoroughly evaluated, and appropriately expressed to patients and healthcare providers through updates to product information, as needed. The EU uses EV as a management and analysis tool for suspected adverse drug reactions (ADRs) to drugs approved or tested in clinical trials (Borg et al. 2015). EU law (Borg et al. 2015) governs the monitoring of EV data. Figure 8.4 summarizes the process while highlighting the three parties' roles and interactions in the six primary monitoring operations (signal identification, verification, approval, analysis, prioritization, assessment, and recommendation) (Borg et al. 2015).

8.6 Major Challenges

Major challenges of the pharmacovigilance system in EU countries have been mentioned in the following:

8.6.1 Insufficient Reporting

The need for more reporting of ADRs is the main obstacle to the effective implementation of Directive 2010/84/EU. Respondents (from the United Kingdom, Poland, Portugal, France, and Germany) emphasize this for every member nation in the sample. The comparative examination of instances chosen in this study based on their variance in terms of the national healthcare systems supports earlier investigations. This is notable given that reporting adverse drug reactions (ADRs) is required by law for healthcare professionals in 22 different countries (79%) and that 26 nations (89%) require obligatory disclosure of ADRs for vaccines (Vermeer et al. 2015).

Even though fewer Member States provide web-based reporting than the Member States offer mail-reporting channels, most ADR reports (38%) are still received via web-based apps. Fewer than half of the French regional drug surveillance centers in our sample have websites and, consequently, web-based reporting forms. In Finland, patients must use ordinary mail even if doctors and chemists can submit reports online. The websites of the national competent authorities in each Member State offer ADR reporting forms (SCOPE) [Annexure 2]. The amount and quality of the information are two crucial factors in underreporting. Quantity is the total number of ADR reports, whereas quality is the worth of the data. The two aspects are sometimes mutually incompatible since quality may decline as quantity rises. While having a lot of information is vital, having the correct information is crucial for efficient pharmacovigilance. Some responders worry that inadequate reports may necessitate follow-up, adding to the effort (Germany). Other respondents expressed mixed feelings about the number of reports submitted (Poland), while they were generally pleased with the standard of ADR reports (Klein et al. 2020).

8.6.2 Data Saturation

Additionally, signal detection may be challenging due to information saturation (Germany).

The fact that the law permits information to be gathered from any sources, including patients and literature reports, only worsens this issue. Additionally, this results in a more extensive data set from which pertinent signals may be evaluated (Felix et al. 2019). In terms of assessment and signal detection, the Member States differ significantly. In the UK, there is no report review before signal discovery; instead, the identification of signals has been automated because of the vast amount of data. The national responsible body, the Medicines and Healthcare Products Regulation Agency (MHRA) sent significant cases to EMA after prioritizing discovered signals.

8.6.3 The Concept of Causality Assessments

The regional units of Portugal and France's two decentralized systems gather and assess ADR reports. However, issues with quantity and quality might need fixing with causality determinations (France). The review, including a causation assessment, is followed by the reports sent to the national responsible authorities. Holders of marketing authorizations submit information to federal authorities directly.

8.6.4 The Capacity of Biological Utilization to Be Identified

Previous research has shown that disclosure of batch numbers and traceability of biologicals is prone to significant variance within Member States. According to many studies on ADR reporting, only a tiny percentage of suspected biologicals had batch numbers accessible (Alvarez et al. 2010). Respondents from various Member States in the sample concur that disclosing batch numbers is still tricky (the UK). In France and Poland, batch numbers are seldom or never provided. Fimea's findings confirm that only in Finland did respondents find the documentation of batch numbers satisfactory.

8.6.5 Increasing Patient Participation

Strengthening patient participation in the safety evaluation of medicines is one of the objectives of Directive 2010/84/EU. Patient reporting systems are in place in all 28 Member States, with the majority putting them in place in 2012–2013 (although the first Member State to establish this procedure did so only beginning in 1968 and followed by another in 1996). During the two-and-a-half-year duration of the reporting period, there has been an overall 50 percent rise in distinct patients reporting from the European Economic Area. This includes ADR reports not filed by other reporters, such as healthcare practitioners, and which contain data that might not have been recorded (Alvarez et al. 2010). Submitting ADRs for biologicals and the corresponding traceability is still difficult when it involves patient reporting. In the UK, serial numbers must be visible on every box. Yet, patients frequently have no access to the package when they receive prescription medication in a hospital environment.

8.6.6 Factors Responsible for Underreporting

The three key "pillars" that make up the optimization of the EU signal system for management are increased transparency, investigation of novel approaches, and ongoing process review. Continuous assessment is required to maintain and enhance the EU signal detection and management process' effective and efficient functioning (de Wit et al. 2019).

The effectiveness of the process to improve public health depends on identifying and controlling aspects where there are chances for Improvement and bolstering elements that operate effectively. The Signal Management Review Technical Working Group (SMART), a subset of the PRAC, was created in recognition of the essential significance of this effort (de Wit et al. 2019). It aims to examine process improvements and promote the invention of innovative approaches in signal detection and monitoring. This group is comprised of professionals from the NCAs, the EMA, PRAC participants, and academic experts in signal detection. Increased monitoring of the pediatric and geriatric populations, better visualization of misuse, abuse, drug overdose mistakes with medication, and workplace exposure, along with faster recognition of new indicates triggered by an unexpected rise in the total number of cases received over a specific timeframe are just a few examples of recent process improvements. Disproportionality metrics were created to aid in quickly identifying emerging safety issues, and it has been shown that they can identify roughly 50% of ADRs earlier than other popular signal detection techniques (Wisniewski et al. 2016).

Improvement in methodology is the second aspect. Signal detection has undergone evidence-based process improvement due to data from the large-scale research project PROTECT (Candore et al. 2015), which examined current approaches and their practical implementations in real-world investigations. By carefully looking at the utility of the reporting odds ratio rather than the corresponding declaring ratio to detect ADRs in pharmacovigilance (Slattery et al. 2013) under PROTECT suggestions on simplicity of implementation and interpretation as well as efficient use of resources, it was possible to introduce a new mathematical technique for signal detection in EV. Additionally, it has been demonstrated that subgroup analysis, made possible by the size of the EV database, improves sensitivity and accuracy while lowering false-positive results, positively affecting the safety evaluation of pharmaceuticals (Lane et al. 2018).

The EMA's ongoing efforts to increase the openness of pertinent information on medicines constitute the third type of process improvement (Santoro et al. 2017). Everyone, from interested consumers and medical professionals to MAHs, may now access up-to-date and comprehensive information on their medications thanks to the PRAC agendas, points of interest minutes, and specific PRAC suggestions for the signal being published on the EMA website. Additionally, the most recent development in 2015 to translate and release the PRAC suggestions into a total of 25 different languages (official EU languages including Norwegian and Icelandic) speeds up the transformation of PRAC suggestions into cautions in product knowledge. It reduces the needless duplication of attempts for NCAs and MAHs. Additionally, it has provided a uniform approach to generating information and decreased the possibility of misinterpretation (Felix et al. 2019).

It is essential to be aware of limitations that might guide future research to more thoroughly validate the impact of the signal management system, even though the data from our analysis demonstrates its significant contribution to disseminating secure knowledge to medicine users through product labeling (Felix et al. 2019). The reliability of the data may be determined, and trends over time might be examined by repeating the research with a more extensive dataset in the future. This would also make it possible to compare the different kinds and patterns of the signals in illuminating ways, such as between various medication classes or phrases from the Medical Dictionary for Legislative Activities (Arlett et al. 2014).

Data collected in 2015 shows that over two-thirds of signals come from ICSRs, which has remained constant. However, a more thorough assessment of the impact of the data sources would be an essential subject for additional study. They are finding out whether there is a greater interest in real-world data, including how these fresh ideas complement one another. Finally, there was no comparison arm because this research was descriptive and focused on the absolute quantity of newly introduced product warnings (Arlett et al. 2014). Future studies may find it interesting to compare the outcomes of the EU data control system to those of other regulators.

8.7 Conclusion

A new age of safeguarding patients and openness regarding the security of EU pharmaceuticals has arrived. A greater level of transparency, including the release of PRAC suggestions and their translations into all EU languages, ensures prompt product information updates and gives patients and healthcare professionals across Europe quick access to reliable information about the safety of their medications.

The EU network is still committed to enhance the effectiveness of the EU signals management and detection procedure. Numerous initiatives are underway to improve signal leadership's effectiveness, including real-world data, a focus on monitoring issues like medication misuse and abuse, elderly safety, drug–drug interactions, and the effect of non-serious suspected ADRs on pharmacovigilance systems. Better and quicker analysis and comprehension of safety problems will be possible with the help of recognizing, assessing, and upgrading the current system. It will also indicate any information gaps that can be filled with risk management planning. In this way, patients who require safe and effective medications may get them, and their faith in their medications is bolstered.

References

Alvarez Y, Hidalgo A, Maignen F, Slattery J (2010) Validation of statistical signal detection procedures in eudravigilance post-authorization data: a retrospective evaluation of the potential for earlier signalling. Drug Saf 33:475–487

Anon (2022) 2022 Annual report on EudraVigilance for the European Parliament, the Council and the Commission. https://www.ema.europa.eu/en/documents/report/2022-annual-report-eudravigilance-european-parliament-council-commission_en.pdf. Accessed on 23 Sept 2023

Arlett P, Portier G, De Lisa R, Blake K, Wathion N, Dogne JM, Spooner A, Raine J, Rasi G (2014) Proactively managing the risk of marketed drugs: experience with the EMA pharmacovigilance risk assessment committee. Nat Rev Drug Discov 13(5):395–397

Arora A, Jalali RK, Vohora D (2017) Relevance of the weber effect in contemporary pharmacovigilance of oncology drugs. Ther Clin Risk Manag 11:1195–1203

Baldo P, De Paoli P (2014) Pharmacovigilance in oncology: evaluation of current practice and future perspectives. J Eval Clin Pract 20(5):559–569

Bilia AR, Corazziari ES, Govoni S, Mugelli A, Racchi M (2021) Medical devices made of substances: possible innovation and opportunities for complex natural products. Planta Med 87(12/13):1110–1116

Borg JJ, Aislaitner G, Pirozynski M, Mifsud S (2011) Strengthening and rationalizing pharmacovigilance in the EU: where is Europe heading to? A review of the new EU legislation on pharmacovigilance. Drug Saf 34:187–197

Borg JJ, Tanti A, Kouvelas D, Lungu C, Pirozynski M, Serracino-Inglott A, Aislaitner G (2015) European union pharmacovigilance capabilities: potential for the new legislation. Ther Adv Drug Saf 6(4):120–140

Candore G, Juhlin K, Manlik K, Thakrar B, Quarcoo N, Seabroke S, Wisniewski A, Slattery J (2015) Comparison of statistical signal detection methods within and across spontaneous reporting databases. Drug Saf 38:577–587

Cohen HP, Blauvelt A, Rifkin RM, Danese S, Gokhale SB, Woollett G (2018) Switching reference medicines to biosimilars: a systematic literature review of clinical outcomes. Drugs 78(4):463–478

Council for International Organizations of Medical Sciences (2010) Practical aspects of signal detection in pharmacovigilance: report of CIOMS Working Group VIII. (No Title)

de Langen J, van Hunsel F, Passier A, den Berg LD, van Grootheest K (2008) Adverse drug reaction reporting by patients in The Netherlands three years of experience. Drug Saf 31:515–524

de Wit M, Cooper C, Tugwell P, Bere N, Kirwan J, Conaghan PG, Roberts C, Aujoulat I, Al-Daghri N, Araujo de Carvalho I, Barker M (2019) Practical guidance for engaging patients in health research, treatment guidelines and regulatory processes: results of an expert group meeting organized by the World Health Organization (WHO) and the European Society for Clinical and Economic Aspects of osteoporosis, osteoarthritis and musculoskeletal diseases (ESCEO). Aging Clin Exp Res 31:905–915

Durand J, Dogné JM, Cohet C, Browne K, Gordillo-Marañón M, Piccolo L, Zaccaria C, Genov G (2023) Safety monitoring of COVID-19 vaccines: perspective from the European medicines agency. Clin Pharmacol Ther 113(6):1223–1234

Edwards BD, Gandhi S (n.d.) Pharmacovigilance for Authorised Human Medicinal Products in the European Union. 129

Esslinger S, Quinn L, Sampat S, Otero-Lobato M, Noël W, Geldhof A, Herijgers N, Reeder SJ (2022) Risk management plans: reassessment of safety concerns based on good pharmacovigilance practices module V (revision 2)—a company experience. J Pharm Health Care Sci 8(1):14

European Commission (2007) Strategy to better protect public health by strengthening and rationalizing EU pharmacovigilance. In: Public Consultation on Legislative Proposals Brussels. European Commission, Brussels

Felix T, Jordan JB, Akers C, Patel B, Drago D (2019) Current state of biologic pharmacovigilance in the European Union: improvements are needed. Expert Opin Drug Saf 18(3):231–240

Guideline IH (2003) Post-approval safety data management: definitions and standards for expedited reporting E2D. Federal Register 68(178):53983–53984

Haycock-Stuart E, James C, McLachlan A, MacLaren J (2014) Identifying good practice in fitness to practise processes in higher education institutes in Scotland. NHS Education, Scotland

Johal H, Niblett HA, Metcalfe NH (2022) Unlicensed medicine prescribing in general practice. InnovAiT 15(10):602–606

Jørgensen KK, Olsen IC, Goll GL, Lorentzen M, Bolstad N, Haavardsholm EA, Lundin KE, Mørk C, Jahnsen J, Kvien TK, Berset IP (2017) Switching from originator infliximab to biosimilar CT-P13 compared with maintained treatment with originator infliximab (NOR-SWITCH): a 52-week, randomised, double-blind, non-inferiority trial. Lancet 389(10086):2304–2316

Kaeding M, Schmälter J, Klika C (2017a) Pharmacovigilance in the European Union: practical implementation across member states. Springer Nature, Singapore

Kaeding M, Schmälter J, Klika C, Kaeding M, Schmälter J, Klika C (2017b) The EU pharmacovigilance system. In: Pharmacovigilance in the European Union: Practical Implementation across Member States. Springer, Singapore, pp 17–34

Klein K, De Bruin ML, Broekmans AW, Stolk P (2015) Classification of recombinant biologics in the EU: divergence between national pharmacovigilance centers. BioDrugs 29:373–379

Klein K, Hazell L, Stolk P, Shakir S (2020) The UK BIO-TRAC study: a cross-sectional study of product and batch traceability for biologics in clinical practice and electronic adverse drug reaction reporting in the UK. Drug Saf 43(3):255–263

Klein K, Scholl JH, Vermeer NS, Broekmans AW, Van Puijenbroek EP, De Bruin ML, Stolk P (2016) Traceability of biologics in The Netherlands: an analysis of information-recording systems in clinical practice and spontaneous ADR reports. Drug Saf 39:185–192

Lane S, Lynn E, Shakir S (2018) Investigation assessing the publicly available evidence supporting postmarketing withdrawals, revocations and suspensions of marketing authorisations in the EU since 2012. BMJ Open 8(1):e019759

Lunddahl B (2016) Reducing the information gap among stakeholders. Inpresentation at the 14th annual biosimilar medicines group conference (London 2016 Apr 28)

McKinnon RA, Cook M, Liauw W, Marabani M, Marschner IC, Packer NH, Prins JB (2018) Biosimilarity and interchangeability: principles and evidence: a systematic review. BioDrugs 32:27–52

Moots R, Azevedo V, Coindreau JL, Dörner T, Mahgoub E, Mysler E, Scheinberg M, Marshall L (2017) Switching between reference biologics and biosimilars for the treatment of rheumatology, gastroenterology, and dermatology inflammatory conditions: considerations for the clinician. Curr Rheumatol Rep 19:1–6

Narayanan AS, Lakshmi KS, Kamaraj R (2020) An overview on good pharmacovigilance practices and new operational plan milestones of Eudravigilance in European Union. Res J Pharm Technol 13(4):1795–1800

Postigo R, Brosch S, Slattery J, van Haren A, Dogné JM, Kurz X, Candore G, Domergue F, Arlett P (2018) EudraVigilance medicines safety database: publicly accessible data for research and public health protection. Drug Saf 41:665–675
Santoro A, Genov G, Spooner A, Raine J, Arlett P (2017) Promoting and protecting public health: how the European Union pharmacovigilance system works. Drug Saf 40:855–869
Siu EC, Tomalin A, West K, Anderson S, Wyatt G (2019) An ever-evolving landscape: an update on the rapidly changing regulation and reimbursement of biosimilars in Canada. GaBI J 8(3):107–119
Slattery J, Alvarez Y, Hidalgo A (2013) Choosing thresholds for statistical signal detection with the proportional reporting ratio. Drug Saf 36:687–692
Sultana J, Zaccaria C, De Lisa R, Rossi F, Capuano A, Ferrajolo C (2019) Good pharmacovigilance practice in paediatrics: an overview of the updated European medicines agency guidelines. Pediatr Drugs 21(5):317–321
Vandenbroucke JP (2008) Observational research, randomized trials, and two views of medical science. PLoS Med 5(3):e67
Vermeer NS, Ebbers HC, Straus SM, Leufkens HG, Egberts TC, De Bruin ML (2016) The effect of exposure misclassification in spontaneous ADR reports on the time to detection of product-specific risks for biologicals: a simulation study. Pharmacoepidemiol Drug Saf 25(3):297–306
Vermeer NS, Giezen TJ, Zastavnik S, Wolff-Holz E, Hidalgo-Simon A (2019) Identifiability of biologicals in adverse drug reaction reports received from European clinical practice. Clin Pharmacol Ther 105(4):962–969
Vermeer NS, Spierings I, Mantel-Teeuwisse AK, Straus SM, Giezen TJ, Leufkens HG, Egberts TC, De Bruin ML (2015) Traceability of biologicals: present challenges in pharmacovigilance. Expert Opin Drug Saf 14(1):63–72
Wisniewski AF, Bate A, Bousquet C, Brueckner A, Candore G, Juhlin K, Macia-Martinez MA, Manlik K, Quarcoo N, Seabroke S, Slattery J (2016) Good signal detection practices: evidence from IMI PROTECT. Drug Saf 39:469–490
World Health Organization (n.d.) HIV self-testing strategic framework: a guide for planning, introducing and scaling up. World Health Organization, Geneva

Pharmacovigilance System in the USA

9

Deepika Pandey, Mukesh Nandave, and Anoop Kumar

Abstract

A multifaceted approach was developed by the Food and Drug Act (FDA) in the USA pharmacovigilance (PV) system, making it robust and well-established with technological advancements. The combined effort of all stakeholders to report and keep track of adverse events assist in effective post-marketing surveillance (PMS) at the national and international level. The PMS program further enables the identification of causal links between medications and adverse events. In this chapter, we have outlined the regulations and database maintenance approaches in the PV system of the USA and how this database helps promote safe drug use in public health benefits. Different databases like FAERS (FDA Adverse Event Report System), VAERS (The Vaccine Adverse Event Reporting System), and MAUDE (Manufacturer and User Facility Device Experience for Medical Devices) form the post-marketing system. The crucial role of the aggregate reporting process in the USA-PV system has been addressed which ensures the safety of pharmaceuticals and abides by the standards set by the FDA to maintain the legality of drug marketing. Data mining is an essential tool in aggregate reporting. Identifying safety risk factors, advantages, challenges, and future directions for advancement in the system's database management is discussed. A wider range of scientific spectrum and new data science technologies might be integrated to establish big data laboratories. Creating novel strategies for using electronic health records, and developing an innovative scientific community is coming up to figure out how to take advantage of the system's core capabilities beyond medication safety.

D. Pandey (✉) · M. Nandave · A. Kumar
Department of Pharmacology, Delhi Pharmaceutical Sciences and Research University, New Delhi, India
e-mail: mukeshnandave@gmail.com; anoopdpsru@dpsru.edu.in

M. Nandave, A. Kumar (eds.), *Pharmacovigilance Essentials*,
https://doi.org/10.1007/978-981-99-8949-2_9

Keywords

Pharmacovigilance system · USA · FDA · Adverse event reporting · Sentinel

9.1 Introduction

The USA PV system is well-established and robust, along with technological advancements that follow a multifaceted technique developed by the FDA. The FAERS (FDA Adverse Event Report System) for pharmaceuticals and biologic products, VAERS (The Vaccine Adverse Event Reporting System), and The MAUDE (Manufacturer and User Facility Device Experience Database for medical devices are the divisions associated with post-marketing systems. These PV databases help update and track adverse event reporting nationally and globally, further recognize causal relationships between drugs and adverse events, and promote drug safety in public health concerns (Jose and Rafeek 2019). Different FDA divisions like CDER (The Center for Drug Evaluation and Research), CBER (The Center for Biologics Evaluation and Research), and CDRH (The Center for Devices and Radiological Health), are developed with the purpose for further evaluation of the reported data to ensure the safety and efficacy of medicinal products for human use. The potential safety signals identified in this process are further investigated (Jose and Rafeek 2019; Qvigilance n.d.; US Food and Drug Administration 2016).

9.2 Role of USA PV System

The responsibility of USA pharmacovigilance is not merely about reporting and addressing the marketed drug's adverse events but also the systematic monitoring of the safety and efficacy of everyday practice medicines throughout the premarket review process and post-market surveillance.

9.2.1 Need to Set up PV System

Although evidence-based information on the safety and effectiveness of the drug is gathered during the clinical trial stage, there are certain gaps due to the small patient population, short trial length, and exclusion of specific demographic groups like children, lactating/pregnant women, etc. Therefore, post-marketing surveillance is crucial in identifying adverse events and continuously assessing the impact of medicinal products in the long term. A strong strategy is required for the Market Authorization Application (MAA) of pharmaceutical products in the USA. As a part of MAA, a key pharmacovigilance document, PSMF (Pharmacovigilance System Master File), is maintained with information about the description of the PV system setup, the SOPs, and the updated PV data (Whopvresources.org n.d.).

9.2.2 Function of the USA PV System

Along with gathering data on adverse events (AEs), a PV system keeps track of other safety-related informations like off-label usage information, prescription errors, drug overdoses, counterfeit items, etc. Furthermore, the PV system also evaluates this data for causality, severity, risk, and potential risk management strategies. These evaluations can also be used to update the product safety profile and labeling. In reaction to regulatory activities, harmful or safe drug interactions, and incorrect medicine prescriptions might be found. Removing an entire product or batch from the market may be necessary in more serious situations (Pitts et al. 2016).

9.2.3 ADR Reporting System in the USA

Healthcare professionals, pharmacists, and patients are expected to report adverse events regularly. Most data is gathered typically through spontaneous and solicited reports. A spontaneous report represents unsolicited communication by a healthcare professional or patient to a competent authority, marketing authorization holder, or other organization, like a regional PV center. The protocol in spontaneous reports is not limited to systematic collections, and this is what medical literature sources, social media, general sources, and non-interventional post-authorization studies could be the source of spontaneous reports. The solicited reports are gathered in organized data collection form, such as clinical trials, non-interventional studies, disease management programs, surveys of patients or healthcare professionals, named patient use, and other patient support.

AE reports, in the form of Individual Case Safety Reports (ICSRs), fulfill the criteria of a good report having the details of an identifiable patient, reporter, drug, and adverse event. An established network of pharmacovigilance personnel with healthcare providers, patient organizations, and Competent Authorities (CAs) is helpful in the collection of ICSRs and data from other sources. They are quite familiar with local languages, regulations, and the relevant national or regional databases (Qvigilance n.d.; Whopvresources.org n.d.).

9.2.4 ADR Coding and Safety Database

Gathering AE data from different sources and areas gives diverging standards and reporting rules. Due to this, ADRs are often coded uniformly using the ICH's MedDRA dictionary (Medical Dictionary for Regulatory Activities), maintaining harmonization. Furthermore, products are tagged to enhance data accuracy and comparability across other countries with different brand names. With all these pieces of information gathered from different ICSRs, an updated safety database is updated frequently. Selecting the appropriate safety database depends partly on the methods used to gather PV data with local and regional regulatory standards (Qvigilance n.d.; Li et al. 2021).

9.2.5 Assessment of Casualty, Seriousness and Expectedness

Any unwanted medical occurrence is an adverse event (AE) associated with a pharmaceutical product administered to a patient but does not necessarily exist a causal link between both. An adverse effect is an event with a suspected causal relationship to the medicinal product, and it could be life-threatening at any dose (US Food and Drug Administration 2015). Additionally, reference documents are needed to decide the expectedness of an adverse reaction. In further action, the frequency of the ADR, which is already established, is expected to be updated on the product label (Qvigilance n.d.; Peyro-Saint-Paul et al. 2021).

9.2.6 Safety Signal Detection

The effective management of signaling involves identifying risks earlier by reviewing ICSRs. It is statistically analyzed, documented well, and communicated better. Not all signals depict risks and do not require additional regulatory actions (US Food and Drug Administration 2015; Anon n.d.-a).

9.2.7 Risk Management Plan (RMP)

US PV system ensures a favorable risk–benefit balance for the target population. Aligned with the aim of pharmacovigilance, an RMP is placed for every product (Peyro-Saint-Paul et al. 2021). The RMP document containing product safety information (risks associated with the product and the strategies to prevent or minimize these risks) is submitted during MAA and is updated throughout the medication's life cycle. The crucial measures adapted toward risk management include product label updates, educational programs for HCPs and patients with better communication, and pregnancy prevention programs (Wilson and Milne 2011; US Food and Drug Administration n.d.).

9.2.8 Reporting to Competent Authorities

The most essential component of safety monitoring is reporting. Reports of suspected adverse reactions received from solicited and unsolicited sources are ensured to be completed accurately, legibly, and consistently because inaccurate and inadequate reporting for their clinical assessment may lead to an incomplete or misinterpreted AE compilation. Hence, false statistical analysis is expected (Qvigilance n.d.).

9.3 Pharmacovigilance Regulation in the USA

Since 2005, the US FDA has been the regulatory body in the US, monitoring the safety and efficacy of medicinal products (including biological vaccines, OTC drugs, and medical devices) for the benefit of human health. The FDA holds the responsibility for setting and implementing regulations, guidelines, and standards for the pharmaceutical industry. It ensures the active conduction of post-marketing surveillance and pharmacovigilance activities (Jose and Rafeek 2019).

9.3.1 The Federal Law Governing the USA PV System

Historical background: On June 30, 1906, the US Federal FDA was formed with the aim of ensuring the drug's purity and contamination-free (Fornasier et al. 2018; Routledge 1998). Consequently, after the Sulfanilamide elixir toxicity in 1937, which caused 107 deaths in the USA, the Federal Food, Drug, and Cosmetic Act (FDCA) in 1938 was established with the purpose of renovating the public health system (Woolf 1998). The Federal Food, Drug, and Cosmetic Act (FDCA) and the FDA Code of Federal Regulations (CFR) Title 21 (with several subchapters) is the law governing this area of drugs and medical devices for human use (Fornasier et al. 2018; Food and Drug Administration (FDA) n.d.).

9.4 ICSRs Reporting Process in the USA PV System

After receiving a new drug application (NDA), abbreviated new drug application (ANDA), or biologic license application (BLA) approval, the FDA needs to receive all the collected and collated AE reports from various sources, including the medical and scientific literature by the MAH (Qvigilance n.d.; PPT PV USA-PharmXL n.d.). The frequency of searches is not explicitly stated by the FDA. Still, it states clearly to file any critical report (as well as any reports resulting from product-specific considerations) within 15 calendar days. Generally, reports of the same medicinal products across other countries with different brand names found severe and expected are encouraged to be reported. For reporting, a report must contain information suggestive of the existence of an individual patient. The license holder must ensure that PV activities like surveillance, processing the ADE data, evaluation, and reporting (15-day reports via Electronic Submission Gateway) are implemented effectively. An adequate written procedure with complete information on patient existence must be documented to report the information (PPT PV USA-PharmXL n.d.).

9.4.1 Flow of Information from FAERS to FDA

FAERS is a publicly available database that contains the safety reports submitted in the form of voluntary reports from healthcare professionals and consumers and mandatory from manufacturers (Fig. 9.1). The FAERS database supports the FDA's post-marketing surveillance program for drug and biologic products. This database structure adheres to the guidelines issued by the International Conference on Harmonisation (ICH E2B) (DrugSafety n.d.).

After FDA approval, the reports in FAERS are evaluated by clinical reviewers in the Center for Drug Evaluation and Research (CDER) and the Center for Biologics Evaluation and Research (CBER) to ensure the safety and efficacy of the medicines in human health (Fig. 9.1). AEs and medication errors are coded using MedDRA terminology. If a potential safety concern is identified in FAERS, further evaluation might be conducted using large database studies, such as those in the Sentinel System. Furthermore, based on evaluation and associated with potential safety concerns, the FDA can restrict the drug use or remove it from the market as a regulatory action and to improve product safety and benefit public health, such as updating a product's labeling information and communicating new safety information to the public (Li et al. 2021).

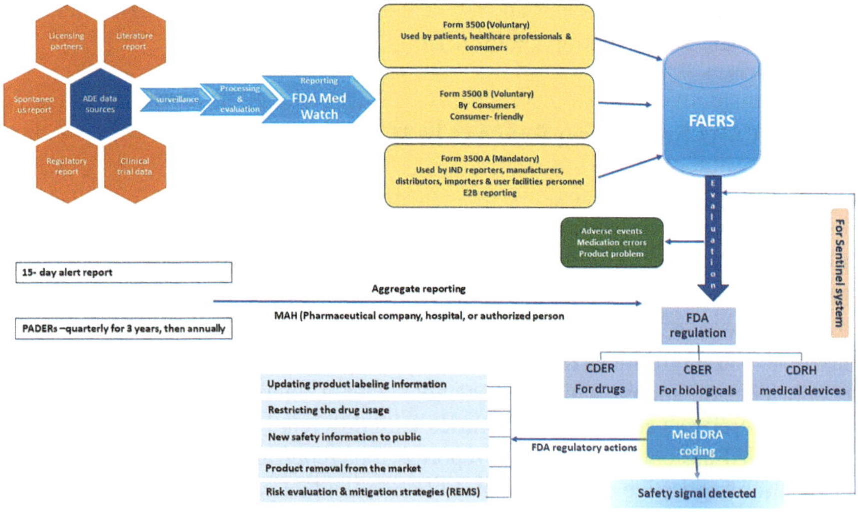

Fig. 9.1 Process of ICSRs reporting in the US FDA pharmacovigilance system

9.4.2 The Sentinel System of the US FDA

With the prime goal of public health safety, the FDA introduced the Sentinel Initiative in May 2008, further to the FDA Amendments Act of 2007. Sentinel is a nationwide electronic system that has revolutionized medical product safety assessment by researchers and scientists, which are subject to FDA regulation. Firstly, introduced as mini-Sentinel phase as a pilot study with the Sentinel's development information, it transformed into the full Sentinel System in September 2014 and formalized in February 2016. Sentinel has developed, over time, the largest multisite database worldwide for product safety and is continually expanding and improving in order to fulfill the FDA's requirements.

In September 2019, the FDA developed a new form of Sentinel and expected participation in a broader range of scientific knowledge. In this view, the FDA expanded the Sentinel into three coordinating centers: Sentinel Operations Center, with the aim to establish organizational partnerships in clinical medicine, health informatics, epidemiology, pharmacy, statistics, data science, exclusively artificial intelligence, machine learning, natural language processing, and network operations for robust post-market safety analyses. Innovation Center aims to develop novel ways to extract and utilize electronic health records information in a better way. The Community Building and Outreach Center is dedicated to improve communication and collaboration among stakeholders and spreading awareness and access toward using Sentinel tools and data infrastructure. Hence, this new design is anticipated to develop laboratories and novel strategies to assess electronic health records. It is expected to develop big data and data science fields and approaches to foster the scientific community for developing innovative ways to engage the system's capacity beyond drug safety (Sentinel n.d.).

9.4.3 Reporting an Adverse Event to FDA: MedWatch (Annexure 4)

The Food and Drug Administration (FDA) has a program called MedWatch that allows users to report serious reactions, product quality issues, therapeutic failure, and any errors in product use. If experiencing a serious reaction to a medical product, such as drugs, biological products, medical devices, dietary supplements, infant formula, or cosmetics, consumers are encouraged to report through the MedWatch forms with clinical information provided by the healthcare provider that can help further FDA in the safety assessment of report (Fda.gov n.d.-a). In circumstances where the form is not processed by the HCP, patients can report to the FDA by completing the online reporting themselves. The MedWatch website is helpful in voluntary and mandatory reporting. Additionally, *MedWatch* receives reports and, as appropriate, publishes safety alerts for FDA-regulated medical products (Medwatch-fda-safety n.d.).

9.4.3.1 Voluntary Reporting

Voluntary reporting can be processed **by consumers, patients, and health professionals** through the online MedWatch portal or by submitting a filled FDA form as follows (MedWatch form n.d.) (Fig. 9.1):

- Form 3500 (reported by a health professional).
- 3500 B (consumer-friendly and can be filled by the patients themselves).

9.4.3.2 Mandatory Reporting

Manufacturers of drug and therapeutic biological products, distributors, packers, and others report the adverse events associated with product launched (Aggregate Reporting n.d.). Electronic submissions of post-marketing ICSRs done to FAERS (Fig. 9.1).

FDA relies on voluntary reporting of the medical products' adverse events to maintain safety monitoring and improve patient safety. The FDA uses these data, which prompts improved safety profiles, ensuring effective and safe products available on the market.

The FDA-regulated other products, such as tobacco products, vaccines, animal drugs, devices, and pet foods, utilize appropriate portals dedicated to these products. All the voluntary and mandatory completed FDA reporting forms are submitted electronically to FAERS. FDA Adverse Events Reporting System (FAERS) electronic submissions guidance can provide help on the electronic submission of post-marketing ICSRs with and without attachments (Fda.gov n.d.-b).

9.5 Aggregate Reporting in the US FDA PV System

Aggregate reporting involves safety data from various sources. A thorough view of an evaluated drug's safety profile is compiled and provided to regulatory authorities. The periodic reporting of aggregate reports covering the collated evidence to date provides a comprehensive overview of the drug safety profile to National Competent Authorities (NCAs). They also assure the critical assessment by MAH toward the benefit–risk balance of the product, and as required, appropriate regulatory actions set by ICH are initiated against risks identified (Aggregate Reporting n.d.; Anon n.d.-b).

9.5.1 Periodic Adverse Experience Report (PADER): Periodic Safety Reporting Requirements

After the US approval for each application, FDA regulations need the submission of post-marketing periodic safety reports in the PADER format, quarterly for the first 3 years after approval and annually thereafter. The PADER is a descriptive summary and safety data evaluation of the received reports and is submitted electronically as an attachment to the electronic Common Technical Document (eCTD). Any periodic report is continually evaluated for its risk–benefit profile with safety and efficacy throughout the product life cycle. Any new or potential risk identified is further investigated. Additionally, non-expedited ICSRs are submitted at the descriptive portion of the PADER to FAERS via the ESG (Qvigilance n.d.; PADER n.d.; Public Safety and Vigilance n.d.).

9.5.2 Aggregate Reporting Regulations

The US FDA mandates periodic safety update reports (PSURs) and specifies their contents and frequency of delivery. This applies to all the medicinal products authorized after the NDA procedure (Aggregate Reporting n.d.). On the demand of regulatory organizations, pharmaceutical businesses are bound to publish aggregate reports regularly, and this prompts the verification of the drug's ongoing safety profile.

9.5.3 Components of Aggregate Report

To fully assess the drug's safety profile, aggregate reports comprise numerous components, depending on regulatory criteria and the development stage of the product (PADER n.d.). Some frequent components of an aggregate report are as follows:

1. **The introduction** outlines the medicine's indication and the dose regimen.
2. **Period of Safety Evaluation** outlines the safety evaluation period of the report and the sources utilized to compile the safety data.
3. **The Adverse Events** section includes the summary of the AE reported during the safety evaluation period.
4. **The Patient Exposure** section details the number of patients taking medicine during the safety monitoring. Furthermore, this data projects the incidence of AE.
5. **The Safety Profile section** includes the maintained drug's safety profile with any safety concerns identified throughout the monitoring period.
6. **Benefit–Risk Assessment:** The collated safety data presents a benefit–risk assessment of the medicinal product.
7. **Conclusion:** Highlights the essential findings of the aggregate report and recommends any additional safety monitoring, if any.

9.5.4 Advantage of Aggregate Reporting

- Safety data collected and collated from various sources in aggregate reporting enables the regulatory authorities to identify potential safety concerns during the monitoring period (Anon n.d.-b). This prompts the implementation of suitable patient health safety measures.

- The standardized format of aggregate reports makes it simpler to conduct safety monitoring procedures by regulatory agencies for various pharmaceuticals (PADER n.d.). Additionally, pharmaceutical companies find it consistent and, hence, easier to adhere to its legal requirements.
- Real-world safety data collected during the post-marketing phase through aggregate reports, which would be in the chance to get unidentified during clinical trials (Anon n.d.-b), ensure the safety monitoring of pharmaceuticals continuously on the market, and regulatory authorities can take the necessary action toward potential safety risks.
- The therapeutic effectiveness and risk stratification calculation of benefit–risk balance for various drugs can also be discovered after gathering post-marketing safety data (Public Safety and Vigilance n.d.). Aggregate reporting data becomes crucial in continuous monitoring and make it available the product's benefit–risk profile regularly over time.
- Aggregate reports' pre-marketing phase data on the drug's safety and efficacy make it possible for a drug to be approved for marketing (Anon n.d.-b).
- Aggregate reports make the post-marketing evaluations of medications reliable to regulatory agencies toward sustained effectiveness and safety (Anon n.d.-b).

9.5.5 Aggregate Reporting Regulatory Requirements

The U.S. FDA requires aggregate reporting with some standards to ensure accurate and timely safety information supplied by pharmaceutical businesses. The most important regulatory requirements outlined for aggregate reporting are as follows:

1. **Timelines for Submission:** The FDA needs pharmaceutical businesses to adhere to timelines and submit aggregate reports regularly (like every 6 months or annually).
2. **Format and Content:** A distinct aggregate report in which the FDA needs the safety and clinical review form summary.
3. **Adverse Event Reporting:** Pharmaceutical companies must promptly disclose all the AE related to their medicinal products.
4. **Signal Detection:** Pharmaceutical companies must conduct signal detection operations to identify potential safety risks.
5. **Risk Management Plans:** Pharmaceutical companies are required to create product risk management plans to take further steps to control and mitigate any safety issues.

9.5.6 Risk Management and Minimization Strategies

Through the REMS (Risk Evaluation and Minimization Strategies), the FDA ensures the continuous safe use of approved medications with a positive benefit–risk ratio in human health safety. The FDA released a list of all approved REMS, which includes any additional safety monitoring steps to be implemented by the license holder. Additional safety monitoring actions may include educational medication guides and better communication plans developed with healthcare providers and patients (Qvigilance n.d.; US Food and Drug Administration n.d.). Also, additional monitoring requirements during the drug administration period.

9.6 Challenges

- The US Government Accountability Office (GAO) reviewed FDA data, and CDER evaluated data in its database, revealing incompleteness, timeliness, and inaccuracy associated with FAERS. The reporting requirements in the US PV system, like no restrictions on proof toward AE and not mandatory to report every AE to the FDA, make the FDA lack the necessary information on the causal link between a product and an adverse event (Anon n.d.-b).
- When both the sponsor and a consumer submit an identical report, it prompts to duplication. All these limitations do not allow us to determine the incidence of an adverse event in the US population merely based on FAERS data.
- Analysis of historical safety data serves as the foundation for aggregate reporting. This implies that signals might not be identified until after the drug has been available on the market for a while. It is then expected by that time, patients may expose to potential safety risks.
- Furthermore, aggregate reporting might not be sufficient for identifying unusual or recurring safety problems (US Government Accountability Office n.d.).
- In aggregate reporting, clinical studies and unprompted complaints are a few of the sources of information to collect, excluding other safety data sources such as electronic health. This restriction may lead to inadequate safety monitoring (Aggregate Reporting n.d.).
- Following the documentation process while producing aggregate reports, compiling aggregate reports, and legally submitting them might be challenging due to several factors like accuracy, timeliness, and submission conforms that add complexity (Aggregate Reporting n.d.; Anon n.d.-b).

9.7 VigiBase Data Flow in the USA PV System

VigiBase is the largest database worldwide, containing more than 30 million potential AE of medicinal products reported since 1968 by WHO-PIDM (Programme for International Drug Monitoring) countries and updated regularly. Since 1978, Uppsala Monitoring Center (UMC) has maintained the VigiBase with the objective of safe clinical practice of therapeutic. Early identification of safety risks and structured data entry and analysis with drug classification tools (Fig. 9.2) linked to the VigiBase system allow effective and accurate evaluation (Vigibase n.d.; WHO n.d.). The automated entry process for VigiBase makes quality checks

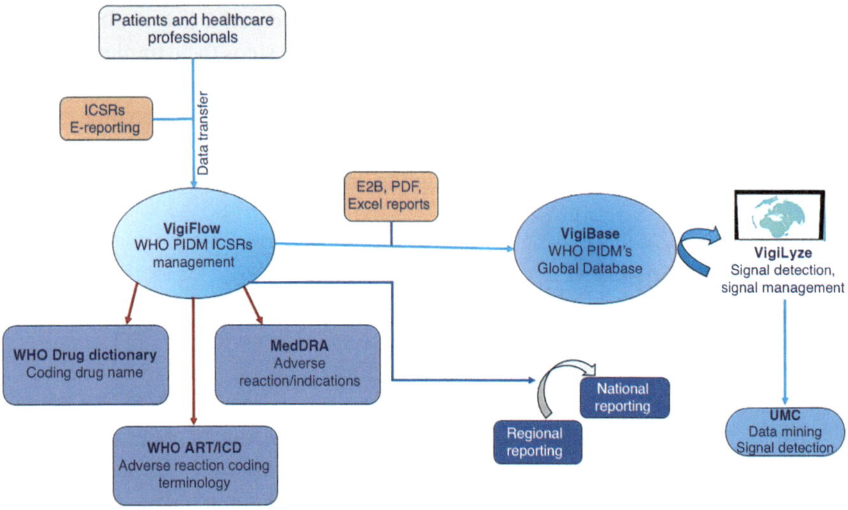

Fig. 9.2 Schematic representation of VigiBase data access through VigiFlow in USFDA (WHO-PIDM). *PIDM* Program for International Drug Monitoring, *ICD* International Classification of disease, *Med DRA* medical drug regulatory activities, *UMC* Uppsala monitoring center

of each incoming report according to predefined criteria. Member countries share these reports in VigiBase, and each PIDM country (WHO Pharmacovigilance 1968) can access the spontaneous reports of suspected adverse effects. Then after, it is reviewed. Detected drug safety signals, if any, may lead to regulatory action. This global database facilitates the probability of detecting rare adverse drug reactions from worldwide data, which would be impossible to detect from single-country data. The heterogeneous data of VigiBase offers opportunities for analyzing differences and comparisons of countries. National PV centers' sincere and disciplined contribution maintains the VigiBase system to a large extent for timeliness, completeness, and report quality (Vigi Base n.d.). The patterns of harm that might emerge during signal analysis from this global database with a large amount of worldwide data might not be evident in smaller national databases (Vogel et al. 2020).

9.7.1 VigiFlow

VigiFlow is a web-based PV management system. VigiFlow has built-in WHODrug Global and MedDRA support to maintain a streamlined workflow in the PV process. This helps optimize the collection and assessment of cases (Fig. 9.2). **Through the E-reporting module of VigiFlow,** national centers can gather information on AE of medicinal products and vaccines from healthcare professionals, consumers, and pharmaceutical companies. E- Reporting offers the instant availability of AE reported in VigiFlow for further review process. The reports, those added via

E-reporting, appear in VigiFlow report lists, that is further coded and assessed (Vigiflow n.d.; E Reporting Vigiflow n.d.).

9.7.2 VigiLyze

VigiBase data is accessed via VigiLyze as a signal detection and signal management tool, and National PV centers regularly use it for PV processing (PV Products/ VigiLyze n.d.). The primary purpose of the Uppsala Monitoring Center (UMC) is signal detection, and it monitors and outlines the potential patient risks related to the consumption of medications. UMC periodically reviews VigiBase for probable adverse effects that have not yet been identified or are only partially documented. Signal identification at UMC uses an array of automated data mining approaches and clinical assessment of reports to sort out medicine-adverse effect combinations. Parallel to this, a qualitative review of the scientific literature offers new approaches that may be used to conduct more focused searches in VigiLyze and decide if more research into potential safety signals is required (Anon n.d.-a).

9.8 Conclusion

The USA has a well-established and robust pharmacovigilance (PV) system, and it follows a multifaceted approach introduced by the Food and Drug Act (FDA). With the primary aim of patient health safety, the US Food and Drug Administration aims to regulate drug quality by ensuring clinically relevant quality standards, monitoring across product lifecycle, applying expertise and techniques effectively, enhancing quality regulation, and open communication. Aggregate reporting periodically plays an important role in database management and ensuring drug safety. Data mining is an important tool for signal detection and management in aggregate reporting for timely identifying potential safety risks and helping to take steps in mitigating the risk. The VigiBase system gives a broad database of global population coverage in terms of identifying the rare AE and establishing the comparison of different regions worldwide. The advancement brought in the sentinel system of database management prompts encouraging innovation with new technologies in a wider array of scientific expertise, data science, developing new approaches to use electronic health records efficiently, and cultivating a robust scientific community to unleash the system's core capabilities beyond drug safety.

References

Aggregate Reporting (n.d.). https://www.qvigilance.com/aggregate-reporting. Accessed 18 Sept 2023

Anon (n.d.-a) How UMC detects signals. https://who-umc.org/signal-work/signal-detection/. Accessed 10 Aug 2023

Anon (n.d.-b) Aggregate reporting. https://drugsafetynest.com/understanding-aggregate-reporting-inpharmacovigilance/#:~:text=Aggregate%20reporting%20is%20the%20process%20of%20gathering%20and,a%20comprehensive%20picture%20of%20the%20drug%E2%80%99s%20safety%20profile. Accessed 10 Sept 2023
DrugSafety (n.d.). https://www.fda.gov/Drugs/DrugSafety/ucm522941.htm/. Accessed 10 July 2023
E Reporting Vigiflow (n.d.). https://who-umc.org/media/ebfgtnpf/ereporting-vigiflow.pdf
Fda.gov (n.d.-a) Medwatch ADR reporting. https://www.fda.gov/safety/medwatch-fda-safety-information-and-adverse-event-reporting-program. Accessed 14 Aug 2023
Fda.gov (n.d.-b) Where do you send completed FDA forms? https://www.fda.gov/safety/reporting-serious-problems-fda/where-send-completed-form-fda-3500a-mandatory-reporting-form. Accessed 18 September 2023
Food and Drug Administration (FDA) (n.d.) History. https://www.fda.gov/AboutFDA/WhatWeDo/History/. Accessed 5 July 2023
Fornasier G, Francescon S, Leone R, Baldo P (2018) A historical overview over pharmacovigilance. Int J Clin Pharm 40(4):744–747
Jose J, Rafeek NR (2019) Pharmacovigilance in India in comparison with the USA and European Union: challenges and perspectives. Ther Innov Regul Sci 53(6):781–786
Li H, Sun X, Sun D et al (2021) Thromboembolic events associated with immune checkpoint inhibitors: a real-world study of data from the Food and Drug Administration adverse event reporting system (FAERS) database. Int Immunopharmacol 98:107818
MedWatch form (n.d.). https://www.fda.gov/safety/medical-product-safety-information/medwatch-forms-fda-safety-reporting. Accessed 14 Aug 2023
Medwatch-fda-safety (n.d.). https://www.fda.gov/safety/medwatch-fda-safety-information-and-adverse-event-reporting-program/reporting-serious-problems-fda. Accessed 14 Aug 2023
PADER (n.d.) PADER all about. pharmacovigilance.org/30-periodic-adverse-drug-experience-report-pader-paer/. Accessed 18 Sept 2023
Peyro-Saint-Paul L, Fedrizzi S, Defer G (2021) Drug safety in multiple sclerosis: from reporting to signal detection and benefit-risk management. Rev Neurol (Paris) 177(5):582–588
Pitts PJ, Louet HL, Moride Y, Conti RM (2016) 21st century pharmacovigilance: efforts, roles, and responsibilities. Lancet Oncol 17(11):e486–e492
PPT PV USA-PharmXL (n.d.). https://www.slideshare.net/PharmXLInternational/pharmacovigilance-sytem-in-unitedstates-of-america-usa/. Accessed 23 July 2023
Public Safety and Vigilance (n.d.). https://publicsafetyandvigilance.com/periodic-adverse-drug-experience-report-pader/. Accessed 18 Sept 2023
PV Products/VigiLyze (n.d.). https://who-umc.org/pv-products/vigilyze/. Accessed 23 Sept 2023
Qvigilance (n.d.). https://www.qvigilance.com/blog/usa-fda-safety-requirements-pharmacovigilance/. Accessed 10 July 2023
Routledge P (1998) 150 years of pharmacovigilance. Lancet 351:1200–1201
Sentinel (n.d.). https://www.fda.gov/safety/fda-sentinel-initiative/ Accessed 10 July 2023
US Food and Drug Administration (2015) Safe use initiative. http://www.fda.gov/Drugs/DrugSafety/SafeUseInitiative/. Accessed 12 July 2023
US Food and Drug Administration (2016) Office of Pharmaceutical Quality. http://www.fda.gov/AboutFDA/CentersOffices/OfficeofMedicalProductsandTobacco/CDER/. Accessed 12 July 2023
US Food and Drug Administration (n.d.) Approved Risk Evaluation and Mitigation Strategies (REMS). http://www.accessdatafdagov/scripts/cder/rems/indexcfm?event/. Accessed 5 July 2023
US Government Accountability Office (n.d.) Drug Safety: FDA Expedites Many Applications, But Data for Postapproval Oversight Need Improvement. https://www.gao.gov/products/gao-16-192/ Accessed 10 Sept 2023
Vigi Base (n.d.). https://who-umc.org/about-the-who-programme-for-international-drug-monitoring/about-the-who-pidm/. Accessed 18 Sept 2023
Vigibase (n.d.). https://en.wikipedia.org/wiki/VigiBase. Accessed 18 Sept 2023

Vigiflow (n.d.). https://who-umc.org/pv-products/vigiflow/. Accessed 18 Aug 2023
Vogel U, van Stekelenborg J, Dreyfus B, Garg A, Habib M, Hosain R, Wisniewski A (2020) Investigating overlap in signals from EVDAS, FAERS, and VigiBase®. Drug Saf 43:351–362
WHO (n.d.). https://who-umc.org/vigibase/ Accessed 18 Sept 2023
WHO Pharmacovigilance (1968) PIDM program in 1968. http://www.who.int/medicines/areas/quality_safety/safety_efficacy/pharmvigi/en/. Accessed 18 Sept 2023
Whopvresources.org (n.d.) Basic steps to setting up PV system. https://whopvresources.org/center.php/. Accessed 10 Aug 2023
Wilson A, Milne CP (2011) FDA's risk evaluation and mitigation strategies (REMS): effective and efficient safety tools or process poltergeist? Food Drug Law J 66:569–585
Woolf AD (1998) The Haitian diethylene glycol poisoning tragedy: a dark wood revisited. JAMA 279:1215–1216

Pharmacovigilance System in Non-EU Countries

10

Divya Shukla, Mukesh Nandave, Anoop Kumar, and Deepali Siwan

Abstract

This chapter explores the landscape of pharmacovigilance systems in non-EU countries, shedding light on pharmacovigilance regulations in non-EU regions. It begins by introducing the role of pharmacovigilance in protecting health and emphasizes the variations between non-EU countries. While the EU has regulations, a harmonized approach, and centralized monitoring through the European Medicines Agency (EMA), non-EU countries have systems influenced by local factors. The following section examines pharmacovigilance systems in EU countries, starting with an overview of their regulatory landscape. It highlights authorities in non-EU regions, such as the FDA in the USA, Health Canada in Canada, TGA in Australia, PMDA in Japan, and CDSCO (Central Drugs Standard Control Organisation) in India, which play a significant role in ensuring drug safety and quality. Furthermore, this chapter outlines the differences in reporting adverse drug reactions (ADRs) pharmacovigilance guidelines, signal detection methods, communication strategies, and collaboration efforts in non-EU countries. These discrepancies arise from legislation, local policies, and international standardization initiatives. Ultimately, this chapter emphasizes that understanding these frameworks is crucial for compliance and effective drug safety monitoring.

Keywords

Regulatory Authorities · Australia · Canada · Japan

D. Shukla (✉) · M. Nandave · A. Kumar · D. Siwan
Department of Pharmacology, Delhi Pharmaceutical Sciences and Research University, New Delhi, India
e-mail: mukeshnandave@gmail.com; anoopdpsru@dpsru.edu.in

M. Nandave, A. Kumar (eds.), *Pharmacovigilance Essentials*,
https://doi.org/10.1007/978-981-99-8949-2_10

10.1 Introduction

The primary goal of pharmacovigilance regulations in non-EU countries is recognizing, evaluating, comprehending, and avoiding any adverse effects or medication-related problems. Although pharmacovigilance systems are used everywhere, it is essential to recognize the distinctions between the European Union (EU) and non-EU nations (Ema. EudraVigilance—European Medicines Agency 2023; WHO Pharmacovigilance 2023). In the EU, pharmacovigilance is supervised by strict laws and standards that apply to all member states. The European Medicines Agency (EMA) works closely with national regulatory agencies to provide a unified approach to drug safety monitoring (Wiktorowicz et al. 2012). The EMA oversees the evaluation and supervision of medications in the consolidated EU pharmacovigilance system.

In contrast, non-EU countries have their unique pharmacovigilance systems that operate based on their specific regulatory frameworks. The regulatory landscape varies considerably across regions and countries, influenced by factors such as healthcare infrastructure, resources, and local regulations. Non-EU countries may have decentralized or semi-centralized pharmacovigilance systems, with individual national regulatory authorities overseeing safety monitoring within their jurisdictions (Elshafie et al. 2018).

The key differences between EU and non-EU pharmacovigilance systems lie in the regulatory processes, reporting mechanisms, and stakeholder coordination. The EU benefits from a centralized system, allowing standardized procedures, unified reporting formats, and a centralized database (EudraVigilance) to collect and analyze safety data. Non-EU countries, however, may have variations in reporting requirements, data collection methods, and the existence of national or regional databases (Xie and Tian 2013).

Moreover, the EU pharmacovigilance system uses tight coordination amongst regulatory bodies to identify signals, manage risks, and provide periodic safety update reports. Non-EU countries may have different approaches to risk management and signal detection based on their specific contexts and available resources (Radecka et al. 2018).

Understanding these differences is crucial for effectively implementing pharmacovigilance systems in non-EU countries. It requires tailoring strategies to address each region's unique challenges and opportunities, considering the local healthcare infrastructure, cultural factors, and resource limitations.

10.2 Role of Regulatory Authorities in Non-EU Countries

Pharmacovigilance is handled by regulatory bodies in non-EU countries responsible for ensuring the quality, safety, and efficacy of medications that fall under their purview. These regulatory agencies all seek to protect the public's health by monitoring and regulating the security of pharmaceutical products, even though their

Table 10.1 Regulatory authorities of major non-EU countries

S. No.	Countries	Regulatory bodies
1.	Australia	Therapeutic goods administration (TGA)
2.	Japan	Pharmaceuticals and medical devices agency (PMDA) Ministry of Health, Labour and Welfare (MHLW)
3.	Canada	Health Canada
4.	Brazil	Agencia Nacional de Vigilancia sanitaria (ANVISA)
5.	New Zealand	The medical Council of new Zealand
6.	Russia	Ministry of health of the Russian Federation
7.	South Africa	South African health products regulatory authority (SAHPRA)
8.	Saudi Arabia	The Saudi Commission for Health Specialties (SCFHS)
9.	Argentina	The Ministry of Health
10.	Korea Republic	The Ministry of Food and Drug Safety (MFDS)
11.	Iran	Medical Council of Iran
12.	Iraq	The Ministry of Health and environment of Iraq

exact titles and organizational structures vary depending on the region (International Federation of Pharmaceutical, Manufacturers,, and Associations 2015). Regulatory authorities of major non-EU countries are mentioned in Table 10.1.

10.2.1 Regulatory Frameworks and Requirements of Non-EU Countries

Non-EU countries have distinct regulatory frameworks and requirements for pharmacovigilance, shaped by national legislation, local guidelines, and international harmonization efforts (Barry et al. 2020; Breckenridge 2012). Here are some key aspects that may differ across regions:

Reporting Requirements: Non-EU countries may have different regulations regarding reporting adverse drug reactions (ADRs) and other safety-related information. This includes variations in the types of events to be reported, timelines for reporting, and the reporting channels utilized.

Pharmacovigilance Guidelines: Each regulatory authority develops its guidelines, outlining the specific requirements and expectations for pharmaceutical companies and healthcare professionals regarding safety monitoring, reporting, and risk management.

Signal Detection and Assessment: The signal detection and assessment methods may vary among non-EU countries. This includes differences in the utilization of data mining techniques, signal validation processes, and risk–benefit evaluations.

Communication and Information Exchange: Non-EU countries may have specific communication channels and requirements for disseminating drug safety information to healthcare professionals, patients, and the public. These can include national drug bulletins, safety advisories, and communication through regulatory websites or portals.

Collaboration and Efforts toward Harmonization: While each regulatory authority operates within its jurisdiction, there are international endeavors to encourage collaboration, exchange of information, and alignment of pharmacovigilance practices. These initiatives involve partnerships between bodies, participation in databases and networks, and adherence to worldwide guidelines such as those issued by the World Health Organization (WHO).

Companies, healthcare professionals, and regulators must understand the frameworks and requirements in non-EU countries. This understanding ensures compliance with regulations and enables effective monitoring of drug safety. At a level, efforts are being made to harmonize practices and standards fostering coordinated pharmacovigilance across the globe. The key points of major non-EU countries like Australia, Canada, and Japan are mentioned in Table 10.2.

10.3 Pharmacovigilance System in Non-EU Countries

Establishing pharmacovigilance centers in non-EU countries is vital in ensuring effective drug safety monitoring and surveillance. These centers act as points for collecting, analyzing, and managing reports on drug reactions (ADR) and other safety-related data (Non-European Medicines Agency 2012). Here is a summary of how national pharmacovigilance centers are established, their roles, integration into healthcare systems, and their collaboration with organizations to share information.

10.3.1 Pharmacovigilance System in Australia

The thalidomide disaster prompted the first safety alert, which opened the door for the National Health Department of Australia to form an Australian Drug Evaluation Committee in 1963 to look into the safety of innovative pharmaceuticals and a program for spontaneous reporting of ADRs. The Australian ADR Reporting System was launched in 1964 with the exchange of reporting forms with prescribers. A "Blue card" form for clinician reporting was developed in 1971. The Australian Adverse Drug Reporting system allows doctors to report any ADR even though these cards are not physically present. In Australia, pharmacovigilance is primarily supported by industry-mandated reporting as well as volunteer reporting from patients and healthcare professionals (HCPs). The reports are kept in the Adverse Event Notifications Database (DAEN). It contains details about adverse drug reactions (ADRs) caused by prescription, over-the-counter, and supplementary medicines and equipment. The Therapeutic Goods Administration posts articles, guidelines, and reports from scientific studies about the safety of medications online (Linger and Martin 2018). Due to a rise in complaints, the Adverse Drug Reactions Advisory Committee (ADRAC), despite its name, became a subcommittee of ADEC by 1970 as shown in Fig. 10.1.

Table 10.2 Key points of pharmacovigilance systems in Australia, Canada, and Japan

Parameter	Australia	Canada	Japan
Regulatory body of pharmacovigilance body	Therapeutic goods administration (TGA)	Health Canada marketed health products, directorate of the health products and food branch	Pharmaceuticals and medical devices agency (PMDA) Ministry of Health, Labour and Welfare (MHLW)
Guidelines	Australian register of therapeutic goods (ARTG), regulated by the TGA. It outlines the mandatory reporting requirements and offers recommendations on pharmacovigilance best practice	GVP guidelines (GUI- 0102)	ICH guidelines for ICSR: E2B, M2, and E2B (R3)
Process for reporting	Australian adverse drug reaction reporting system. In this system, you can report a case of a suspected adverse reaction in association with a medicine (including complementary, OTC, or prescription) or a vaccine. For general privacy information, go to http://www.tga.gov.au/about/website-privacy.htm	Via online, fax/mail, or telephone at Canada vigilance regional Office for Canada Vigilance Program (MedEffect Canada)	Via e-mail, fax, post via websites creates ICSR files
Master file for pharmacovigilance system	Not mentioned	Not mentioned	Not mentioned
Pharmacovigilance inspection	TGA publishes annual inspection program Metrices reports	GVP inspection program, inspection strategy for GVP for drugs (POL-0041)	In Japan, regulatory authorities conduct pharmacovigilance inspections to ensure pharmaceutical companies comply with safety regulations. These inspections assess if companies monitor and report adverse events effectively and take appropriate actions to ensure product safety

(continued)

Table 10.2 (continued)

Parameter	Australia	Canada	Japan
Pharmacovigilance audit	Not mentioned	In accordance with the GVP guidelines (GUI-0102)	Not mentioned
Risk management system	Not mentioned	Mentioned in the guidance document—Submission of risk management plans and follow-up commitments	Not mentioned
The time period for the ADR reporting database	Within 30 calendar days of the occurrence of ADR	Within 15 calendar days of the occurrence of ADR	For serious adverse event—15 days For non-serious adverse events—30 days
Different types of ADR reporting form	Blue card adverse reaction reporting form	Canada vigilance adverse reaction online database; two: Form for suspected adverse drug reaction to marketed products by industry; form for suspected adverse drug reaction reporting by consumers	Direct patient reporting system (DPRS) for direct patient reporting through the internet
Submission of PSUR	To submit PSUR as an eCTD/NeeS sequence, as a standalone sequence with sequence type "periodic safety update report"	To submission and information policy division therapeutic products directorate Health Canada	According to ICH E2C, all PSURs in Japan for all marketed items must be filed to the MHLW and must contain all foreign data
PSUR data lock point	Either 6 months or 1 year from date of approval letter	70/90 days	Within 70 calendar days
Safety communication	Communicated via the TGA website	Communicated via the Health Canada website	Communicated via the PMDA and MHLW website
Risk minimization measures	Not mentioned	Guidance document—Submission of risk management plans and follow-up commitments	Not mentioned
Contact number for help	Yes, 1800 555,677	Yes, 1–866–337-7705	+81 3–3506-9400
UMC connection	Not mentioned	Yes, via the med effect program	Not mentioned

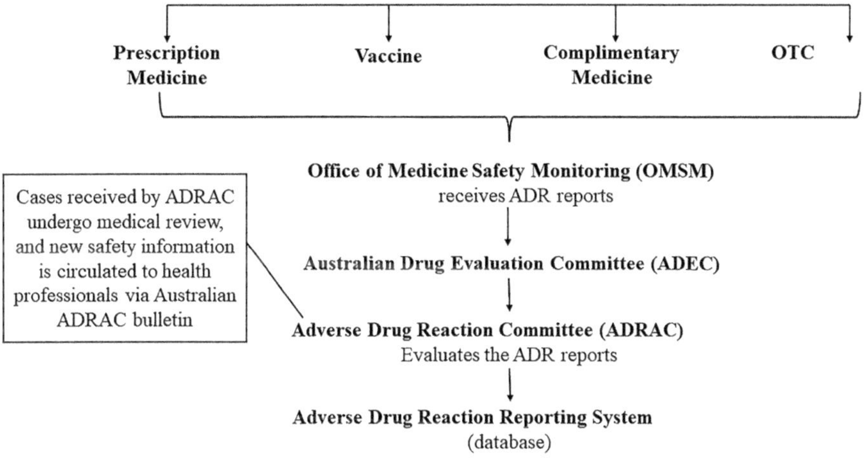

Fig. 10.1 Pharmacovigilance system in Australia

The Department of Health received guidance from ADEC and, via it, ADRAC. An examination of impromptu reports has produced several warnings on new safety issues and verification of issues found in other Australia, likewise experiencing these nations (McEwen and Therapeutic Goods Administration 2007). The Therapeutic Goods Administration (TGA), administratively a division of the Department of Health and Ageing, was responsible for overseeing all national operations relating to drugs and medical devices in August 1989. The only sources of funding for the TGA are assessments, registration fees, and license fees collected from the industry. The TGA established a new organizational structure on July 1, 2010. The establishment of distinct pre-marketing and post-marketing groups was a crucial aspect pertinent to pharmacovigilance. The Market Authorisation Group is in charge of the pre-marketing assessment of pharmaceuticals and medical devices. The Advisory Committee on Prescription Medicines, which replaced ADEC, provides advice to this group with regard to prescription medications. The Monitoring and Compliance Group's Office of Product Review (OPR) is responsible for conducting pharmacovigilance and monitoring device issue reporting. The Advisory Committee on the Safety of Medicines (ACSOM) and the Advisory Committee on the Safety of Vaccines (ACSOV) provide advice to this agency about medications and vaccines. It is significant to note that the Medicines Safety Advisory Committee is no longer reporting through the assessment committee. ACSOM and ACSOV are now formed as statutory expert committees directly reporting to the TGA. Every two months, the Australian Prescriber magazine publishes the Medicines Safety Update, which is produced by OPR.

10.3.1.1 The Reporting System in Australia

Even a mere suspicion that a medicine could have a negative impact might prompt a report. The task of investigating and establishing causation falls to the TGA. The TGA can continue to develop a drug's "safety profile" by receiving reports of adverse occurrences that are already well-known or frequent. Physicians and others in the community are free to report. Contrarily, sponsors of registered and listed pharmaceuticals are legally required to notify the TGA of any suspected adverse events they learn about or receive from any source, even if the sponsor does not accept responsibility for the event's occurrence.

The Therapeutic Goods Administration posts articles about medication safety online, including reviews, recommendations, and findings from scientific reviews. 57,771 reports of medication and vaccine adverse events were accepted by TGA during the 2020–2021 fiscal year. The number of reports is up 59% from the previous year. HCPs provided 4744 (20%) in 2019–2020 and 7960 (13%) in 2020–2021, whereas the pharmaceutical sector contributed 14,418 (24%) in 2019–2020 and 14,128 (61%) in 2020–2021. Among all HCPs, chemists excelled at reporting adverse events (AEs) (Therapeutic Goods Administration 2020).

The TGA is primarily interested in adverse events involving recently listed or registered medications, drug or vaccine interactions, incidents resulting in death or hospitalization, and occurrences not described in the literature or product information. In order to distinguish between newly registered medications and those that have already been registered but are being used in novel ways that call for increased attention, Australia adopted the Black Triangle method from Europe (TGA Black Triangle n.d.; Linger and Martin 2018).

10.3.1.2 Post-Marketing Activities in Australia

With the provisional approval procedure used in Canada, a procedure similar to that suggested in Australia, post-marketing safety issues have been highlighted. Compared to pharmaceuticals authorized through a regular review procedure, there is a statistically substantial probability that those approved using this technique may get a severe safety warning or be taken off the market (Pharmacovigilance and expedited drug approvals—PMC (nih.gov) n.d.).

10.3.1.3 Latest Regulatory Trends in Australia

The Therapeutic Goods Administration's (TGA) Office of Medicines Safety Monitoring (OMSM), also known as the Adverse Drug Reaction Advisory Committee, is responsible for overseeing drug safety in Australia. Applying a framework that provides advantages in the use of therapeutic items while minimizing the possible hazards helps regulatory agencies fulfill their duty. They work with other national monitoring centers, have their own pharmacovigilance regulations, and use the WHO's International Drug Monitoring Program's database.

The Australian Adverse Drug Reactions Reporting System receives all data submitted to the TGA. Additionally, information is provided to VigiBase, a global database of adverse drug events maintained by the World Health Organization. These databases are studied to look for signs that might point to previously undiscovered safety issues, a rise in the frequency or severity of adverse events, or patient populations who are more vulnerable to them.

Through the online Database of Adverse Event Notifications, which was launched in October 2012, the public may access adverse event data that has been reported to the TGA since 1971. The fact that this database does not include all known adverse events and cannot be used to calculate adverse event rates should be noted. Clinicians can also learn about new safety issues and adverse occurrences through the Medicines Safety Update publication or TGA notifications. International data contributed to VigiBase may be accessed online through VigiAccess (vigiaccess.org) (Therapeutic Goods Administration 2010).

The early detection of negative occurrences has been made possible through Australian reporting. A few examples are acute kidney damage from the "triple whammy" (combination of ACE inhibitor, non-steroidal anti-inflammatory, and diuretic) and liver failure risk from lumiracoxib, black cohosh, and flucloxacillin. Recent reports have revealed the possibility of QT prolongation when using denosumab. The table lists additional important safety problems that the TGA has identified since 2010 (Therapeutic Goods Administration 2016; Thomas 2000).

10.3.1.4 Limitations

The reporting of adverse events in Australia has severe constraints. The inability to estimate the sample size, like other observational research techniques, makes estimating the rate of occurrences difficult. The general public's and physicians' reporting is also a major source of data for the numerator. Negative incidents are significantly underreported as a result of voluntary reporting. Reports in the UK are thought to reflect fewer than 10% of actual incidents (Hazell and Shakir 2006). Comorbidity information is not available. The capacity to identify contributing and confounding elements to an adverse occurrence is constrained by these criteria.

10.3.2 Pharmacovigilance System in Canada

The Canada Vigilance Program is the name of Health Canada's post-marketing surveillance system. To collect the probable ADRs of the marketed products, this initiative was established in 1965. The ADRs in the database can be searched online. There is an optional ADR reporting mechanism for HCPs and consumers, similar to those in many other nations. Market authorization holders (MAHs) are required by the Canadian Food and Drugs Act and regulations to report severe ADRs involving their marketed goods. Serious ADRs linked to Canadian items sold abroad are also included in the MAHs. The Canada Vigilance web database, which may be accessed for information, houses the gathered ADRs (Anon n.d.-a).

There are seven regional vigilance centers in Canada, which HCPs and consumers may use to communicate and which also provide data to the Canada Vigilance National Office (centralized database) as mentioned in Fig. 10.2. The quantity of ADRs has grown yearly since the start of the Canada Vigilance program. Increased marketing of goods, hospital reporting requirements, industry patient safety programs, active surveillance programs, etc. are all significant causes (Health Canada Canada Vigilance Program n.d.). In 2019, Health Canada received 96,559 domestic reports, up 4 times over the previous 10 years, from 22,211 in 2010 to 96,559 in

2019. In 1 year, 93.6% of reports came from required reporters, compared to 90% over the previous 10 years (Anon 2019).

Canada has made it clear that it intends to change the rules governing medical devices and food and drugs in 2022. A risk management strategy will be necessary for applicants for the authorization of drugs and medical devices, among other planned changes and the information of ADRs are transferred in proper manner as shown in Fig. 10.2 (Anon n.d.-b).

- In Canada, a preferred method of reporting ADRs is electronically.
- Electronic Reporting—Trading Partner Management Office.
- For Non-Electronic Reporting of ADRs, sent to Canada Vigilance Program, Health Canada, 250 Lanark Avenue Address Locator 2004D Ottawa, Ontario K1A 0 K9.

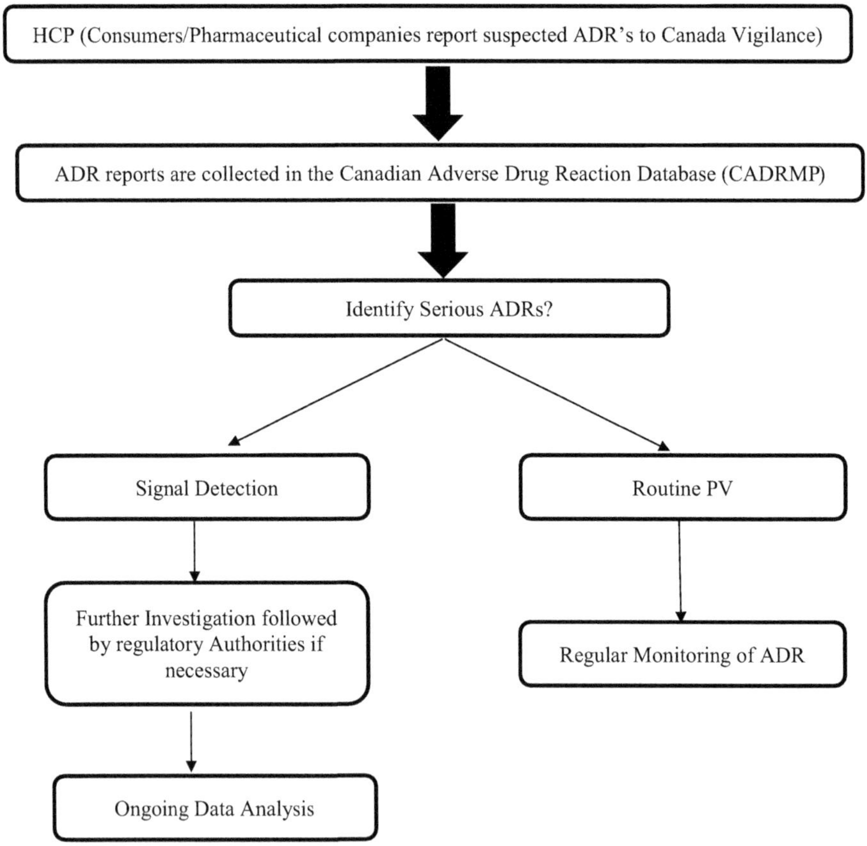

Fig. 10.2 Pharmacovigilance system in Canada

10.3.3 Pharmacovigilance System in Japan

Japan's pharmacovigilance system is considered the most complicated post-approval safety procedure due to its many functions, such as collecting suspected adverse drug reactions and reporting them to the regulatory body. The drug company has long had the legal duty to conduct a "drug use investigation" (DUI), in which physicians have to register thousands of patients with a newly launched product to monitor and report suspected ADRs (Tanaka et al. 2002).

Japan began conducting pharmacovigilance operations from medical facilities in 1967. It joined the WHO's international drug monitoring program in 1972. A post-marketing mechanism was set up in Japan in 1979 to evaluate the efficacy and safety of drugs that had already been sold. By establishing three systems—the ADR collecting and reporting system, the re-examination system, and the re-evaluation system—Japan is regarded as the first nation in the world to require pharmaceutical companies to carry out pharmacovigilance activities. Early-phase post-marketing vigilance (EPPV) was instituted as an additional criterion in 2001. Japan delivered international recommendations on pharmacovigilance planning (PVP) at the International Conference on Harmonisation of Technical Requirements for Registration of Pharmaceuticals for Human Use (ICH). However, DUIs take more time to reinvestigate according to the scientific standards of PVP guidelines. In April 2012, Japan also combined the risk management action plan (risk MAP) with risk management plan (RMP) guidance. It also endorsed the Pharmaceutical Affairs Law (PAL) revisions to strengthen pharmacovigilance and revolutionize other regulatory events for drugs and medical devices. Pharmacovigilance system of Japan is shown in Fig. 10.3 (Anon n.d.-c).

10.3.3.1 The Reporting System in Japan

Japan followed the spontaneous reporting system operation from 1967, in which its performance was poor till the 1990s. The total amount of reports from medical professionals was fewer than 2000 each year, mostly because the reports were sent by just a few "designated" medical facilities and pharmacies prior. During the year 1997, the Ministry of Health and Welfare (MHW) and The Ministry of Health, Labour and Welfare (MHLW) revised the policy in 2000 and obtained around 5000 reports yearly from every physician and chemist. In the 2002 PAL Amendment, pharmacists, nurses, and other health professionals were required by law to report any ADRs when deemed essential to stop the onset or the increase in the danger to the public's health and hygiene. Until 1979, when a ministerial ordinance required drug firms to transmit ADR reports to the MHW, the number of domestic reports produced by pharma companies was similarly quite low (less than 500 annually). In 1994, the number of reports received from pharmaceutical firms approached 10,000 annually. Since 2007, the number has steadily hovered around 30,000 annually (PMDA 2011a).

Following the 2002 PAL modification, the definition and requirements for post-approval ADR reporting hastened by pharmaceutical firms were altered in 2005 as

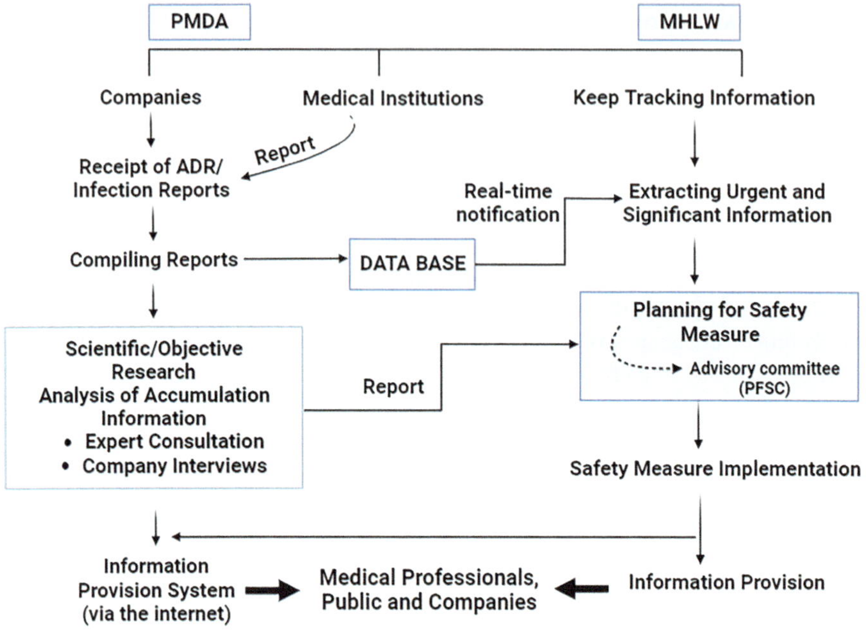

Fig. 10.3 Pharmacovigilance system in Japan

greater focus was placed on documenting the significant responses in accordance with the ICH-E2D guideline's introduction in April 2005. Non-serious reactions are no longer included among those that call for rapid reporting under the new standards. In contrast, the response must be disclosed within 15 calendar days if the marketing authorization holder (MAH) is aware that a domestic patient has had an anticipated and fatal ADR. Additionally, after the EPPV and for the first 2 years following the approval of a novel chemical entity, all anticipated significant reactions must be reported within 15 calendar days. The 2005 revision mandated that all expected and unexpected serious cases of infection due to the use of any drug be reported within 15 calendar days, as well as non-serious unexpected domestic cases of infection. This was done in accordance with the enhancement of the safety measures for biological products in the 2002 PAL amendment, which is discussed in the next section (PMDA 2011a).

A pilot project was launched in January 2011 to see if spontaneous reports sent directly from patients over the Internet may be successful in Japan (PMDA, 2011b). A total of 716 suspected ADRs were reported by 160 patients during the course of the pilot study's first 6 months. Beginning in early 2012, the patient report system was formally included in Japanese regulatory actions (PMDA 2011b).

10.3.3.2 Post-Marketing Activities in Japan

Japan began "re-examining "commercially available medications in 1971 and has continued to do so ever since. The re-examination procedure involves reevaluating the efficacy of every new medicine after a certain amount of time (8 years for common goods, 4–10 years for some other treatments) has passed after the first approval. It is customarily necessary to provide the results of the DUI at the re-examination. The producer is no longer permitted to market the product until the re-examination outcomes show no significant issues with the product. Conversely, when medical and pharmaceutical sciences improve, it may be necessary to reevaluate the quality, efficacy, and safety of an already authorized medicine. Since April 1997, the initial post-marketing study plan was needed to be submitted as part of the new product approval process.

In April 1997, the ICH-E2C guideline's periodic safety update report (PSUR) was introduced to Japan, where the manufacturer was required to submit a PSUR to the MHW along with a synopsis of the current post-marketing investigations and other documentation. The EPPV, which is exclusive to Japan, was implemented as an extra regulation in 2001. For the first 6 months after product introduction, the MAHs must urge medical practitioners to report ADRs in accordance with this rule.

New rules to guarantee the security of biological products were included in the PAL amendment of 2002. It was discovered in the 1990s that many hemophiliacs with HIV acquired the virus via plasma products made in the 1980s.

In a similar vein, a large number of hepatitis C patients got the virus via blood and plasma preparations created circa 1980. For specific blood and plasma preparations needing particular rules, such as long-term record keeping pertaining to production, distribution, and administration, "specified biological products" were defined in the 2002 PAL amendment.

The Law of the Incorporated Administrative Agency-Pharmaceutical and Medical Devices Agency, passed in December 2002, allowed for the establishment of the Pharmaceutical and Medical Device Agency (PMDA) in April 2004. Subsequently, the PMDA's current responsibility for ensuring drug safety includes gathering, evaluating, and disseminating drug safety information received through spontaneous reports and medical databases (Anon n.d.-c).

10.3.3.3 Latest Regulatory Trends in Pharmacovigilance in Japan

Although there have been occasional exceptions, such as gathering spontaneous reports directly from medical professionals, the regulatory body's contribution to drug safety has traditionally been mostly done through the regulation of drug firms. However, during the past several years, certain pharmacovigilance and risk management operations have been carried out directly by the regulatory agency. For instance, as was already indicated, the PMDA began managing the web-based patient reporting system in early 2012 after a one-year pilot research period in 2011 (PMDA 2007). The creation of the "Japan Drug Information Institute in Pregnancy" (www.ncchd.go.jp/kusuri/index.html), which is managed by the National Center for Child Health and Development (NCCHD) in partnership with the "Motherisk program" at the hospital for sick children in Toronto, Canada, is among the other activities (MHLW 2006). 75 manuals in 19 system organ classes are presently accessible to the general public following the 4-year project of compiling the "ADR manuals" from 2005 to deliver the information connected to the major ADRs to health professionals and patients (Endo et al. 2010). The regulatory

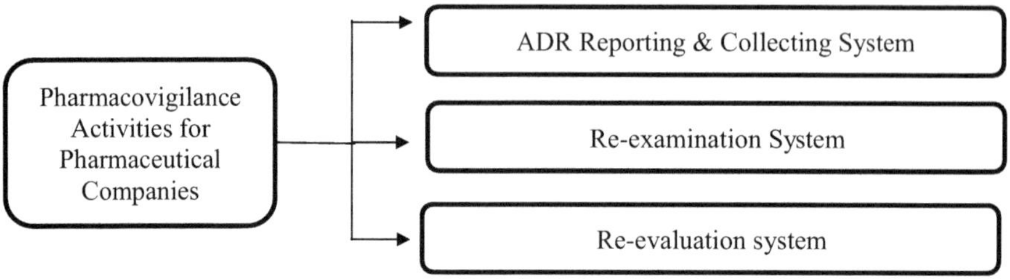

Fig. 10.4 Pharmacovigilance activities for pharmaceutical companies in Japan

body oversaw the development of medication guides for patients regarding the drugs that require special care.

The "Medical Information for Risk Assessment Initiative" project, often known as MIHARI (meaning monitoring or watching in Japanese) project, is another recent development inside the PMDA (Al-Zubiedi et al. 2023). The project develops pharmacoepidemiologic tools to assess the risk of ADRs and ways to quantify regulatory measures' effects using various electronic health information forms. Pharmacovigilance activities for pharmaceutical companies in Japan are shown in Fig. 10.4.

10.4 Setting up National Pharmacovigilance Center in Non-EU Countries

Non-European Union countries usually establish pharmacovigilance centers or units to oversee drug safety monitoring within their jurisdictions. These centers receive, evaluate, and handle reports of drug reactions (ADRs) from healthcare professionals, patients, and other stakeholders (Suwankesawong et al. 2023). National pharmacovigilance centers often work closely with authorities and other relevant healthcare organizations to ensure drug safety monitoring.

10.4.1 Roles of National Pharmacovigilance Centers

Receipt and Evaluation of ADR Reports: These centers serve as the primary recipients of ADR reports and play a crucial role in assessing their severity, causality, and implications for patient safety.

Data Management and Analysis: Pharmacovigilance data, such as ADR reports, medication mistakes, and other safety-related data, are collected and managed by national pharmacovigilance centers. They examine this information to find potential safety indicators and add to our understanding of drug safety profiles.

Risk Assessment and Management: These facilities evaluate the dangers linked to certain pharmaceuticals and help create and implement risk management plans. They are essential in ensuring that drugs are used safely in their nations.

Education and Communication: National pharmacovigilance centers participate in communication efforts to encourage reporting adverse drug reactions (ADRs) and increase public knowledge of drug safety. To ensure patient safety and improve learning, they might work with patients, healthcare professionals, and the general public (Jeetu and Anusha 2010).

10.4.2 Integrating with Healthcare Systems

Non-EU nations understand how crucial it is to incorporate pharmacovigilance into their larger healthcare systems. To encourage the reporting of ADRs and maintain patient safety, national pharmacovigilance centers work with healthcare providers, hospitals, and other healthcare organizations. Pharmacovigilance activities are incorporated into healthcare protocols, medical instruction, and patient care pathways as part of integration efforts. This improves the overall drug safety culture throughout the healthcare system.

10.4.3 Collaboration with International Organizations and Networks

National pharmacovigilance organizations from non-EU countries actively collaborate with international networks and organizations to share knowledge and expand capabilities. These relationships make sharing information about safety, skills, and expertise more superficial.

Non-EU nations can access support, direction, and training opportunities from international organizations like the World Health Organization (WHO), the Uppsala Monitoring Centre (UMC), and regional pharmacovigilance networks. They are essential in increasing the global harmonization of pharmacovigilance procedures ([CIOMS] C for IO of MS 2005; Prakash et al. 2021).

Non-EU nations can create vital national pharmacovigilance centers, incorporate pharmacovigilance into healthcare systems, and work with international organizations to improve drug safety monitoring capacities. As a result, possible safety issues are promptly identified, risks are effectively managed, and patient outcomes are enhanced.

10.5 Reporting of ICSRs in Non-EU Countries

Adverse drug reaction (ADR) reporting is a cornerstone of pharmacovigilance systems in non-EU countries. It involves systematically gathering, analyzing, and assessing information related to the safety of medicinal products (Anon 2012; Strandell and Wahlin 2011). Here, we will examine the processes and mechanisms of ADR reporting in non-EU countries, the challenges and barriers they encounter, and the strategies to promote ADR reporting and improve data collection.

10.5.1 Processes and Mechanisms for ADR Reporting

Non-EU countries have established various ADR reporting methods, including voluntary and mandatory systems. These systems rely on active participation from healthcare professionals, patients, consumers, and other stakeholders to report suspected adverse events related to medication use (Khan et al. 2022). Reporting mechanisms range from traditional paper-based forms to electronic platforms and online reporting portals. Non-EU countries may employ dedicated reporting forms or mobile applications or integrate ADR reporting within existing healthcare information systems.

10.5.2 Obstacles and Challenges in ADR Reporting

Underreporting, or failing to disclose or recognize many ADRs, is a significant problem in ADR reporting. This could result from needing more knowledge, time restraints, perceived difficulty reporting, or worries about legal repercussions (Valinciute-Jankauskiene and Loreta 2021).

Healthcare personnel, patients, and consumers frequently need more awareness and education about ADR reporting mechanisms and their importance. As a result, drug safety profiles still need to be completed (Adenuga et al. 2020).

Reporting systems need to be more cohesive and integrated into the healthcare system in some non-EU nations. This leads to consistent data collection, better coordination, and data analysis and interpretation difficulties.

10.5.3 Strategies for Promoting ADR Reporting and Enhancing Data Collection

Educational and awareness campaigns can be developed to raise awareness among healthcare professionals, patients, and consumers about the importance of ADR reporting. These campaigns can emphasize the role of reporting in enhancing patient safety and overall healthcare quality.

Streamlining the ADR reporting process by implementing user-friendly reporting forms, online portals, or mobile applications can overcome barriers and encourage reporting. Simplifying the process, making it accessible and time-efficient can boost participation and engagement.

Comprehensive training programs for healthcare professionals on ADR recognition, reporting, and documentation can enhance their knowledge and skills. This enables accurate identification and reporting of ADRs, contributing to robust data collection and analysis.

Non-EU countries can foster collaboration between regulatory authorities, healthcare professionals, and other stakeholders involved in pharmacovigilance. Establishing feedback loops, promptly acknowledging reported ADRs, and communicating the outcomes of ADR investigations can motivate continued reporting (Gautier et al. 2003).

By implementing these strategies to address challenges and barriers, non-EU countries can promote ADR reporting, enhance data collection, and strengthen the overall pharmacovigilance system. Engaging healthcare professionals, patients, and consumers in the reporting process, along with education and streamlined reporting mechanisms, can bolster the safety monitoring of medicinal products (Holm et al. 2013)."

In the upcoming section, we will explore the methods and tools utilized for signal detection and risk assessment in non-EU countries, including the role of data mining, signal validation, and epidemiological studies. Stay tuned to delve into this critical aspect of pharmacovigilance beyond the EU borders.

10.6 Risk Assessment and Signal Detection

In non-EU countries, signal detection and risk assessment are crucial elements of pharmacovigilance systems. These techniques aim to identify and evaluate potential pharmaceutical safety issues (Almenoff et al. 2005; Holm et al. 2013). The methods for risk assessment and management, data mining, signal validation, and epidemiological studies in non-EU countries, as well as the methods and tools for signal detection, are shown below.

10.6.1 Methods and Tools for Signal Detection (Abiri and Johnson 2019; Kumar et al. 2018)

Outside the European Union, countries utilize techniques and resources to identify signals and signs indicating safety concerns or emerging risks linked to medications. Some of these methods are mentioned in Table 10.3.

Table 10.3 Procedures for the detection of signals

1	Reporting	Examining data from systems that collect reports of suspected adverse events submitted by healthcare professionals, patients, and consumers
2	Data mining	Using databases and advanced statistical techniques to identify patterns, trends, and potential associations between drugs and adverse events
3	Signal detection in clinical trials	Monitoring safety data generated during clinical trials to identify signals that may not have been previously recognized
4	Signal detection in real-world data	Data from real-world settings, including electronic health records, insurance claims databases, and disease registries, is analyzed to identify potential safety signals
5	Literature review	Evaluation of scientific literature, case reports, and published studies to identify safety signals related to specific medications

10.6.2 Approaches to Risk Assessment and Management (Hauben et al. 2005)

Non-EU countries adopt various approaches to assess and manage risks associated with medicinal products. These approaches include:

Benefit–Risk Evaluation: An assessment of the balance between the therapeutic benefits of a medication and its potential risks. This evaluation involves considering the severity of the disease, available treatment alternatives, and the overall risk profile of the drug.

Regulatory Measures: Implement regulatory actions such as labeling changes, contraindications, warnings, restrictions, or withdrawals of medications to mitigate identified risks.

Risk Minimization Strategies: Develop and implement strategies to minimize the occurrence or impact of identified risks, such as additional warnings, educational materials, or specific monitoring requirements.

Post-Marketing Surveillance Studies: Conducting additional studies or trials to gather more information on the safety profile of a medication, especially for newly approved drugs or in specific patient populations.

10.6.3 Utilization of Data Mining, Signal Validation, and Epidemiological Studies

Non-EU countries leverage data mining techniques, signal validation processes, and epidemiological studies to strengthen signal detection and risk assessment. These approaches involve (Olsson and Harrison-Woolrych 2018; Trifirò et al. 2018).

Data Mining: Analysis of large volumes of data using statistical methods, machine learning, and data visualization tools to identify significant safety signals and patterns.

Signal Validation: Conducting in-depth evaluations of identified signals to determine their clinical relevance, potential causality, and impact on patient safety.

Epidemiological Studies: Using epidemiological research methods to investigate the relationship between drug exposure and adverse events in larger populations provides valuable insights into safety concerns.

By employing these methods and tools, non-EU countries can enhance their ability to detect signals, assess risks, and make informed decisions regarding the safety of medicinal products. Integrating data mining, signal validation, and epidemiological studies into pharmacovigilance practices strengthens the evidence base for risk assessment and facilitates effective risk management strategies.

10.7 Communication and Information Exchange

Effective communication and information exchange are vital in pharmacovigilance systems in non-EU countries. These processes ensure the dissemination of drug safety information to healthcare professionals, patients, and the public (Jeetu and Anusha 2010; Monteagudo 1996). Here's an exploration of the dissemination strategies, practical communication approaches, and collaboration with international databases and networks for global information exchange in non-EU pharmacovigilance systems.

10.7.1 Dissemination of Drug Safety Information

Non-EU countries employ various channels and platforms to disseminate drug safety information to key stakeholders:

Healthcare Professionals: Pharmacovigilance centers collaborate with healthcare professional organizations, medical associations, and academic institutions to provide drug safety updates, alerts, and educational materials. This can include organizing training programs, webinars, and conferences to enhance healthcare professionals' awareness and knowledge of drug safety.

Patients and Consumers: Non-EU countries develop patient-oriented resources, including brochures, leaflets, and websites, to provide information on medication safety, potential adverse effects, and reporting mechanisms. Empowering patients and consumers with accurate and accessible information encourages their active participation in pharmacovigilance efforts.

Public Awareness Campaigns: Non-EU countries may launch public awareness campaigns through various media channels, including television, radio, social media, and print. These campaigns aim to raise awareness about the importance of reporting adverse drug reactions and promote the safe and rational use of medications.

10.7.2 Strategies for Effective Communication

National Drug Bulletins: Non-EU countries often publish national drug bulletins that update drug safety, regulatory changes, and emerging safety concerns. These bulletins are essential references for healthcare professionals, offering evidence-based information to support informed decision-making.

Dedicated Websites and Portals: Non-EU pharmacovigilance systems maintain dedicated websites and portals to disseminate drug safety information, promote

ADR reporting, and provide resources for healthcare professionals and the public. These platforms serve as centralized hubs for accessing up-to-date information and reporting tools.

Helpline Services: Some non-EU countries establish helpline services or hotlines to address inquiries related to medication safety, adverse events, and reporting procedures. These services directly assist healthcare professionals, patients, and consumers, promoting timely and accurate communication.

10.7.3 Collaboration with International Databases and Networks

Non-EU pharmacovigilance systems actively collaborate with international databases and networks to enhance global information exchange and harmonization efforts (Andersen et al. 2013; Holm et al. 2013; Olsson et al. 2010):

World Health Organization (WHO): Non-EU countries collaborate with the WHO to align their pharmacovigilance practices with global standards. The WHO provides guidance, technical support, and capacity building initiatives to strengthen pharmacovigilance systems worldwide.

International Databases: Non-EU countries contribute data to international pharmacovigilance databases such as the WHO Global Individual Case Safety Report Database (VigiBase) and the Uppsala Monitoring Centre's (UMC) VigiFlow. These databases facilitate sharing safety information globally and support signal detection and analysis.

Regional Pharmacovigilance Networks: Non-EU countries actively participate in regional networks, fostering collaboration, information sharing, and capacity building. These networks facilitate regional cooperation, harmonization of practices, and the exchange of expertise and resources.

Through effective communication strategies and collaboration with international databases and networks, non-EU countries can ensure the timely dissemination of drug safety information, enhance public awareness, and promote a culture of pharmacovigilance. The exchange of information on a global scale facilitates the identification and management of safety concerns, leading to improved patient safety and healthcare outcomes.

The following section will delve into the challenges and future perspectives of pharmacovigilance systems in non-EU countries, addressing the evolving landscape, emerging technologies, and the importance of international cooperation. Stay tuned for an in-depth analysis of these critical aspects beyond the EU borders.

10.8 Training and Capacity Building

Initiatives to build capacity and train people are essential for improving pharmacovigilance skills in non-EU nations. Through these initiatives, healthcare practitioners, regulators, and pharmacovigilance employees should have better knowledge, abilities, and competencies (Kalaiselvan et al. 2022; Maiga et al. 2010).

Here is a look at the numerous initiatives made, training programs provided, and the significance of ongoing education and awareness campaigns in pharmacovigilance systems outside the EU:

10.8.1 Enhancing Pharmacovigilance Capabilities

Non-EU nations invest in capacity building to improve their capacities because they understand the value of constructing robust pharmacovigilance systems.

National pharmacovigilance centers collaborate with regulatory agencies, healthcare organizations, and international organizations to develop strategic plans, guidelines, and standard operating procedures to streamline pharmacovigilance activities. This involves strengthening the infrastructure, resources, and expertise required for efficient drug safety monitoring and surveillance.

10.8.2 Healthcare Professionals, Regulators, and Pharmacovigilance Staff Can all Benefit from Training Programs

Healthcare practitioners, regulators, and pharmacovigilance employees can improve their knowledge and abilities in pharmacovigilance practices by enrolling in extensive training programs offered by non-EU nations. These courses cover various subjects, such as ADR recognition, reporting, causality evaluation, signal detection, risk evaluation, and risk management techniques. Workshops, seminars, online courses, and interactive sessions led by knowledgeable pharmacovigilance specialists can all be used to conduct training programs. They want to ensure that pharmacovigilance procedures are applied uniformly and consistently in all healthcare settings.

10.8.3 The Significance of Ongoing Awareness and Education Campaigns

It is critical to keep pharmacovigilance employees, regulators, and medical experts current on the latest advancements, legal changes, and safety concerns. The dissemination of current information and best practices is aided via newsletters, seminars, webinars, and ongoing professional development programs.

Campaigns to raise awareness are necessary to support a pharmacovigilance culture and increase involvement in ADR reporting. These initiatives spread knowledge about the significance of reporting suspected adverse events and the function of pharmacovigilance in protecting patient safety among healthcare professionals, patients, and the general public.

Non-EU nations can strengthen their pharmacovigilance skills, increase patient safety, and support international efforts to ensure the safety of drugs by investing in capacity building and training. Campaigns for constant education and awareness encourage a culture of alertness.

10.9 Ideal Techniques

Optimal Methods Promoting a Culture of Pharmacovigilance entails encouraging a mindset that values attentiveness and prioritizes safety through education and awareness programs involving patients, healthcare workers, and the general public.

Establishing frameworks, standards, and SOPs to ensure uniform pharmacovigilance practices and effective risk management will increase regulatory oversight.

Strengthening Collaborative Partnerships: Collaborating with regional pharmacovigilance networks, international organizations, and healthcare facilities to share knowledge, expertise, and resources. Holding regular training sessions for healthcare professionals, regulators, and pharmacovigilance staff to enhance their skills, stay updated on expertise, and promote practices.

Imposing Advanced Technologies: Using data mining techniques, detecting tools, and information systems to streamline data collection activities while facilitating analysis and signal validation.

Active Involvement of Patients and Consumers: Encouraging participation from patients and consumers in reporting suspected events and promoting their role in improving medication safety.

Other regions can learn from pharmacovigilance systems implemented in EU countries to enhance their pharmacovigilance efforts further. By adopting lessons learned from these experiences and globally shared practices by various stakeholders within the field of pharmacovigilance, we can collectively advance patient safety standards leading to improved healthcare outcomes.

10.10 Key Challenges

Creating pharmacovigilance systems in countries outside of the European Union poses challenges. Recognizing and tackling these obstacles is vital for progress and the future development of pharmacovigilance endeavors (Khan et al. 2023; Liu et al. 2021). Below, we delve into the difficulties encountered by EU countries and explore potential avenues to strengthen their pharmacovigilance systems.

(a) **Limited Resources:** Non-European Union (EU) nations frequently encounter challenges related to resource limitations, such as restricted resources, inadequate infrastructure, and a scarcity of personnel. These limitations can impact the implementation and effectiveness of pharmacovigilance activities.
(b) **Underreporting of Adverse Events:** Underreporting adverse drug reactions (ADRs) remains a significant challenge in non-EU countries. Barriers such as

lack of awareness, fear of consequences, and inadequate reporting systems contribute to low ADR reporting rates.

(c) **Diverse Healthcare Systems:** Non-EU countries encompass diverse healthcare systems, which can challenge standardizing pharmacovigilance practices and harmonizing data collection and analysis.

(d) **Regulatory Harmonization:** Achieving regulatory harmonization among non-EU countries can be complex due to variations in regulatory frameworks, requirements, and capacities. Harmonization efforts are essential to ensure consistent pharmacovigilance practices and facilitate global information exchange.

10.10.1 Future Perspectives and Areas of Improvement

(a) **Utilization of Digital Technologies:** Non-EU countries can illuminate digital technologies, such as electronic health records, mobile applications, and data analytics, to enhance pharmacovigilance activities. These technologies enable efficient data collection, signal detection, and real-time medication safety monitoring.

(b) **Real-World Evidence:** Non-EU pharmacovigilance systems can utilize real-world evidence from data sources like electronic health records, insurance claims databases, and social media platforms. This data can provide valuable insights into drug safety profiles, patient outcomes, and safety concerns.

(c) **Strengthening Pharmacovigilance Education:** Continued education and training programs should be strengthened for healthcare professionals, regulators, and staff. This includes raising awareness about the importance of ADR reporting, promoting pharmacovigilance as a career path, and incorporating pharmacovigilance modules into healthcare curricula.

(d) **International Cooperation:** Non-EU nations should encourage more cross-border cooperation and sharing of knowledge, expertise, and best practices. Collaboration can improve regulatory harmonization, strengthen international drug safety initiatives, and improve pharmacovigilance capabilities.

(e) **Public–private partnerships:** By bringing together public health agencies, regulatory bodies, pharmaceutical companies, and academic institutions, these partnerships can foster innovation, resource sharing, and knowledge exchange in pharmacovigilance. Public–private partnerships can advance data collection, analysis, and risk management methods.

By addressing these problems and looking toward the future, pharmacovigilance systems in non-EU nations will be enhanced. By increasing resources, expanding ADR reporting methods, developing regulatory harmonization, implementing digital technologies, and encouraging international collaboration, non-EU countries may strengthen their pharmacovigilance capabilities and ensure their populations' safe and effective use of pharmaceuticals.

10.11 Importance of Pharmacovigilance in Non-EU Countries

The significance of pharmacovigilance in non-EU countries includes the following reasons:

Patient Safety: A robust pharmacovigilance system plays a crucial role in ensuring the safety of patients by detecting and managing adverse reactions to drugs, ultimately minimizing potential harm.

Public Health: Effective pharmacovigilance contributes to health by monitoring and addressing safety concerns related to medications, promoting the use of medicines, and preventing public health crises caused by medication-related issues.

Regulatory Compliance: Pharmacovigilance enables non-EU countries to adhere to international regulatory standards, ensuring that their healthcare systems align with global requirements for drug safety.

Global Collaboration: Active participation in pharmacovigilance makes information exchange and practice harmonization possible. In the end, this is advantageous to patients and global healthcare systems.

10.12 Conclusion

This chapter has concluded by thoroughly reviewing the pharmacovigilance framework in non-EU nations. We looked at several things, such as the regulatory environment, the pharmacovigilance infrastructure, ADR reporting, signal identification, risk assessment, communication, capacity building, success stories, difficulties, and prospects for the future (Khan et al. 2023). Here, we summarize the key ideas raised and stress the significance of pharmacovigilance in non-EU nations for patient safety and general health.

References

[CIOMS] C for IO of MS (2005) Current Challenges in pharmacovigilance: pragmatic approaches. Report CIOMS Work Gr V, Geneva CI- OMS. (4):345. http://www.sciencedirect.com/science/article/B6VC6-45F5X02-. Accessed 12 Sept 2023

Abiri OT, Johnson WCN (2019) Pharmacovigilance systems in resource-limited settings: an evaluative case study of Sierra Leone. J Pharm Policy Pract 12:13

Adenuga BA, Kibuule D, Bamitale KDS, Rennie TW (2020) Effective integration of pharmacovigilance systems at public health facilities in resource-limited settings: a qualitative study. Res Social Adm Pharm 16(8):1111–1116

Almenoff J, Tonning JM, Gould AL, Szarfman A, Hauben M, Ouellet-Hellstrom R et al (2005) Perspectives on the use of data mining in pharmacovigilance. Drug Saf 28(11):981–1007

Al-Zubiedi SA, Younus M, Al-Khalidi S, Ekilo M, Alshammari TM (2023) Pharmacovigilance regulatory actions by national pharmacovigilance centers in Arab countries following COVID-19 pandemic. Expert Opin Drug Saf 22(2):165–174

Andersen M, Bergman U, Choi NK, Gerhard T, Huang C, Jalbert J et al (2013) The Asian Pharmacoepidemiology network [AsPEN]: promoting multi-national collaboration for pharmacoepidemiologic research in Asia. Pharmacoepidemiol Drug Saf 22(7):700–704

Anon (2012) Publicly accessible pharmacovigilance databases. Prescrire Int 21(126):99

Anon (2019) Health Canada Adverse Reactions, Medical Device Incidents and Health Product Recalls in Canada: 2019 Summary Report. https://www.canada.ca/en/health- canada/services/drugs-health-products/reports-publications/medeffect-canada/adverse-reactions-incidents-recalls-2019-summary.html. Accessed 24 Sept 2023

Anon (n.d.-a) Health Canada Search the Canada Vigilance Adverse Reaction Online Database. https://cvp-pcv.hc-sc.gc.ca/arq-rei/. Accessed 3 Sept 2023

Anon (n.d.-b) Health Canada Notice of Intent to Amend the Food and Drug Regulations and the Medical Devices Regulations to Support Regulatory Agility. https://gazette.gc.ca/rp-pr/p1/2021/2021-07-31/html/notice-avis-eng.html#na2. Accessed 2 Sept 2023

Anon (n.d.-c) https://doi.org/10.1002/9781118820186. Accessed 10 Sept 2023

Barry A, Olsson S, Minzi O, Bienvenu E, Makonnen E, Kamuhabwa A et al (2020) Comparative assessment of the National Pharmacovigilance Systems in East Africa: Ethiopia, Kenya, Rwanda and Tanzania. Drug Saf 43(4):339–350

Breckenridge A (2012) Development and delivery of clinical pharmacology in regulatory agencies. Br J Clin Pharmacol 73(6):866–869

Elshafie S, Zaghloul I, Roberti AM (2018) Pharmacovigilance in developing countries (part I): importance and challenges. Int J Clin Pharm 40(4):758–763

Ema. EudraVigilance—European Medicines Agency (2023). https://www.ema.europa.eu/en/human-regulatory/researchdevelopment/pharmacovigilance/eudravigilance#:~:text=EudraVigilance is the system for European Economic Area [EEA]. Accessed 20 Aug 2023

Endo A, Ishiguro C, Tada E et al (2010) Utilization of medical information databases in drug safety evaluation process in PMDA. Pharmacoepidemiol Drug Saf 19:S180

Gautier S, Bachelet H, Bordet R, Caron J (2003) The cost of adverse drug reactions. Expert Opin Pharmacother 4(3):319–326

Hauben M, Madigan D, Gerrits CM, Walsh L, Van Puijenbroek EP (2005) The role of data mining in pharmacovigilance. Expert Opin Drug Saf 4(5):929–948

Hazell L, Shakir SA (2006) Under-reporting of adverse drug reactions: a systematic review. Drug Saf 29:385–396. https://doi.org/10.2165/00002018-200629050-00003

Health Canada Canada Vigilance Program (n.d.). https://www.canada.ca/en/health-canada/services/drugs-health-products/medeffect-canada/canada-vigilanceprogram.html. Accessed 20 Sept 2023

Holm G, Snape JR, Murray-Smith R, Talbot J, Taylor D, Sörme P (2013) Implementing ecopharmacovigilance in practice: challenges and potential opportunities. Drug Saf 36(7):533–546

International Federation of Pharmaceutical, Manufacturers & Associations (2015) Pharmacovigilance Good Pharmacovigilance Principles and Considerations for Biotherapeutic Medicines. https://www.ifpma.org/wp- content/uploads/2016/02/IFPMA-PV-Brochure.pdf. Accessed 20 Sept 2023

Jeetu G, Anusha G (2010) Pharmacovigilance: a worldwide master key for drug safety monitoring. J Young Pharm 2(3):315–320

Kalaiselvan V, Shukla S, Arora S, Shrivastava TP, Raghuvanshi RS (2022) Public-private partnership [3Ps] in ensuring safe use of medicines: an Indian experience. Front Public Heal 10:930696

Khan MAA, Hamid S, Babar ZU (2023) Pharmacovigilance in high-income countries: current developments and a review of literature. Pharmacy [Basel, Switzerland] 11(1):10. https://doi.org/10.3390/pharmacy11010010

Khan MAA, Hamid S, Khan SA, Sarfraz M, Babar ZUD (2022) A qualitative study of stakeholders' views on pharmacovigilance system, policy, and coordination in Pakistan. Front Pharmacol 13:891954

Kumar A, Ahuja J, Shrivastava TP, Kumar V, Kalaiselvan V (2018) Statistical signal process in R language in the pharmacovigilance programme of India. Ther Innov Regul Sci 52(3):329–333

Linger M, Martin J (2018) Pharmacovigilance and expedited drug approvals. Aust Prescr 41:50–53

Liu Z, Roberts RA, Lal-Nag M, Chen X, Huang R, Tong W (2021) AI-based language models powering drug discovery and development. Drug Discov Today 26(11):2593–2607

Maiga AS, Diakite M, Diawara A, Sango HA, Coulibaly CO (2010) Pharmacovigilance and impact of intermittent preventive treatment with sulfadoxine-pyrimethamine in pregnant women in Sélingué, Mali. Mali Med 25(3):41–48

McEwen J (2007) In: Therapeutic Goods Administration (ed) A history of therapeutic goods regulation in Australia, Canberra, Australia. ISBN 9780980422900

MHLW (2006) Manuals for serious adverse drug reactions. http://www.mhlw.go.jp/topics/2006/11/%20tp1122-1.html. Accessed 28 Sept 2023

Monteagudo JL (1996) Data exchange in the European pharmacovigilance. Stud Health Technol Inform 28:69–77

Non-European Medicines Agency (2012) Guideline on good pharmacovigilance practices [GVP]—Module IX—Signal Management, EMA/827661/2011 [superseded version]. 2011[June 2012]:3,5,6. http://www.ema.europa.eu/docs/en_GB/document_library/Scientific_guideline/2012/06/WC500129138.pdf. Accessed 5 Sept 2023

Olsson S, Harrison-Woolrych M (2018) The role and strategy of ISoP in global pharmacovigilance. Int J Clin Pharm 40(4):740–743

Olsson S, Pal SN, Stergachis A, Couper M (2010) Pharmacovigilance activities in 55 low- and middle-income countries: a questionnaire-based analysis. Drug Saf 33(8):689–703

Pharmacovigilance and expedited drug approvals—PMC (nih.gov) (n.d.) Pharmacovigilance and expedited drug approval. Accessed 5 Sept 2023

PMDA (2007) Pharmaceuticals and medical devices safety information, No. 235. https://www.pmda.go.jp/english/%20service/pdf/precautions/PMDSI-235.pdf. Accessed 31 Aug 2023

PMDA (2011a) An achievement of PMDA enterprise [in Japanese]. www.pmda.go.jp/guide/hyougikai/23/h231220gijishidai/file/siryo2-1.pdf. Accessed 31 Sept 2023

PMDA (2011b) Pharmaceuticals and medical devices safety information, No. 276. Accessed 29 Aug 2023

Prakash J, Sachdeva R, Shrivastava TP, Jayachandran CV, Sahu A (2021) Adverse event reporting tools and regulatory measures in India through outcome of pharmacovigilance Programme of India. Indian J Pharmacol 53(2):143–152

Radecka A, Loughlin L, Foy M, de Ferraz Guimaraes MV, Sarinic VM, Di Giusti MD et al (2018) Enhancing pharmacovigilance capabilities in the non EU regulatory network: the SCOPE joint action. Drug Saf 41(12):1285–1302

Strandell J, Wahlin S (2011) Pharmacodynamic and pharmacokinetic drug interactions reported to VigiBase, the WHO global individual case safety report database. Eur J Clin Pharmacol 67(6):633–641

Suwankesawong W, Dhippayom T, Tan-Koi WC, Kongkaew C (2023) Pharmacovigilance activities in ASEAN countries. Pharmacoepidemiol Drug Saf 29(9):1061–1069

Tanaka K, Morita Y, Kawabe E, Kubota K (2002) Drug use investigation (DUI) and prescription-event monitoring in Japan (J-PEM). Pharmacoepidemiol Drug Saf 10:653–658

TGA Black Triangle (n.d.). https://www.tga.gov.au/black-triangle-scheme. Accessed 2 Sept 2023

Therapeutic Goods Administration (2010) Medicines safety update. Australian Government Department of Health, Canberra

Therapeutic Goods Administration (2016) Denosumab and QT prolongation. Medicines Safety Update 7:2. www.tga.gov.au/publication-issue/medicines-safety-update-volume-7-number-4-august-2016#a2

Therapeutic Goods Administration (2020) Annual performance statistics reports. Therapeutic Goods Administration, Woden

Thomas MC (2000) Diuretics, ACE inhibitors and NSAIDs--the triple whammy. Med J Aust 172:184–185

Trifirò G, Sultana J, Bate A (2018) From big data to smart data for pharmacovigilance: the role of healthcare databases and other emerging sources. Drug Saf 41(2):143–149

Valinciute-Jankauskiene A, Loreta K (2021) Qualitative study of general public views towards adverse drug Reactions in Lithuania. Healthcare (Basel, Switzerland) 9(3):303

WHO Pharmacovigilance (2023). https://www.who.int/teams/regulation-prequalification/regulation-and-safety/pharmacovigilance. Accessed 23 Aug 2023

Wiktorowicz M, Lexchin J, Moscou K (2012) Pharmacovigilance in Europe and North America: divergent approaches. Soc Sci Med 75(1):165–170

Xie YM, Tian F (2013) Interpretation of guidelines on good pharmacovigilance practices for European Union. China J Chinese Mater Med 38(18):2963–2968

Vaccine Safety Surveillance

11

Mohd Amir, Mukesh Nandave, and Anoop Kumar

Abstract

Vaccine safety surveillance is an essential component of public health initiatives to assure the safety and effectiveness of vaccination programs. This chapter looks into the fundamentals of vaccination safety monitoring, emphasizing its importance, methods, and results. The objective of vaccine safety monitoring is to detect and analyze adverse events that occur after immunization, which might range from minor local responses to uncommon, serious adverse events. Active and passive surveillance systems gather data from a variety of sources, including patients, healthcare professionals, and electronic health records. There are many well-established worldwide and national vaccine safety monitoring systems, such as the Vaccine Adverse Event Reporting System (VAERS) in the USA and the Vaccine Safety Datalink (VSD) initiative. Vaccine safety monitoring is critical in ensuring the integrity of vaccination programs across the globe, thanks to an innovative combination of modern technology and coordinated efforts among researchers, healthcare practitioners, and regulatory agencies.

Keywords

VAERS · AEFI · Causality assessment · Vaccine Safety Datalink

M. Amir (✉) · M. Nandave · A. Kumar
Department of Pharmacology, Delhi Pharmaceutical Sciences and Research University, New Delhi, India
e-mail: mukeshnandave@gmail.com; anoopdpsru@dpsru.edu.in

M. Nandave, A. Kumar (eds.), *Pharmacovigilance Essentials*,
https://doi.org/10.1007/978-981-99-8949-2_11

11.1 Introduction

Immunization stands as one of the most beneficial and affordable public health treatments that help in preventing disease by providing immunity (US Public Health Service 1999; Budhiraja and Akinapelli 2010). Extensive research has been conducted on vaccines, establishing them as among the safest medical interventions globally, with notable achievements such as the worldwide eradication of smallpox and the elimination of poliomyelitis in specific regions (Joshi et al. 2018). Vaccine pharmacovigilance is "the science and activities associated with the detection, assessment, understanding, prevention, and communication of AEFI or any other vaccination or immunization-related problems (Heininger et al. 2017)."

The World Health Organization (WHO) working group, along with the Council for International Organizations of Medical Sciences (CIOMS) has defined "adverse event following immunization (AEFI) as any untoward medical occurrence that occurs after immunization and does not necessarily have a causal relationship with vaccine use. The adverse event may be any unfavorable or unintended sign, an abnormal laboratory result, symptom or disease (Heininger et al. 2017)."

In order to guide future safety assessments, gather information for vaccine recommendations, and take regulatory action, CDC and FDA analyze VAERS data using a variety of procedures and statistical techniques. Because passive surveillance has inherent limitations, VAERS data must be examined carefully. The main function of VAERS is safety signal identification and hypothesis generation (Hause et al. 2022). Robust vaccine safety surveillance systems are crucial for monitoring and analyzing the possible adverse effects of immunization, allowing for early detection and reaction to any emergent safety issues (Verstraeten et al. 2003). To monitor, respond, and detect any possible adverse events associated with immunization, vaccine safety surveillance plays an important role (Hinrichsen et al. 2007).

11.2 Vaccine Safety Concerns

Vaccine safety concerns refer to apprehensions or doubts regarding the safety of vaccines. These concerns can arise from various factors such as perceived risks associated with vaccine ingredients, potential adverse effects, controversies surrounding specific vaccines, or uncertainty about long-term effects (Piltch-Loeb et al. 2021). Vaccine safety concerns are often divided into two categories: potential adverse effects and vaccine-related issues.

Potential adverse effects refer to the possibility of unintended side effects following vaccination. However, vaccine-related issues involve vaccine preventable diseases, vaccine side effects, vaccine effectiveness, and vaccine policy (Nuwarda et al. 2022).

11.3 Vaccine Pharmacovigilance Methods

11.3.1 Passive Surveillance

Passive surveillance is referred to as spontaneous reporting of adverse events delivered to a central database or health authority (U.S. Food and Drug Administration 2021).

11.3.1.1 Spontaneous Reports

Spontaneous reporting is basically an affordable, flexible, and highly active method of gathering information in which medical professionals submit case reports of ADR voluntarily, consumers to national pharmacovigilance centers, or pharmaceutical companies for evaluation in order to reduce the societal impact of ADR (Asiamah et al. 2022). It plays an important role in identification of safety signals once the drug is marketed. It also provides updates on unusual AEs that were previously not observed in premarketing studies or previous clinical trials. It provides important information on clinical features, risk groups, and risk factors of known serious ADRs. However, other related information regarding risk factors, clinical components, and risk groups of known serious ADRs is provided (Edwards 1999).

11.3.1.2 Case Series

A case series is a descriptive method of study that involves collection and analysis of extensive information on a group of people who have comparable qualities or experiences. In a case series, individuals with particular medical condition or exposure are identified and their demographic or clinical features, interventions received, as well as outcomes are recorded. They are primarily used for generating hypotheses, providing insights into treatment outcomes, identifying potential adverse effects of interventions, or describing rare conditions (Dekkers et al. 2012).

11.3.1.3 Stimulated Reporting

Stimulated reporting can be defined as the phenomena in which more awareness or attention to a certain occurrence or situation causes an increase in the reporting of related cases or events. It happens when consumers, healthcare practitioners, or the media become more aware or sensitive to a certain health condition, resulting in an increase in the frequency with which such instances are reported. It may have implications for disease monitoring due to the fact that it might cause an apparent rise in the prevalence of a certain condition even if the actual occurrence remains constant (Daley et al. 2017; Wong et al. 2017).

Stimulated reporting has significant consequences for the usefulness of post-marketing AE data, since alert-driven alterations in reporting may impair the accuracy of comparative research and associated analytical methodologies like disproportionality analysis (Hoffman et al. 2014).

11.3.1.4 Active Surveillance

A systematic and continuing practice of actively obtaining data and information about particular events or conditions is referred to as active surveillance. Unlike passive surveillance, which includes consumers or healthcare professionals passively reporting data, active surveillance involves drastic steps to actively seek and gather relevant information. This strategy includes routine follow-up, data gathering from specified sources, or the use of specialized surveillance devices to monitor and track incidents or events of interest (van den Bergh et al. 2012).

11.3.1.5 Cohort Event Monitoring

Cohort event monitoring (CEM) represents a form of prospective, observational research conducted during the initial stages of a novel drug's post-marketing period. It aims to systematically gather data on all adverse events that manifest within a specific group of individuals, referred to as the cohort, who are being exposed to a newly approved medication as part of routine clinical practice. Its purpose is to oversee the safety profile of a recently introduced chemical compound during the initial phase following its market approval, but it may also be used to monitor older drugs with new indications (World Health Organization 2008). Its objective is to evaluate medication safety and efficacy in real-world settings, specifically by tracking adverse events and other significant outcomes over time (Strom 2019).

11.3.1.6 Sentinel Surveillance

Sentinel surveillance is a public health surveillance system that involves the collection and analysis of data from a representative sample of healthcare facilities or individuals in a specific population. It focuses on monitoring a limited number of selected sites or participants to detect and track specific health events or conditions of interest, providing an early warning system for public health threats (Arita et al. 2004).

11.4 Databases

11.4.1 Vaccine Adverse Event Reporting System (VAERS)

The Vaccine Adverse Event Reporting System (VAERS) is a surveillance system jointly administered by the U.S. Food and Drug Administration (FDA) and the Centers for Disease Control and Prevention (CDC). Its major goal is to monitor and gather data on adverse events after immunization. VAERS is an essential tool for post-marketing monitoring for ensuring vaccination safety (Varricchio et al. 2004). VAERS is a passive reporting database that allows healthcare practitioners, manufacturers, and people to report any adverse events they think are related to vaccines. These adverse events might vary from minor, temporary side effects to serious or rarely found complications. VAERS reports contain adverse event descriptions, patient data, vaccination details, and any relevant medical history (Institute of Medicine (US) Committee on Health Effects Associated with Exposures During the Gulf War et al. 2000).

VAERS data aids in the identification of possible vaccination safety problems, patterns, or signals. While the method fails to establish a clear cause-and-effect link between vaccinations and reported adverse effects, it does serve as an early warning system for additional research. VAERS data is analyzed on a regular basis in order to detect possible safety signals and to guide vaccination safety research and policy choices (Shimabukuro et al. 2015).

11.5 Other Vaccine Monitoring System

11.5.1 Vaccine Safety Datalink

The Vaccine Safety Datalink (VSD) initiative commenced in 1990 through a collective research endeavor involving the Centers for Disease Control and Prevention (CDC) and four health maintenance organizations (HMOs) to enable investigations into major adverse events after immunization (McNeil et al. 2014). The number of participating HMOs increased from eight to ten, with an enclosed population of more than nine million people enrolled at any particular time (and more than 24 million persons overall during the project's duration) (Baggs et al. 2011).

The Vaccine Safety Datalink (VSD) project was established by the CDC Immunization Safety Office to undertake post-marketing reviews of vaccine safety in a specific population. Rapid cycle analysis (RCA) is a primary analytic approach for VSD post-marketing surveillance, in which the observed number of adverse events is compared to the expected number of events, with the predicted number of incidents based on historical data, a contemporary comparison control group, or control approaches. Weekly VSD comparisons analyze various safety outcomes of relevance; as such, the statistical significance criterion is changed to account for multiple outcomes and multiple assessments (Blumenthal et al. 2021).

The VSD is a type of active safety surveillance system that was designed to solve the shortcomings of passive surveillance systems such as VAERS. As a passive surveillance system, VAERS gathers reports of incidents that are freely reported by persons who encounter them, caretakers, or others (Ball et al. 2003).

11.5.2 Post-Licensure Rapid Immunization Safety Monitoring System (PRISM)

The Post-Licensure Rapid Immunization Safety Monitoring System (PRISM) was instituted by the CDC with the primary objective of real-time safety monitoring for newly licensed vaccines. PRISM serves as a complementary addition to pre-existing vaccine safety monitoring systems, including the Vaccine Adverse Event Reporting System (VAERS), by immediately identifying and investigating possible adverse events after immunization using electronic health data from participating healthcare organizations (Baker et al. 2013).

The major purpose of PRISM is to improve knowledge of vaccine safety profiles and identify any possible safety problems that may occur after a vaccine is licensed and introduced into the community. It offers continuous monitoring and analysis of vaccination safety data from varied patient groups by using electronic health records (EHRs) and other healthcare databases (Schuemie et al. 2022).

PRISM has a dispersed data approach, which means that participant healthcare organizations maintain control of their data, while the CDC manages and enables aggregated data analysis. This method enables fast monitoring of vaccination safety across various locations and populations while avoiding the need to transmit or centralize individual patient data. Overall, PRISM is an important component of the post-licensure vaccine safety monitoring infrastructure, contributing to the ongoing assessment and confirmation of the safety of recently licensed vaccines (Nguyen et al. 2012).

11.5.3 Clinical Immunization Safety Assessment Project (CISA)

The Centers for Disease Control and Prevention (CDC) collaborates with six different academic medical centers to provide support for immunization safety evaluation and research through the Clinical Immunization Safety Assessment (CISA) Network. The CDC established the CISA Network in 2001 with four key purposes:

1. develop clinical assessment, diagnostic, and treatment strategies for adverse events after immunization (AEFI);
2. increase individual knowledge of AEFI, including identifying probable genetic and other predisposing risk factors for specific people and high-risk subpopulations;
3. crafting vaccination protocols rooted in evidence for individuals who are at an elevated risk of experiencing significant AEFI; and,
4. serving as authoritative sources of expertise regarding clinical inquiries related to vaccine safety.

   CISA Network experts offer extensive clinical, pathophysiologic, and epidemiologic knowledge to the task of determining causal links between vaccinations and adverse events as well as comprehending the origins of AEFI. Network researchers undertake expert opinions of clinically relevant adverse events and use clinical and laboratory criteria to verify the validity of documented diagnosis. They also perform specific research to examine possible causes of adverse events, evaluate vaccine-adverse-event connections, and maintain a centralized repository for clinical samples. The CISA Network offers particular clinical recommendations to both vaccination providers and those who examine and treat individuals with suspected AEFI. It is vital in delivering critical immunization safety information and expertise to vaccine policymakers. It is an exclusive resource for the CDC's vaccination safety monitoring operations (Williams et al. 2011; LaRussa et al. 2011).

11.5.4 Global Vaccine Safety Initiative (GVSI)

The Global Vaccine Safety Initiative (GVSI) by the World Health Organization (WHO) is a program designed to ensure the safety of vaccines and foster public trust in vaccination programs worldwide. To enhance vaccine safety systems, GVSI encourages and supports worldwide cooperation in vaccine safety monitoring, capacity development, research, and communication (World Health Organization 2011). The Global Vaccine Safety Initiative focuses on several key areas:

1. Strengthening national vaccine safety systems.
2. Promoting research and innovation.
3. Enhancing communication and public trust.
4. Building capacity.

The Global Vaccine Safety Initiative is crucial in developing global vaccine safety systems and providing continued vaccine safety monitoring and review. It strives to sustain public faith in immunization and protect public health by promoting worldwide collaboration and knowledge exchange (Amarasinghe et al. 2013).

11.6 Adverse Event Following Immunization (AEFI)

According to the World Health Organization (WHO), "Adverse event following immunization (AEFI) is any untoward medical occurrence which follows immunization and which does not necessarily have a causal relationship with the usage of the vaccine." Any unfavorable or unexpected sign, abnormal test result, symptom, or illness might be considered an unpleasant event. Reported adverse events might be either actual adverse events, i.e. those caused by the vaccine or immunization process, or coincidental occurrences, which are not caused by the vaccine or immunization process but are temporally related to immunization (World Health Organization 2016). Concerning the causes of AEFI, it is divided into the five broad categories of AEFI as per WHO classification. These encompass reactions related to the vaccine product itself, reactions related to vaccine quality defects, reactions associated with the process of immunization, reactions influenced by anxiety related to immunization, and coincidental reactions or events (World Health Organization 2016; Bonhoeffer et al. 2002). Categories of AEFI are provided in Table 11.1 (CIOMS 2012).

11.7 Causality Assessment of AEFI

The investigation of the association between vaccination and an adverse event to determine if the vaccine caused the reported event is known as vaccine causality assessment. It aims to assess the strength of the relationship and establish a causal link using available evidence and standardized criteria. It is essential in vaccine safety monitoring since it enables the identification of actual vaccine-related adverse events and assists in distinguishing them from coincidental or unrelated occurrences. It helps with the ongoing assessment of vaccination safety and the implementation of risk-mitigation methods (World Health Organization 2017).

Causality assessment consists of four steps: (World Health Organization 2015).

Step 1. Eligibility: The first step is to determine whether the AEFI case meets the minimal requirements for causation evaluation, which are detailed below.

Table 11.1 Definitions of AEFIs by cause according to CIOMS

Vaccine product related reaction	An AEFI that is caused or precipitated by a vaccine due to one or more of the inherent properties of the vaccine product
Vaccine quality defect reaction	An AEFI that is caused or precipitated by a vaccine that is due to one or more quality defects of the vaccine product including its administration device as provided by the manufacturer
Immunization-related reaction	An AEFI that is caused by inappropriate vaccine handling, prescribing, or administration and thus by its nature is preventable
Immunization anxiety related reaction	An AEFI arising from anxiety about the immunization
Coincidental reaction/event	An AEFI that is caused by something other than the vaccine product, immunization error, or immunization anxiety

Step 2. Checklist: The second step is thoroughly analyzing all relevant and accessible information to address potential AEFI causative elements.

Step 3. Algorithm: The final phase uses the information acquired in the checklist to establish a pattern of causality.

Step 4. Classification: The fourth step classifies the AEFI's relationship with the vaccine/vaccination based on the algorithm's trend.

11.8 Steps for Causality Assessment of an AEFI

11.8.1 Eligibility

The tool is versatile and applicable to any AEFI for which the diagnosis can be confirmed using widely accepted definitions, such as those provided by the Brighton Collaboration or other established epidemiological and clinical criteria (Brighton Collaboration 2013). The AEFI inquiry needs to be reasonably finished in order to use the tool. Before utilizing the tool, it is essential to ensure that all data gathered during the case investigation, including autopsy results, laboratory findings, or clinical assessments, are readily accessible. If more pertinent information becomes available in the future, the evaluation might be reviewed again. Eligibility for causality evaluation as depicted in Fig. 11.1.

11.8.2 Checklist

The causality assessment checklist is used to review the data gathered during the AEFI investigation. This checklist contains specific items pertinent to the process, such as evidence against a causal vaccine-event correlation, confirming evidence for a cause other than vaccination, and evaluation of all potential causes of the AEFI as appropriate in the case. The checklist also encompasses factors such as the previous medical history on the occurrence, background rate of the event within the general population, the potential impact of the individual's health status, and any potential exposures that might have contributed to the event. Regarding the published evidence suggesting that a vaccination might be linked to the reported incident, WHO

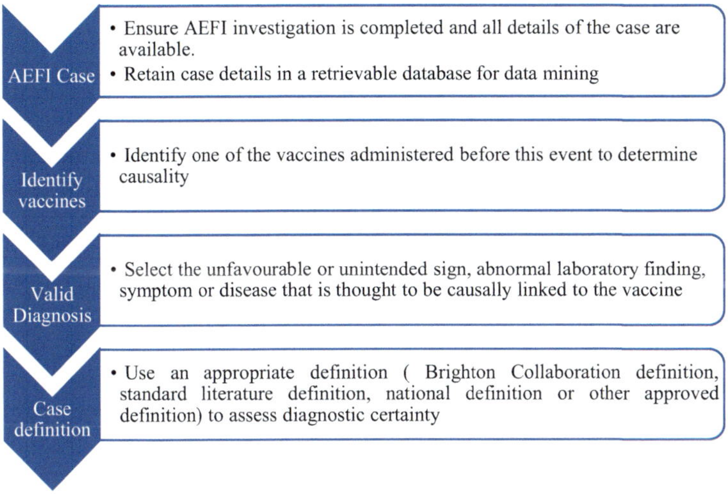

Fig. 11.1 Causality assessment eligibility

has established and continuously updates informational sheets detailing the occurrence rates of adverse events and evidence associated with various vaccines (World Health Organization 2020).

Causality assessment checklist is provided in Table 11.2.

11.8.3 Algorithm

The algorithm is then fed summarized information from each of the checklist's four domains (established causal links with vaccines or vaccinations, evidence for other potential causes, compelling evidence refuting a causal connection, and any additional relevant criteria for classification), and reviewers are directed to assess deductive reasoning to interpret all available data. The assessor is required to systematically go through all the four steps, from I to IV, to classify the information collected in each section of the checklist. It is important to acknowledge that the results obtained through this approach may indicate either a consistent or inconsistent association with a causal relationship to vaccination (World Health Organization 2017). The details are shown in Fig. 11.2.

11.8.4 Classification

The ultimate categorization is determined based on the definition and utilization of terminology within the field of vaccine pharmacovigilance, as outlined in the CIOMS Working Group on Vaccine Pharmacovigilance Report. The cause-specific definitions make it easier to understand "A. Consistent causal association to immunization" and "C. Inconsistent causal association to immunization" (coincidence).

Table 11.2 Causality assessment checklist

I. Is there strong evidence for other causes?	Y	N	UK	NA	Remarks
1. In this patient, does the medical history, clinical examination, and/or investigations confirm another cause for the event?	☐	☐	☐	☐	
II. Is there a known causal association with the vaccine or vaccination?					
Vaccine product					
1. Is there evidence in published peer reviewed literature that this vaccine may cause such an event if administered correctly?	☐	☐	☐	☐	
2. Is there a biological plausibility that this vaccine could cause such an event?	☐	☐	☐	☐	
3. In this patient, did a specific test demonstrate the causal role of the vaccine?	☐	☐	☐	☐	
Vaccine quality					
4. Could the vaccine given to this patient have a quality defect or is substandard or falsified?	☐	☐	☐	☐	
Immunization error					
5. In this patient, was there an error in prescribing or non-adherence to recommendations for use of the vaccine (e.g. use beyond the expiry date, wrong recipient, etc.)?	☐	☐	☐	☐	
6. In this patient, was the vaccine (or diluent) administered in an unsterile manner?	☐	☐	☐	☐	
7. In this patient, was the vaccine's physical condition (e.g. color, turbidity, presence of foreign substances, etc.) abnormal when administered?	☐	☐	☐	☐	
8. When this patient was vaccinated, was there an error in vaccine constitution/preparation by the vaccinator (e.g. wrong product, wrong diluent, improper mixing, improper syringe filling, etc.)?	☐	☐	☐	☐	
9. In this patient, was there an error in vaccine handling (e.g. a break in the cold chain during transport, storage, and/or immunization session, etc.)?	☐	☐	☐	☐	
10. In this patient, was the vaccine administered incorrectly (e.g. wrong dose, site, or route of administration; wrong needle size, etc.)?	☐	☐	☐	☐	
Immunization anxiety (immunization stress related responses, ISRR)					
11. In this patient, could this event be a stress response triggered by immunization (e.g. acute stress response, vasovagal reaction, hyperventilation, dissociative neurological symptom reaction, etc.)?	☐	☐	☐	☐	
II (time): Was the event in section II within the time window of increased risk (i.e. "yes" response to questions from II 1 to II 11 above)					
12. In this patient, did the event occur within a plausible time window after vaccine administration?	☐	☐	☐	☐	
III. Is there strong evidence against a causal association?					
1. Is there a body of published evidence (systematic reviews, GACVS reviews, Cochrane reviews, etc.) against a causal association between the vaccine and the event?	☐	☐	☐	☐	

(continued)

Table 11.2 (continued)

IV. Other qualifying factors for classification					
1. In this patient, did such an event occur in the past after administration of a similar vaccine?	☐	☐	☐	☐	
2. In this patient, did such an event occur in the past independent of vaccination?	☐	☐	☐	☐	
3. Could the current event have occurred in this patient without vaccination (background rate)?	☐	☐	☐	☐	
4. Did this patient have an illness, pre-existing condition, or risk factor that could have contributed to the event?	☐	☐	☐	☐	
5. Was this patient taking any medication prior to the vaccination?	☐	☐	☐	☐	
6. Was this patient exposed to a potential factor (other than vaccine) prior to the event (e.g. allergen, drug, herbal product, etc.)?	☐	☐	☐	☐	

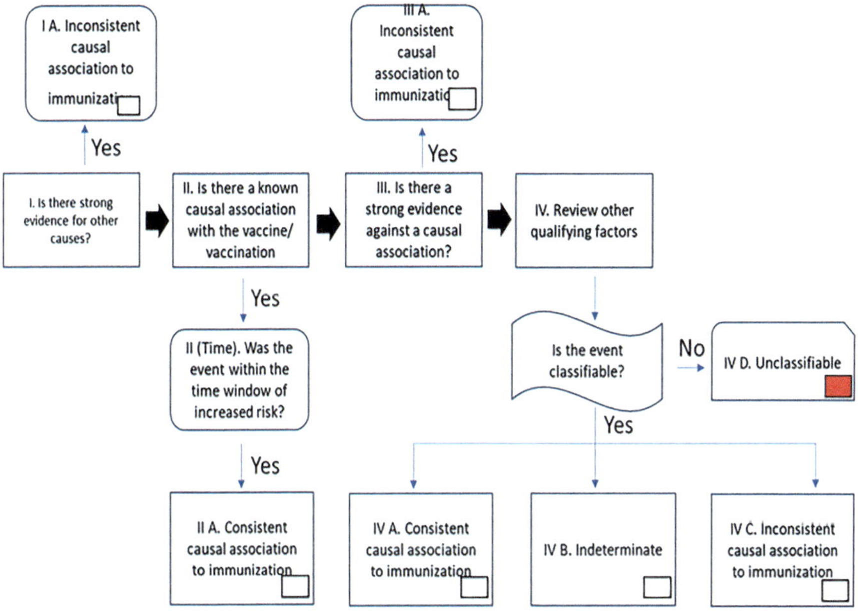

Fig. 11.2 Causality assessment algorithm

The association is classified as "B. indeterminate" when appropriate information on the AEFI is available but it cannot be assigned to one of the preceding groups (Report of the CIOMS/WHO Working Group on Vaccine Pharmacovigilance 2012). The details are shown in Fig. 11.3.

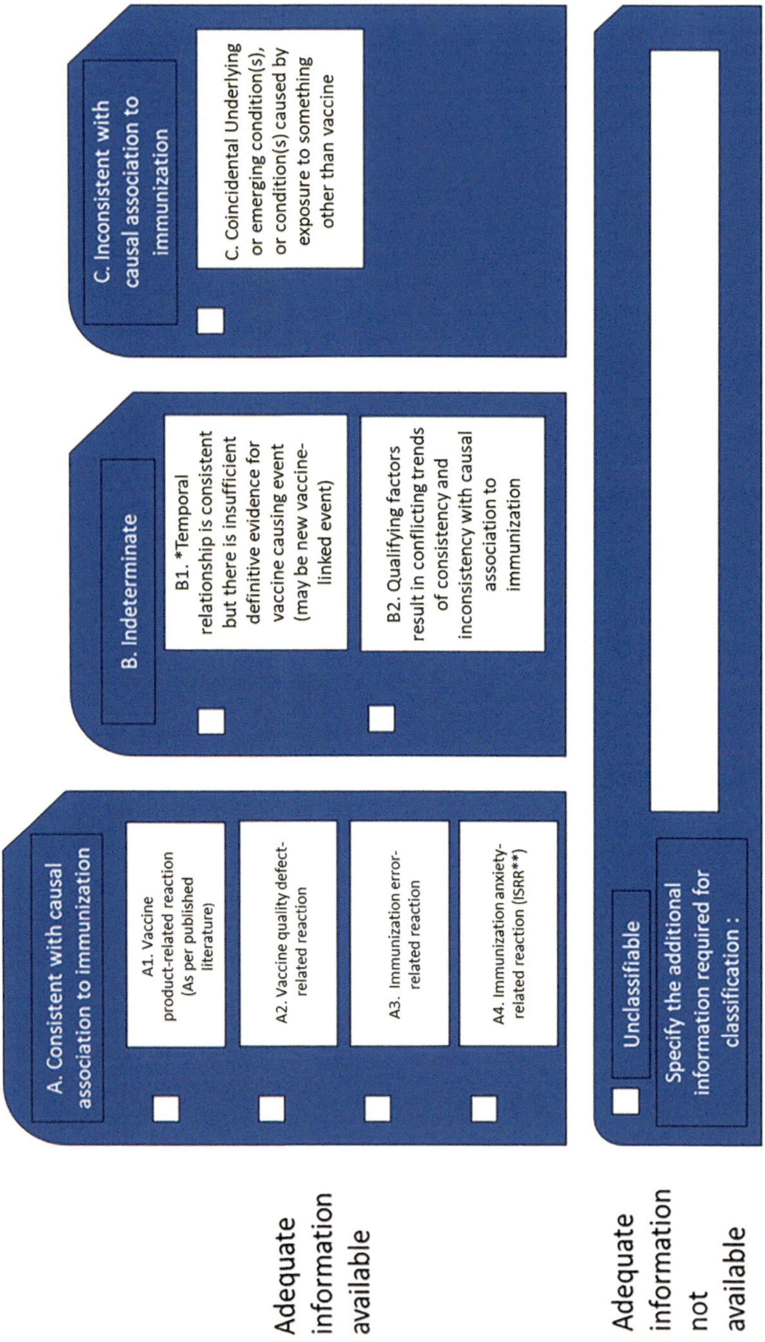

Fig. 11.3 Causality assessment classification

11.9 Conclusion

Vaccine surveillance is an important and continuing process that serves a critical role in protecting public health. We can assure the safety and efficacy of immunization programs by conducting systematic monitoring and evaluation of vaccine-related adverse events. Transparent communication and coordination among healthcare professionals, international health organizations, the general public, and governments are critical for maintaining public trust in vaccines and maximizing global immunization efforts. Vaccine safety surveillance helps in safeguarding people and communities from avoidable illnesses, eventually contributing to a better and safer world with ongoing vigilance and evidence-based practices.

References

Amarasinghe A, Black S, Bonhoeffer J, Carvalho SMD, Dodoo A, Eskola J, Sato Y (2013) Effective vaccine safety systems in all countries: a challenge for more equitable access to immunization. Vaccine 31:B108–B114. https://doi.org/10.1016/j.vaccine.2012.10.119

Arita I, Nakane M, Kojima K, Yoshihara N, Nakano T, El-Gohary A (2004) Role of a sentinel surveillance system in the context of global surveillance of infectious diseases. Lancet Infect Dis 4(3):171–177. https://doi.org/10.1016/S1473-3099(04)00942-9

Asiamah M, Akuffo KO, Nortey P, Donkor N, Danso-Appiah A (2022) Spontaneous reporting of adverse drug reaction among health professionals in Ghana. Arch Public Health 80(1):1–11. https://doi.org/10.1186/s13690-021-00783-1

Baggs J, Gee J, Lewis E, Fowler G, Benson P, Lieu T, Weintraub E (2011) The Vaccine Safety Datalink: a model for monitoring immunization safety. Pediatrics 127(Supplement_1):S45–S53

Baker MA, Nguyen M, Cole DV, Lee GM, Lieu TA (2013) Post-licensure rapid immunization safety monitoring program (PRISM) data characterization. Vaccine 31:K98–K112. https://doi.org/10.1016/j.vaccine.2013.04.088

Ball R, Braun MM, Chen RT, Ellenberg SS, English-Bullard R, Haber P, Zhou W (2003) Surveillance for safety after immunization; vaccine adverse event reporting system (VAERS)-United States 1991–2001. https://stacks.cdc.gov/view/cdc/13491

Blumenthal KG, Phadke NA, Bates DW (2021) Safety surveillance of COVID-19 mRNA vaccines through the vaccine safety datalink. JAMA 326(14):1375–1377. https://doi.org/10.1001/jama.2021.14808

Bonhoeffer J, Kohl K, Chen R, Duclos P, Heijbel H, Heininger U, Brighton Collaboration (2002) The Brighton collaboration: addressing the need for standardized case definitions of adverse events following immunization (AEFI). Vaccine 21(3–4):298–302. https://doi.org/10.1016/S0264-410X(02)00449-8

Brighton Collaboration (2013) Case definitions. Brighton Collaboration, Basel. https://brighton-collaboration.us/category/pubs-tools/case-definitions/. Accessed 18 July 2023

Budhiraja S, Akinapelli R (2010) Pharmacovigilance in vaccines. Indian J Pharmacol 42(2):117. https://doi.org/10.4103/0253-7613.64488

CIOMS (2012) Definition and application of terms for vaccine pharmacovigilance. Report of CIOMS/WHO working group on vaccine pharmacovigilance. CIOMS, Geneva, p 2013. https://cioms.ch/wp-content/uploads/2017/01/report_working_group_on_vaccine_LR.pdf. Accessed 16 July 2023

Daley MF, Glanz JM, Newcomer SR, Jackson ML, Groom HC, Lugg MM et al (2017) Assessing misclassification of vaccination status: implications for studies of the safety of the childhood immunization schedule. Vaccine 35(15):1873–1878. https://doi.org/10.1016/j.vaccine.2017.02.058

Dekkers OM, Egger M, Altman DG, Vandenbroucke JP (2012) Distinguishing case series from cohort studies. Ann Int Med 156(1_Part_1):37–40. https://doi.org/10.7326/0003-4819-156-1-201201030-00006

Edwards IR (1999) Spontaneous reporting—of what? Clinical concerns about drugs. Br J Clin Pharmacol 48(2):138. https://doi.org/10.1046/j.1365-2125.1999.00000.x

Hause AM, Baggs J, Marquez P, Myers TR, Su JR, Hugueley B et al (2022) Safety monitoring of Pfizer-BioNTech COVID-19 vaccine booster doses among children aged 5–11 years—United States, may 17–July 31, 2022. Morb Mortal Wkly Rep 71(33):1047. https://doi.org/10.15585/mmwr.mm7133a3

Heininger U, Holm K, Caplanusi I, Bailey SR, Abdoellah SA, Arellano F et al (2017) Guide to active vaccine safety surveillance: report of CIOMS working group on vaccine safety–executive summary. Vaccine 35(32):3917–3921. https://doi.org/10.1016/j.vaccine.2017.06.033

Hinrichsen VL, Kruskal B, O'Brien MA, Lieu TA, Platt R (2007) Using electronic medical records to enhance detection and reporting of vaccine adverse events. J Am Med Inform Assoc 14(6):731–735. https://doi.org/10.1197/jamia.M2232

Hoffman KB, Demakas AR, Dimbil M, Tatonetti NP, Erdman CB (2014) Stimulated reporting: the impact of US food and drug administration-issued alerts on the adverse event reporting system (FAERS). Drug Saf 37:971–980. https://doi.org/10.1007/s40264-014-0225-0

Institute of Medicine (US) Committee on Health Effects Associated with Exposures During the Gulf War (2000) In: Fulco CE, Liverman CT, Sox HC (eds) Gulf War and health: depleted uranium, sarin, pyridostigmine bromide, vaccines, vol 1. National Academies Press (US), Washington, DC. https://www.ncbi.nlm.nih.gov/books/NBK222854/. Accessed 13 July 2023

Joshi J, Das MK, Polpakara D, Aneja S, Agarwal M, Arora NK (2018) Vaccine safety and surveillance for adverse events following immunization (AEFI) in India. Indian J Pediatr 85:139–148. https://doi.org/10.1007/s12098-017-2532-9

LaRussa PS, Edwards KM, Dekker CL, Klein NP, Halsey NA, Marchant C, Slade BA (2011) Understanding the role of human variation in vaccine adverse events: the clinical immunization safety assessment network. Pediatrics 127(Supplement_1):S65–S73

McNeil MM, Gee J, Weintraub ES, Belongia EA, Lee GM, Glanz JM, DeStefano F (2014) The vaccine safety datalink: successes and challenges monitoring vaccine safety. Vaccine 32(42):5390–5398. https://doi.org/10.1016/j.vaccine.2014.07.073

Nguyen M, Ball R, Midthun K, Lieu TA (2012) The Food and Drug Administration's post-licensure rapid immunization safety monitoring program: strengthening the federal vaccine safety enterprise. Pharmacoepidemiol Drug Saf 21:291–297. https://doi.org/10.1002/pds.2323

Nuwarda RF, Ramzan I, Weekes L, Kayser V (2022) Vaccine hesitancy: contemporary issues and historical background. Vaccine 10(10):1595. https://doi.org/10.3390/vaccines10101595

Piltch-Loeb R, Harriman NW, Healey J, Bonetti M, Toffolutti V, Testa MA et al (2021) COVID-19 vaccine concerns about safety, effectiveness, and policies in the United States, Canada, Sweden, and Italy among unvaccinated individuals. Vaccine 9(10):1138. https://doi.org/10.3390/vaccines9101138

Report of the CIOMS/WHO Working Group on Vaccine Pharmacovigilance (2012) Definition and application of terms for vaccine pharmacovigilance. Council for International Organizations of Medical Sciences, Geneva. https://cioms.ch/wp-content/uploads/2017/01/report_working_group_on_vaccine_LR.pdf. Accessed 19 July 2023

Schuemie MJ, Arshad F, Pratt N, Nyberg F, Alshammari TM, Hripcsak G et al (2022) Vaccine safety surveillance using routinely collected healthcare data—an empirical evaluation of epidemiological designs. Front Pharmacol 13:893484. https://doi.org/10.3389/fphar.2022.893484

Shimabukuro TT, Nguyen M, Martin D, DeStefano F (2015) Safety monitoring in the vaccine adverse event reporting system (VAERS). Vaccine 33(36):4398–4405. https://doi.org/10.1016/j.vaccine.2015.07.035

Strom BL (2019) What is pharmacoepidemiology? In: Pharmacoepidemiology. Wiley, Hoboken, pp 1–26. https://doi.org/10.1002/9781119413431.ch1

U.S. Food and Drug Administration (2021) COVID-19 vaccine safety surveillance. U.S. Food and Drug Administration, Silver Spring, MD. https://www.fda.gov/vaccines-blood-biologics/safety-availability-biologics/covid-19-vaccine-safety-surveillance. Accessed 13 July 2023

US Public Health Service (1999) Centers for Disease Control and Prevention: ten great public health achievements: United States 1900-1999. MMWR 48:241–243. https://cir.nii.ac.jp/crid/1572261549196027776

van den Bergh RC, Korfage IJ, Bangma CH (2012) Psychological aspects of active surveillance. Curr Opin Urol 22(3):237–242. https://doi.org/10.1097/MOU.0b013e328351dcb1

Varricchio F, Iskander J, Destefano F, Ball R, Pless R, Braun MM, Chen RT (2004) Understanding vaccine safety information from the vaccine adverse event reporting system. Pediatr Infect Dis J 23(4):287–294. https://journals.lww.com/pidj/toc/2004/04000

Verstraeten T, DeStefano F, Chen RT, Miller E (2003) Vaccine safety surveillance using large linked databases: opportunities, hazards and proposed guidelines. Expert Rev Vaccines 2(1):21–29. https://doi.org/10.1586/14760584.2.1.21

Williams SE, Klein NP, Halsey N, Dekker CL, Baxter RP, Marchant CD, Edwards KM (2011) Overview of the clinical consult case review of adverse events following immunization: clinical immunization safety assessment (CISA) network 2004–2009. Vaccine 29(40):6920–6927. https://doi.org/10.1016/j.vaccine.2011.07.044

Wong CK, Marshall NS, Grunstein RR, Ho SS, Fois RA, Hibbs DE, Saini B (2017) Spontaneous adverse event reports associated with zolpidem in the United States 2003–2012. J Clin Sleep Med 13(2):223–234. https://doi.org/10.5664/jcsm.6452

World Health Organization (2008) A practical handbook on the pharmacovigilance of antimalarial medicines. World Health Organization, Geneva

World Health Organization (2011) The global vaccine safety initiative. World Health Organization, Geneva. https://www.who.int/vaccine_safety/initiative/en/. Accessed 15 July 2023

World Health Organization (2015) Immunization safety surveillance. Guidelines for immunization programme managers on surveillance of adverse events following immunization, 3rd edn. World Health Organization, Geneva. https://apps.who.int/iris/rest/bitstreams/1247061/retrieve. Accessed July 17 2023

World Health Organization (2016) Global manual on surveillance of adverse events following immunization [internet]. WHO, Geneva. http://apps.who.int/iris/bitstream/10665/206144/1/9789241507769_eng.pdf. Accessed 15 July 2023

World Health Organization (2017) Causality assessment of an adverse event following immunization (AEFI): user manual for the revised WHO classification, 2nd edn. World Health Organization, Geneva. https://www.who.int/publications/i/item/9789241516990. Accessed 17 July 2023

World Health Organization (2020) WHO vaccine reaction rates information sheets. World Health Organization, Geneva. https://www.who.int/teams/regulation-prequalification/regulation-and-safety/pharmacovigilance/health-professionals-info/reaction-rates-information-sheets. Accessed 18 July 2023

Herbovigilance

12

Prabhakar Kumar, Mukesh Nandave, Anoop Kumar, and Dipali Nandave

Abstract

Herbal medicines have been used for treating a wide variety of diseases and illnesses since ancient times. There are still issues concerning the use of herbal treatments and the adverse pharmacological responses that can occur because of them. Herbovigilance is the practice of monitoring herbal treatments for safety. It is critical to analyze safety and discover potential threats and eliminate the instances resulting from inferior-quality products and improper consumption. In territories where herbal medicine is widely utilized, integrating herbovigilance into contemporary healthcare systems and gaining collaboration between practitioners and regulatory bodies can be challenging. Harmonizing these processes can make it easier to monitor the safety of herbal medications. A lack of detailed evidence and information regarding the effectiveness and safety of herbal drugs hinders herbovigilance programs. Substantial evidence is needed to identify and evaluate adverse effects, pharmacological interactions, and potential risks associated with herbal treatments. It is crucial to remember that these potential difficulties are not all-inclusive and that herbovigilance is a field that is continually changing. Regulatory agencies, healthcare practitioners, scientists, and herbal medicines must work together to address these difficulties to ensure herbal remedies' long-term safety and efficacy.

P. Kumar (✉) · M. Nandave · A. Kumar
Department of Pharmacology, Delhi Pharmaceutical Sciences and Research University, New Delhi, India
e-mail: mukeshnandave@gmail.com; anoopdpsru@dpsru.edu.in

D. Nandave
Department of Dravyaguna Vigyan, All India Institute of Ayurveda, New Delhi, India

M. Nandave, A. Kumar (eds.), *Pharmacovigilance Essentials*,
https://doi.org/10.1007/978-981-99-8949-2_12

This Chapter Contains: Introduction, Concept of Herbovigilance in PV, Sources of Reporting ADRs, Reporting of ADRs related to Herbal medicines, Regulatory aspects of herbal medicines, WHO Guidelines for Safety Monitoring in Herbovigilance, Current Scenario of Herbovigilance in India, Herbovigilance Overview Worldwide, Future Prospects, Future Obstacles and Conclusion.

Keywords

Herbovigilance · Pharmacovigilance · Healthcare · Herbal treatments · Adverse effects and Herbal medicines

12.1 Introduction

Monitoring and assuring the safety of traditional medications is called "herbovigilance." Various illnesses and health concerns have been treated with conventional therapies and their formulations for a long time. However, there is a universal misconception that traditional remedies are safe and have no side effects. Multiple studies in scientific research demonstrating the incidence of adverse drug reactions connected to herbal medications have cast doubt on this myth (Bhimaneni et al. 2021).

For the safety of herbal medicines, pharmacovigilance, the procedures involved in the detection, assessment, awareness, and prevention of side effects or any additional drug-associated issues, is essential. Whereas the pharmacovigilance platforms now functioning were effectively created and implemented for synthesized medicines, adjustments are required to account for the unique characteristics and consequences related to natural products (Bhimaneni et al. 2021).

12.1.1 History and Background

The history and background for pharmacovigilance, which covers a broader range of drug safety surveillance, can shed light on how herbovigilance came to be. About 170 years have passed since the beginning of organized pharmacovigilance in professional healthcare. It all started with practitioners informing the authors of scientific literature about negative impacts and safety issues. These earliest reports, which frequently took the shape of warnings or cautions, set the stage for systematic surveillance of the risk-to-benefit ratio of pharmaceuticals and enhanced the safety of patients and their standard of life (Fornasier et al. 2018).

Pharmacovigilance has transformed continuously because of the emergence of distinct benchmarks. In the past, strategies, including the establishment of committees including the cooperation of healthcare professionals and research publication authors, have been utilized to gather reports about adverse effects. These initiatives progressively developed toward more official and organized procedures involving the development of computerized records (Fornasier et al. 2018).

The need for surveillance of adverse effects of drugs has been increasingly recognized, which has led to an expansion of pharmacovigilance operations. The concept of "adverse drug reactions" appears directly related to pharmacovigilance; it refers to instances where medications are used appropriately, wrongly, or even in a way that differs from what is specified on the label or instructions. Pharmacovigilance monitors and evaluates adverse responses to improve patient safety and avoid injury.

12.1.2 Herbal Medicine and Herbovigilance

The approach of using plants and phyto-extracts from them for medicinal use to treat a wide range of health problems is referred to as herbal medicine or conventional therapy. This has been used extensively worldwide for decades and is still in use today. The use of herbal remedies is becoming increasingly common, linked to its presumed security, availability, and faith in the effectiveness of herbal therapies.

As the consumption of herbal remedies escalates, questions concerning safety and adverse outcomes are raised. ADRs (adverse drug reactions) and interactions with other drugs are possible with herbal medicines since they are complex combinations of bioactive components. These worries have sparked the establishment of a dedicated industry called "herbovigilance," which concentrates on tracking the security of herbal medications and spotting possible adverse effects.

Pharmacovigilance for herbal remedies is a framework for monitoring and assessing the safety of drugs throughout their entire shelf life, mainly herbal medicine. ADR data must be collected, analyzed, and appropriate action must be taken to ensure the safety of patients. Since post-marketing safety monitoring standards for herbal drugs were published in the latter part of the twentieth century, pharmacovigilance for herbal therapies has developed and grown (Choudhury et al. 2023). Herbal treatments are being used more frequently due to an increase in the percentage of individuals who decide to turn to these remedies for their primary healthcare needs. Despite this, pharmacovigilance in this market is challenging since herbal drugs occur in various formulations, and no established regulations exist (Ahmad Khan and Ahmad 2018).

Herbovigilance is required while utilizing herbal remedies to ensure the safety of conventional medicines at both the national and international levels (Choudhury et al. 2023). The goal is to improve patient safety by detecting and minimizing risks related to herbal medication use. As the use of herbal medicine develops in recognition, there is an increased requirement of a reliable herbovigilance system (Ahmad Khan and Ahmad 2018). Herbovigilance monitors adverse effects and allows for the use of safe herbal medicine.

12.1.3 Need for Herbovigilance

Herbovigilance, which assures the safety and monitoring of herbal medicines, is becoming increasingly crucial because the utilization of herbal remedies spreads around the world. With a rising popularity of herbal remedies, there are main concerns about their safety and potential side effects, such as combinations with prescribed pharmaceutical medicines (Skalli et al. 2022). Because herbal therapies are not often subjected to extensive regulations and assessment, it is critical to build reliable pharmacovigilance protocols. Several causes contribute to the expanding global requirement for herbovigilance. Pharmacovigilance comprises identifying, assessing, raising awareness about and dealing with potential adverse drug responses (Hassan 2014). It is essential to assess the efficacy of herbal treatments and detect potential hazards. Pharmacovigilance programs enable early detection of adverse reactions that could enhance the safety of patients and assist informed decision-making (Hugman and Skalli 2022).

Due to the potential side effects of herbal remedies and their combinations with other treatments, herbal care is necessary. While herbal remedies have historically been used to treat various illnesses, it is crucial to understand that they may additionally exhibit adverse effects and even be toxic (Gruszycki Kisiel et al. 2017). Herbal remedy's fundamental safety could lead consumers to overlook the possible adverse effects (Toklu 2016).

Although herbal medications are frequently used to treat various illnesses, some safety issues exist. A popular misconception is that they are risk-free and may be eaten without adverse effects. However, numerous reports and studies have emphasized adverse drug interactions and reactions linked to herbal remedies (Bhimaneni et al. 2021). It is essential to monitor the safety of herbal medications using herbovigilance to spot any hazards, treat them, and guarantee the well-being of people taking these products.

Herbal medicines are specific in that their composition, manufacture, and mode of action differ from synthetic drugs. They frequently contain intricate combinations of active substances, which can give rise to specific safety problems. As a result, it is necessary to adapt current pharmacovigilance systems created for synthetic medicines to consider the unique properties of herbal medicines (Bhimaneni et al. 2021).

Interactions between herbal goods and contemporary drugs are possible since herbal treatments are frequently taken in addition to prescription medications. These interactions may impact the effectiveness and safety of the herbal and prescribed medicines. Herbovigilance assists in recognizing and comprehending herb–drug interactions, ensuring that patients and healthcare providers have access to the necessary information (Divakar 2022).

Recently, high-profile safety issues involving herbal medications have increased public awareness of their dangers. Establishing pharmacovigilance systems explicitly designed to track and assess the safety of herbal medicines is crucial to ease these worries and safeguard the public's health (Rahman and Rashid 2020).

Herbovigilance is required to address the safety issues with herbal medications, track adverse effects, spot herb–drug interactions, and guarantee these goods' general reliability and caliber. It is possible to deliver accurate information and encourage the safe use of herbal medicines in healthcare practices by implementing efficient herbovigilance systems.

12.1.4 Herbovigilance in India

Herbovigilance is the process of monitoring and ensuring the safety of herbal items within India. It is an essential component of pharmacovigilance, which concentrates on identifying, evaluating, comprehending, and avoiding adverse effects and other drug-related issues connected with pharmaceuticals, including herbal remedies.

The importance of developing pharmacovigilance procedures specifically for herbal medications is becoming increasingly recognized in India. Herbal formulations are used as medicinal agents for various conditions, including diabetes, arthritis, hepatoprotection, cough relief, memory improvement, and adaptogens. However, a widespread misconception about herbal medications is that they are perfectly safe and may be taken without a doctor's prescription. This idea has encouraged many people to self-medicate, which frequently has disappointing results, adverse reactions, or other consequences (Wal et al. 2011).

Herbovigilance aims to address these safety concerns and ensure the safe use of herbal medicines in India. It involves monitoring adverse reactions, assessing the quality of herbal products, identifying herb–drug interactions, and promoting the rational use of herbal drugs (Wal et al. 2011). By implementing effective herbovigilance systems, the Indian healthcare system can gather data on adverse events related to herbal medicines, evaluate their safety profiles, and take appropriate measures to ensure public health and safety.

The establishment of herbovigilance practices in India has evolved. Pharmacovigilance activities related to herbal medicines were initiated before introducing the National Pharmacovigilance Program of India (PvPI). Efforts have been made to develop and enhance pharmacovigilance systems tailored explicitly for herbal products through training and teaching in medical and allied health science colleges (Rahman and Ruknuddin 2022).

It is significant to remember that herbovigilance is a component of India's larger pharmacovigilance framework. The Pharmacovigilance Program of India (PvPI) was formed in 2010 to monitor the safety of all drugs in India, including herbal products (Kalaiselvan et al. 2019). The PvPI, governed by the Indian Pharmacopoeia Commission (IPC), works to protect the health of the Indian populace by making sure that the advantages of medications outweigh any potential hazards (Kalaiselvan et al. 2019).

12.1.5 Problems with Herbal Therapies

For thousands of years, different civilizations have employed herbal remedies, sometimes known as herbal medicines or phytomedicines, to treat illnesses and promote health. They originate from plants and are frequently found in lotions, teas, vitamins, and other preparations. While herbal remedies are widely used and have historically been seen as safe and effective, some difficulties and problems come with their use, as listed below.

12.1.6 The Absence of Standards and Regulations

Herbal supplements are not as strictly controlled by the FDA or other governing bodies as prescription medications are. This lack of control may result in variations in the quality, strength, and safety of herbal products. Due to the complexity and non-uniformity of the substances used in herbal medicines, standardization is necessary to assure consistent quality and efficacy, but it can be challenging (Zhang et al. 2012).

12.1.7 Adverse Effects and Interactions

Misusing herbal remedies in excess amounts or in conjunction with other treatments can all have adverse effects. Some herbal medicines may also interact negatively or less effectively with prescription medications, resulting in side effects. However, the entire scope of these interactions is only sometimes well understood due to the absence of thorough scientific studies (Barkat et al. 2019).

12.1.8 Adulteration and Contamination

During cultivation or processing, hazardous metals, pesticides, or bacteria may find their way into herbal products. Additionally, certain herbal products could be tampered with to lose effectiveness and possibly present health hazards (Tsutani and Takuma 2008).

12.1.9 Limited Scientific Evidence

Although anecdotal evidence and a long history of use suggest the efficacy of traditional herbal treatments, many assertions need to be backed up by solid scientific proof. The intricacy of herbal preparations and the requirement for standardization can make it difficult to conduct high-quality clinical studies for herbal medicines (Thillaivanan 2014).

12.1.10 Adverse Reactions and Safety Concerns

Like any other form of therapy, herbal remedies might have adverse reactions or side effects in some people. It might be challenging to spot possible safety risks with herbal products due to the need for thorough monitoring and standardized testing (Ekor 2014).

12.1.11 Lack of Knowledge and Education

The appropriate usage, dose, and possible hazards of herbal medicines may only sometimes be widely known to the public. This ignorance may result in abuse or unsatisfactory treatment.

Due to its long-standing cultural relevance, perceived safety, and accessibility as a substitute for traditional medications, herbal medicine continues to interest many despite these obstacles. These problems are being addressed, and initiatives are being taken to raise herbal treatments' caliber, security, and effectiveness. Integrative medicine is becoming more popular as a strategy to improve patient care and safety since it blends traditional medicine with evidence-based supplementary therapies like herbal medicine.

To ensure safe and appropriate use based on individual health needs and potential interactions with other medications or health conditions, individuals considering herbal therapies must consult with qualified healthcare professionals (HCPs), such as herbalists or integrative medicine practitioners, as with any medical treatment. Additionally, it is critical to purchase herbal goods from reliable sources to reduce the possibility of contamination or adulteration.

12.2 Concept of Herbovigilance in PV

Herbovigilance is a term that combines pharmacovigilance and herbal therapy. Pharmacovigilance, commonly referred to as medication safety, is the process of gathering, identifying, evaluating, monitoring, and preventing unfavorable outcomes related to pharmaceutical goods. Adverse drug reactions (ADRs), characterized as any unpleasant and unexpected response to medicine, including lack of efficacy, are the article's main subject.

Herbovigilance is the term used to describe the use of pharmacovigilance concepts to monitor the safety of herbal and conventional drugs (Barnes 2022; Bhimaneni et al. 2021; Toklu 2016). Herbal remedies are frequently used to treat various medical ailments, so confirming their safety and pinpointing potential side effects is critical.

Pharmacovigilance systems for synthetic drugs have been successfully created and put into place; however, due to the unique adaptations and procedures needed for herbal medicines given their qualities (Bhimaneni et al. 2021), herbal medication's safety profiles may differ from those of synthetic drugs because they are made from natural sources and contain complex combinations of bioactive chemicals. To record adverse occurrences connected to herbal medicines, rigorous reporting protocols and laws are also required (Skalli et al. 2022).

The development of herbovigilance systems aims to improve the safety oversight of herbal medications, identify and evaluate side effects, and mitigate any potential risk from their use. It entails gathering and analyzing information on adverse events, such as adverse drug reactions, negative drug–herb interactions, and negative herb–herb interactions (Divakar 2022). Regulators, medical professionals, and consumers can all make knowledgeable choices about the security and effective use of herbal medications by applying herbovigilance.

12.3 Sources of Reporting ADRs

The various sources of reporting ADRs are shown in Fig. 12.1.

12.3.1 Reports from Health Care Professionals (HCPs)

On a global scale, most adverse drug reaction reporting systems in post-marketing safety surveillance rely on medical practitioners' voluntary reporting, preferably those actively involved in the patient's treatment. This is appropriate because medical expertise is necessary to comprehend adverse drug responses, and healthcare practitioners should be familiar with the patient's medical history and sensitive to the nuances of clinical differential diagnosis (WHO 2004).

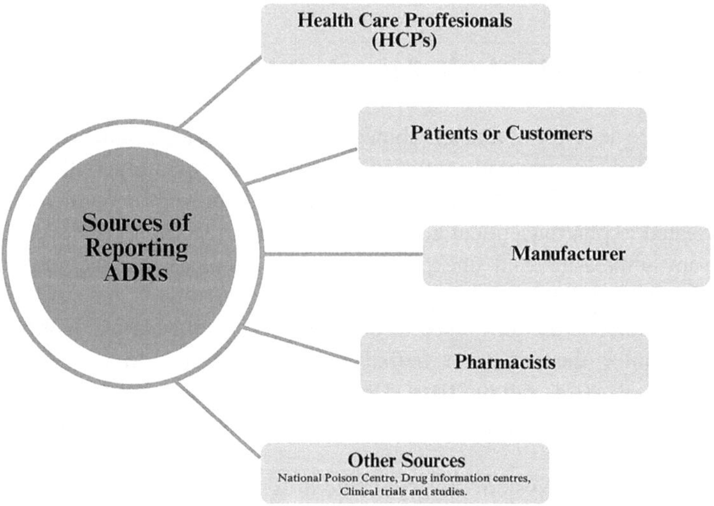

Fig. 12.1 Sources of reporting ADRs

12.3.2 Feedback from Patients and Customers

Customer involvement in using herbal medications and herbal products in healthcare and their worry over potential side effects should be regarded favorably. Consumer complaints about side effects should be taken seriously as a source of information that might help researchers spot warning signs of potential consequences of herbal medications (WHO 2004).

12.3.3 Manufacturers

Herbal medicine producers can provide information about side effects connected to their medications. Some nations' regulatory frameworks require producers to report any unfavorable events. Consumers have the option of reporting businesses or their representatives directly. Still, other factors besides worry about an adverse outcome could influence a customer to contact a company. Legal issues and, most typically, requests for further product information are among them. Consumer reports can also come from a few industry programs where details about adverse reactions may be requested; these cases are not considered spontaneous reports (WHO 2004).

12.3.4 Information from Other Sources

Toxicities to the following may be reported in connection with herbal medicine issues.

- National poison centers may be crucial in the pharmacovigilance and safety monitoring of herbal medicines in countries with inadequate resources and no formal pharmacovigilance centers.
- Drug information centers are the first point of contact and a potential source of clinical data. The communication between these centers and national pharmacovigilance centers should be good.
- National guidelines on good clinical practice for trials on pharmaceutical products (GCP) should apply to clinical trials and studies that report adverse events that occur during clinical trials (WHO 2004).

12.3.5 ADRs Reported Herbal Drugs

The various herbal–drug interactions are shown in Table 12.1.

Table 12.1 Herbal–drugs interactions

Herbal drug	Herb–drug interaction	Main outcome	References
St. John's wort *(Hypericum perforatum)*	This substance induces CYP1A2, increasing drug metabolism. It also induces CYP3A4 and P-gP	Warfarin and its anticoagulant action, protease inhibitors, and atorvastatin will be less effective when co-administered with cyclosporine, which may also result in transplant graft rejection	Markowitz et al. (2000)
Ginger *(Zingiber officinalis)*	It inhibits thromboxane synthetase, prolonging bleeding time	Ginger may interact with warfarin-like drugs and cause an excess of bleeding while also extending the bleeding time	Nutescu et al. (2006)
Garlic *(Allium sativum)*	Induces CYP3A4, reducing drug metabolism, and inhibits CYP2C9 and P-gP	Decreased saquinavir metabolism can cause adverse drug reactions, increased bleeding risk with warfarin, and reduced docetaxel clearance	Piscitelli et al. (2002)
Tea *(Camellia sinensis)*, coffee *(Coffea arabica)*	Significantly increase the acidity in stomach	Consuming tea or coffee can reduce the effectiveness of penicillin and erythromycin due to increased stomach acidity, leading to antibiotic degradation	Dent et al. (2005); El-Serag (2007)
Liquorice *(Glycyrrhiza glabra)*	Glycyrrhizin in liquorice, an 11-keto steroid, can affect CYP2C9 and 3A4 induction and mimic corticosteroid actions	Warfarin and lidocaine reduce actions, while corticosteroids enhance effects via synergy. Spironolactone effects are increased	Penninkilampi et al. (2017)
Gingko *(Ginkgo biloba)*	It blocks the activity of a liver enzyme CYP2C9	The metabolism of drugs such as celecoxib, glipizide, tolbutamide, piroxicam, and tamoxifen may be significantly decreased	Robertson et al. (2008)
Tulsi *(Ocimum sanctum)*	The active compounds in tulsi, such as eugenol, carvacrol, and linalool inhibit CYP1A1&1B1. This prevents the conversion of the procarcinogen benzo [a] pyrene to toxic diol epoxide	Benzo[a]pyrene becomes toxic when converted to diol epoxides by CYP1A1 and CYP1B1 in the liver. Repeated exposure can cause skin darkening, thickening, and pimples	Uma Devi (2001); Kim et al. (1998)

(continued)

Table 12.1 (continued)

Herbal drug	Herb–drug interaction	Main outcome	References
Grapefruit juice *(Citrus ×paradisi)*	Grapefruit juice inhibits drug-metabolizing enzymes (CYP1A2, CYP3A4, CYP2C9), leading to higher drug levels in the bloodstream and potential toxicity	The intake of this medication can lead to an increase in the blood levels of saquinavir, acyclovir, lovastatin, atorvastatin, nifedipine, amiodarone, clomipramine, and carbamazepine	Bailey et al. (1998)
Pippali *(Piper longum L.)*	The blocking of CYP3A4, CYP2D6, and CYP1A2 enzymes	The effectiveness of drugs such as verapamil, digoxin, and propranolol is reduced	Shaikh et al. (2020)
Coneflower *(Echinacea angustifolia)* Purple coneflower *(Echinacea purpure)*	Antagonistic effects	Echinacea's immunostimulant properties can reduce the efficacy of immunosuppressive medications	Mamindla et al. (2016)
Aloe vera *(Aloe barbadensis miller.)*	There is a possibility of developing hypokalemia	When taken in combination with corticosteroids or diuretics	Boudreau and Beland (2006)
Amla *(Phyllanthus emblica)*	Amla is rich in tannins which bind with iron. Raw amla powder is recommended due to degradation of ascorbic acid at high temperature. Additionally, amla contains high levels of calcium	Consuming raw amla powder can lower iron levels and reduce the effect of iron tonics. However, excessive intake of amla may lead to kidney stones	Gowri et al. (2001)
Sweet flag *(Acorus calamus)*, tomato *(Solanum lycopersicum)* (melatonin), and pomegranate *(Punica granatum)*	Additive effects	Taking carbamazepine together with these herbs can enhance its anti-epileptic effects	Sharma et al. (2022)
Ashwagandha *(Withania somnifera)*	Ashwagandha induces the activity of CYP3A4, and it also exhibits synergistic effects	When administered with ritonavir, ashwagandha protects blood cells and liver from drug-induced damage. Additionally, when combined with benzodiazepines, it may enhance the sedative effects of drugs like clonazepam, diazepam, or lorazepam	Nagaraj and Veeresham (2018)

(continued)

Table 12.1 (continued)

Herbal drug	Herb–drug interaction	Main outcome	References
Turmeric *(Curcuma longa L.)*	Inhibition of CYP3A4, CYP1A2, CYP2B6, CYP2C19, CYP2C9	The effects of losartan, rosuvastatin, warfarin, and clopidogrel will be decreased	Shaikh et al. (2020)
Passion flower *(Passiflora incarnata)*	Additive effects	Increase the potency of CNS depressant drugs	Ernst (2003)
Peppermint *(Mentha piperita L.)*	Inhibition of CYP3A4	The effect of felodipine will be increased	Costache et al. (2019)
Pepper *(Piper nigrum)*	Enhance absorption	To improve the absorption and effectiveness of phenytoin and propranolol	Bano et al. (1991)
Garden heliotrope *(Valeriana officinalis),* Sugandhbala *(V. Wallichii)*	Synergistic effect	It enhances the impact of central nervous system depressants	Houghton (1988)
Kava (*Piper methysticum*) Bromelain pineapple (*Ananas comosus*), saw palmetto (*Serenoa repens*)	Induce CYP2C9	The efficacy of the anticoagulant medication, warfarin, will be notably decreased	Nutescu et al. (2006); Almeida and Grimsley (1996)
Flax seeds, marshmallow, and aloes	Preventing certain drugs from being absorbed into the body	These herbs contain large amounts of mucilage, which can inhibit drug absorption	Kuhn (1999)

12.4 Reporting of ADRs Related to Herbal Medicines

An essential component of pharmacovigilance, which involves monitoring and assessing the safety of herbal medications, is reporting adverse drug reactions (ADRs). The process flow of ADR reporting is shown in Fig. 12.2. Despite their widespread use and perceived safety, herbal medicines can nonetheless have adverse effects because of their complicated chemical makeup, hazy pharmacology, and toxicity (Chang et al. 2021). Reporting and analyzing ADRs related to these products are crucial for ensuring the proper and safe use of herbal medications. Like pharmacovigilance for conventional drugs, herbovigilance uses a reporting method for adverse drug reactions. Healthcare professionals and patients should notify the appropriate regulatory agency or pharmacovigilance center when they notice or have an adverse reaction to an herbal drug. Regulatory authorities offer online reporting platforms as well as specialized forms for reporting. These reports are essential for identifying, evaluating, comprehending, and avoiding adverse effects or other drug-related issues related to herbal medicines (Sharma and Kellarai 2014).

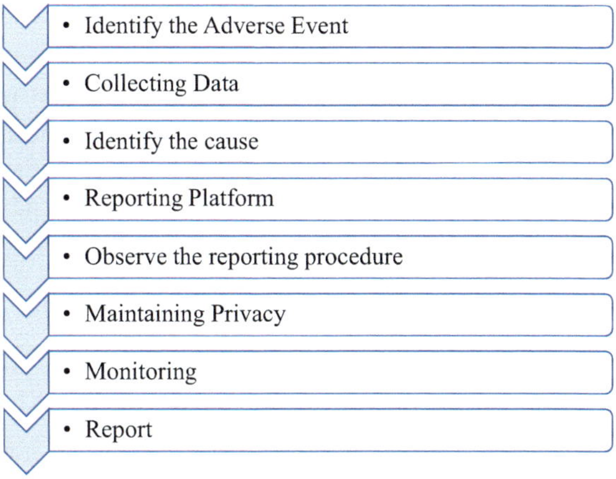

Fig. 12.2 Process flow of ADRs reporting

Overcoming the difficulties of underreporting ADRs is crucial in the context of herbovigilance. Underreporting occurs for various reasons, including lack of knowledge, the belief that herbal remedies are safe, insufficient training of healthcare workers, and a need for a well-established reporting culture (Walji et al. 2009). Educating medical professionals, herbalists, and consumers about the significance of reporting adverse drug reactions (ADRs) related to herbal medicines is essential if herbovigilance is to enhance ADRs reporting. Healthcare personnel's knowledge and abilities in recognizing and reporting ADRs can be improved by education and training programs that can be put in place (Al-Worafi et al. 2017).

Effective herbovigilance requires close coordination between regulatory agencies, medical experts, herbalists, and consumers. The safety profile of herbal medications can be enhanced by establishing reliable reporting mechanisms, carrying out post-marketing monitoring studies, and encouraging active participation in ADRs reporting (Hadi et al. 2017). It is important to note that different nations or areas may have different rules and laws for writing ADRs in herbovigilance, so it is essential to adhere to the precise instructions given by the relevant regulatory authorities.

Regulatory agencies and healthcare organizations publish the general reporting standards for adverse events to report adverse drug reactions (ADRs) in herbovigilance. Although there might not be specific guidelines for herbovigilance, the fundamentals of writing ADRs apply to all classes of medicinal drugs. The following is a thorough method for reporting ADRs in herbovigilance.

12.4.1 Identify the Adverse Event

Reporting herbal medications with unanticipated, severe, or adverse effects is essential. This includes adverse effects inconsistent with the product package insert or labeling and those related to using new herbal products that have been on the market for under 5 years (Chang et al. 2021).

12.4.2 Collecting Data

Collect all pertinent details regarding the herbal product and the adverse event before filing an ADR. The minimal information needed to file a report varies but is often composed of data on the patient's demographics, the name of the herbal product, the batch number, the dosage, the mode of administration, the start and end dates of usage, a description of the adverse event, and its seriousness (Martin and Lucas 2021).

12.4.3 Identify the Cause

Examine the link between using the herbal product and the occurrence of the unfavorable event. Healthcare practitioners should make an initial assessment when reporting severe ADRs, but businesses can refrain from concurring with that opinion. ADRs reporting form in India has been shown in Fig. 12.3.

12.4.4 Reporting Platforms

Several regulatory agencies and nations have their reporting systems. In Singapore, the Health Sciences Authority (HSA) can be notified of adverse incidents involving therapeutic items, including herbal medications. In Australia, reports may be reported to the Database of Adverse Event Notifications (DAEN), which keeps track of adverse drug events, including those involving herbal remedies (Martin and Lucas 2021).

12.4.5 Observe the Reporting Procedure

There might be unique procedures and paperwork for each reporting system. Make sure the adverse event is reported accurately and entirely by familiarizing yourself with the reporting requirements of the relevant authorities (Martin and Lucas 2021).

12.4.6 Maintaining Privacy

Patient confidentiality is a top priority for adverse event reporting systems. Ensure patient data is safeguarded and registered securely, adhering to data protection laws and standards.

Patient/consumer identification (please complete or tick boxes below as appropriate)

Last name	**First name(s)**	**Patient/record number**
Ethnicity		
Address (place and region, or health facility may be used)		**Date of birth**
		Sex ☐M ☐F

List of all medicines/vaccines/herbal medicines used by the patient. Please indicate suspected medicines with an asterisk (*) (please complete boxes below)

Medicine(s)Vaccine(s) + batch no.	Daily dose	Route of administration	Date started	Date stopped	Reason for use

For herbal medicines please give detailed information on the product

Product name:

How was the product obtained?

List of product ingredients; attach product label if available:

Name and address of the manufacturer;

Name and address of the distributor:

Other relevant information:

Description of the suspected adverse reaction (please complete boxes below)

Date of onset of reaction (dd/mm/yy):
Description of reaction (please include results of laboratory tests if available):

Outcome of the suspected adverse reaction (please tick boxes as appropriate)

Recovered ☐	Not yet recovered ☐	Unknown ☐	Fatal ☐	Date of death
Severe? Yes ☐ No ☐		Rechallenge? Result:	Yes ☐	No ☐
Was the patient admitted to hospital? If yes, give name and address of hospital:			Yes ☐	No ☐

Other factors (please tick box or describe as appropriate)

Kidney disease ☐	Liver disease ☐	Allergy (please describe) ....
Other illnesses (please describe):		Malnutrition ☐

Reporter identification

Type (please circle): nurse/doctor/pharmacist/other health worker /manufacturer/ distributor/supplier
Name:
Address: Telephone:
E-mail address:

Signature of reporter: .... Date: ....

Please send completed form to: ....

Fig. 12.3 ADRs reporting form in India

12.4.7 Monitoring

The regulatory body or healthcare organization may occasionally ask for more details or explanations. Be cooperative and prompt in providing any follow-up data required to support the investigation and assessment of the reported ADRs.

Reporting adverse drug reactions (ADRs) in herbovigilance enables healthcare authorities and organizations to take the necessary steps to protect public health and safety as well as the overall safety monitoring and assessment of herbal medications.

12.5 Regulatory Aspects of Herbal Medicines

Regulatory aspects of herbal medicines vary across different countries and regions. The classification and regulations surrounding herbal medicines can differ based on the national and regional frameworks in place. The global trade in medicinal plants and their derivatives is substantial and expected to increase in the coming years. Different countries and regions have distinct regulatory frameworks and categories for herbal medicines. These classifications include medicines (Australia), herbal medical products (European Union), botanicals (USA), natural health products (Canada), traditional Chinese medicine (China), Ayurveda, Unani, and Siddha (India), and others (Bilia et al. 2022).

Due to patients' potential for treatment and acceptance, herbal remedies have become more critical in healthcare. Different plant components or their separated phytoconstituents are used when using herbal remedies. In the search for innovative medicines, there has been interest in studying herbal medications made from natural resources. Most medications utilized in contemporary treatment are natural products (Barkat et al. 2020).

The regulatory environment is not uniform because of the many regulatory standards for herbal goods worldwide. The worldwide trade and expansion of herbal goods need to be more consistent due to the absence of uniformity and problems with herb availability and preservation (Sharma 2015).

The regulatory environment surrounding nutritional supplements and herbal medications is a global concern. The growing use of these items has sparked discussions regarding the goods' quality, effectiveness, and safety. Due to the various public perceptions and classifications of these goods, regulatory authorities need to help ensure herbal treatments' safety and effective monitoring (Thakkar et al. 2020).

Drugs made from plants must undergo rigorous clinical trials, which bring unique hurdles. Clinical trials are crucial given that traditional medicine is the primary source of healthcare for approximately 80% of the world's population. Certain nations, such as China, Japan, and Germany, have national policies for conventional medicine and laws governing herbal medications (Parveen et al. 2015).

Herbal medications are included in the legal definition of alternative and complementary medicine, which has gained acceptance worldwide. They must be preserved and made available, which requires international collaboration and coordination. Guidelines from the World Health Organization (WHO) and the European Union establish standards for analyzing herbal remedies' effectiveness, safety, and quality (Ajazuddin and Saraf 2012).

More scientific information has become available to support both the efficacy and safety of herbal remedies. Even though natural herbs have long been used extensively, many herbal products need more scientific support. Although complementary and herbal therapy is still being researched, Western medicine has limits when treating complicated chronic disorders (Zhang et al. 2015).

The safety, effectiveness, and overall quality of herbal medicine are difficult for regulatory bodies to ensure, particularly during pregnancy. The public frequently views herbal items as traditional treatments or healthy dietary supplements, making regulation less necessary. However, laws governing foods, medications, and cosmetics are commonplace, including provisions for herbal medicines (Rousseaux and Schachter 2003).

Regulatory science has advanced in the pharmaceutical industry but has not progressed significantly in nutritional supplements and herbal medicines. These fields frequently need to pay more attention to risk identification, assessment, and supervision. Regulatory science must be improved to ensure the safety and quality of herbal remedies and nutritional supplements (Tsutani and Takuma 2008).

In the case of Traditional Indian Medicines (TIM), regulatory aspects are vital in both the Indian and international contexts. Regulatory affairs are crucial in controlling the safety and efficacy of various products, including herbal medicines. Governments implement policies to protect public health by establishing approval criteria for pharmaceuticals, complementary treatments, veterinary drugs, medical devices, food products, and cosmetics (Sharma and Pundarikakshudu 2019).

12.6 WHO Guidelines for Safety Monitoring in Herbovigilance

The World Health Organization (WHO) issued recommendations regarding pharmacovigilance networks that keep track of the security of herbal treatments. These recommendations give advice and detailed ways to monitor the safety of herbal drugs. Some key concepts are outlined below regarding the connection with pharmacovigilance and the safety surveillance for herbal medicines. On its website, the World Health Organization provides a document with guidelines for the safety surveillance of herbal medications in pharmacovigilance networks. The rules seek to ensure the security of using herbal drugs and offer direction on ensuring their security. The 18-page set of instructions is available in three languages: English, Spanish, and Chinese (WHO 2004). The research and practices involved in identifying, assessing, comprehending, and preventing adverse effects of drugs and associated issues are referred to as pharmacovigilance (Shetti et al. 2011).

The safety of pharmaceuticals and vaccines is ensured via pharmacovigilance, according to the WHO (World Health Organization 2002). Pharmacovigilance includes collecting, analyzing, and reporting information for adverse drug reactions

(ADRs) to monitor and control medication-related risks. Digital health technology can help with writing, gathering, and analyzing data on adverse events and the safety of drugs, which can assist in pharmacovigilance and risk surveillance. The WHO also offers recommendations for general safety monitoring of pharmaceuticals, including guidance for the public to use when documenting adverse reactions (World Health Organization 2012).

12.7 Current Scenario of Herbovigilance in India

Herbovigilance is the term used to describe the surveillance and reporting of adverse effects or problems involving herbal remedies in India. The data shows no specific details or inquiries regarding the herbovigilance scenario in India exist. The data collected through online resources focuses primarily on the pharmacovigilance program in India and pharmacovigilance in general.

In India, pharmacovigilance ensures the monitoring of and assessment of adverse drug reactions (ADRs) by pharmaceuticals. To improve the system for drug safety monitoring in the nation, the National Programme of Pharmacovigilance, subsequently known as the Pharmacovigilance Programme of India (PvPI), became operational in 2005. The initiative aims to identify, analyze, recognize, and prevent adverse drug reactions related to drugs. The Indian Pharmacopoeia Commission (IPC) manages PvPI coordination (Kalaiselvan et al. 2019).

Herbovigilance, connected explicitly to herbal remedies, might not be a unique or specialized program in India. The current pharmacovigilance system includes surveillance of adverse reactions associated with pharmaceutical and herbal medicines. The regulatory authority responsible for pharmacovigilance activities, including those related to herbal products, is the Central Drugs Standard Control Organization (CDSCO) (Pansare et al. 2021). However, the available information should provide further details regarding the current status and specific activities related to herbovigilance in India.

12.8 Herbovigilance Overview Worldwide

Herbovigilance is the term used to describe the monitoring and surveillance of adverse reactions related to herbal remedies and products. It also covers detecting, assessing, comprehending, and preventing other possible drug-related problems related to herbal and conventional treatments. Herbovigilance seeks to ensure the efficacy and security of these products while safeguarding the general public's health.

The current scenario with herbal vigilance globally reveals specific difficulties and causes for concern. Most reported side effects from using herbal medicines result from misusing them or using low-quality products. Inadequate regulatory controls, feeble quality assurance procedures, and unrestrained distribution channels, such as mail order and online sales, make such situations more likely. Reduce or minimize incidents brought on by these circumstances to increase knowledge about natural adverse reactions to herbal medications and prevent resource waste (Shetti et al. 2011).

To improve the monitoring of herbal medicines' safety, the World Health Organization (WHO) has developed guidelines for their safety monitoring in pharmacovigilance systems. The existing pharmacovigilance systems can use these principles to enhance monitoring and widen the area of safety monitoring for herbal medications.

Although there is a need for more information about herbovigilance globally, some nations and regions are putting their pharmacovigilance systems in place to monitor the safety of herbal drugs. For instance, herbovigilance has received attention on the Indian subcontinent, and attempts have been made to fully identify, evaluate, comprehend, and prevent harmful effects associated with herbal, traditional, and complementary therapies. Herbovigilance attempts to ensure the secure and efficient utilization of herbal remedies, much to pharmacovigilance methods for conventional medication (Verma and Shah 2018).

It is crucial to remember that "herbovigilance" may not be generally accepted or developed as a separate field in all geographical areas. The emphasis on monitoring and guaranteeing the safety of herbal medications may come under the more general category of pharmacovigilance, which includes the monitoring and evaluation of adverse drug responses for many medicines (Felix et al. 2019). However, attempts are being made to address the unique characteristics and difficulties related to herbal and conventional drugs in pharmacovigilance systems.

12.9 Future Prospects

Future prospects for herbovigilance involve addressing concerns and improving patient safety related to the use of herbal medicines. Herbovigilance, also known as pharmacovigilance for herbal medicines, focuses on monitoring and assessing the safety of herbal products to identify any adverse effects or interactions that may occur when these medicines are consumed.

The following factors should be considered while evaluating the prospects for herbovigilance in the future.

Growing acceptance of herbal medicines: Due to the assumption that herbal medications are safer than traditional allopathic therapies, their use is expanding globally. Despite this impression, specific herbal formulations have been linked to documented toxicity incidents and unfavorable medication interactions if administered improperly (Choudhury et al. 2023).

Improved safety monitoring is required. As the use of herbal medications increases, a strong and thorough pharmacovigilance system tailored to herbal products is needed. To protect patients, a system like this should be able to record and analyze adverse drug reactions, herb–drug interactions, and herb toxicity (Divakar 2022).

The complete scientific assessments are essential in identifying the challenges and safety concerns associated with herbal medications. This approach uses data from several scientific platforms to analyze information about pharmacovigilance, conventional medicine, adverse drug reactions, underreporting, and other pertinent topics (Choudhury et al. 2023).

Using herbal medicines worldwide requires international cooperation to build effective pharmacovigilance protocols. Information and data on the safety of herbal medications can be shared, which could lead to better patient outcomes and a fuller understanding of potential risks and advantages (Choudhury et al. 2023).

Integration of Herbovigilance with Current Systems includes the pharmacovigilance system, which focuses primarily on monitoring contemporary drugs. This method requires expansion and reorientation to have specific considerations for herbal medicines. This might make it easier to collect data on clinically critical herb–drug interactions and improve our understanding of the safety profiles of herbal treatments (Divakar 2022).

Utilizing Digital Health Technologies with the growth of social media, mobile apps, and digital health tools, it is possible to proactively monitor patient health and identify adverse events connected to herbal medications at an early stage. Information on the interactions and safety of pharmaceuticals can be learned by watching social media and digital health data (Sollers Edu 2021).

Addressing challenges involves underreporting adverse effects, and the limited degree of patient and healthcare professional awareness may make it challenging to adopt herbal vigilance. Education and awareness campaigns are required to encourage reporting and improve safety monitoring to overcome these challenges (Pubrica-Academy 2021).

It includes developing a targeted and complete pharmacovigilance system specifically for herbal medications. International collaboration, digital health tools, and problem-solving are crucial to ensure the safe use of herbal medicines and enhance patient outcomes. Healthcare systems may make educated judgments and give patients and practitioners evidence-based recommendations by consistently assessing the safety of herbal products.

12.10 Future Obstacles

Future obstacles to herbovigilance may arise from various factors. Here are some potential challenges that could impact the monitoring and regulation of herbal medicines.

Inadequate regulatory measures, such as adverse incidents involving herbal items, may occur due to insufficient oversight and restrictions. It may be difficult to guarantee product quality and safety if distribution channels, including online sales, are unmanaged and have weak quality control procedures (Shetti et al. 2011).

The need for standardized guidelines makes establishing standardized regulations for pharmacovigilance challenging since herbal medicines have a wide range of uses and are traded and regulated through various channels and formats. The application of efficient monitoring systems needs to be improved by this complexity (Rasmussen 2022).

Limited resources for identifying and analyzing adverse events: The limited resources may make it challenging to identify and examine adverse occurrences linked to herbal medications. Reduce or minimize incidents brought on by subpar product quality and inappropriate use to ensure effective herbovigilance (Shetti et al. 2011).

Lack of knowledge, education, and effective herbovigilance might be hampered by healthcare professionals and the public needing to be sufficiently informed on herbal medications' possible dangers and interactions. It is crucial to improve instruction and spread knowledge about using herbal products responsibly (Divakar 2022).

Integrating herbovigilance into current healthcare systems and securing cooperation between traditional medicine practitioners and regulatory agencies can be difficult in areas where conventional medicine is widely practiced. The monitoring of the security of herbal medicines can be facilitated by harmonizing these procedures (Rasmussen 2022).

Lack of comprehensive data and evidence: The herbovigilance initiatives are hampered by the need for more thorough information on the safety and efficacy of herbal medicines. Substantial evidence is required to identify and assess adverse events, drug interactions, and possible dangers related to herbal medicines (Toklu 2016).

It is crucial to understand that the list of potential obstacles in herbovigilance field is not exhaustive and is constantly changing. To overcome these challenges, regulatory agencies, healthcare practitioners, investigators, and the herbal drug industry must collaborate to ensure that patients can safely and effectively use herbal remedies in the future.

12.11 Conclusion

Conventional medicine commonly depends on herbal therapies that are essential to public health. Herbovigilance is gathering, evaluating, and analyzing information about the potential risk factors and adverse impacts of herbal medicines. Herbovigilance's primary objective is to ensure that citizens are informed of the risk assessment of herbal remedies and to actively watch and report any potential risks, which might assist in the establishment of adequate specifications. The herbovigilance in India has several obstacles, including absence of regulation of herbal medicines and insufficient reporting of adverse occurrences. As a result, establishing an effective platform for the surveillance and control of herbal medicines is essential for encouraging ethical consumption and protecting the well-being of the public. A nationwide database of adverse occurrences should be created, post-marketing surveillance should be implemented, and guidelines should be developed for both herbal medicine producers and medical practitioners. Herbovigilance can successfully assure the potency as well as security of conventional herbal treatments while encouraging responsible usage by employing these strategies.

References

Ahmad Khan MS, Ahmad I (2018) Herbal medicine: current trends and future prospects. In: New look to phytomedicine: advancements in herbal products as novel drug leads. Academic, Cambridge, MA. https://doi.org/10.1016/B978-0-12-814619-4.00001-X

Ajazuddin, Saraf S (2012) Legal regulations of complementary and alternative medicines in different countries. Pharmacogn Rev 6(12):154. https://doi.org/10.4103/0973-7847.99950

Almeida JC, Grimsley EW (1996) Coma from the health food store: interaction between kava and alprazolam [7]. Ann Intern Med 125(11):940. https://doi.org/10.7326/0003-4819-125-11-199612010-00023

Al-Worafi YM et al (2017) Pharmacovigilance and adverse drug reaction reporting: a perspective of community pharmacists and pharmacy technicians in Sana'a, Yemen. Ther Clin Risk Manag 13:1175. https://doi.org/10.2147/TCRM.S140674

Bailey DG, Malcolm J, Arnold O, Spence JD (1998) Grapefruit juice-drug interactions. Br J Clin Pharmacol 46(2):101. https://doi.org/10.1046/j.1365-2125.1998.00764.x

Bano G, Raina RK, Zutshi U, Bedi KL, Johri RK, Sharma SC (1991) Effect of piperine on bioavailability and pharmacokinetics of propranolol and theophylline in healthy volunteers. Eur J Clin Pharmacol 41(6):615. https://doi.org/10.1007/BF00314996

Barkat MA, Goyal A, Barkat HA, Salauddin M, Pottoo FH, Anwer ET (2020) Herbal medicine: clinical perspective and regulatory status. Comb Chem High Throughput Screen 24(10):1573. https://doi.org/10.2174/1386207323999201110192942

Barkat A, Goyal A, Harshita A, Pottoo FH, Beg S, Ahmad FJ (2019) Herbal medicine: current progress, and challenges. Curr Bioact Compd 15. https://doi.org/10.2174/1573407215666191111114853

Barnes J (2022) Pharmacovigilance for herbal and traditional medicines: advances, challenges and international perspectives. Springer, Cham. https://doi.org/10.1007/978-3-031-07275-8

Bhimaneni S, Sharma R, Dey P, Kumar A (2021) Pharmacovigilance of herbal medicines: an overview. In: Evidence based validation of traditional medicines: a comprehensive approach. Springer, Cham. https://doi.org/10.1007/978-981-15-8127-4_25

Bilia AR et al (2022) Editorial: drug development of herbal medicines: regulatory perspectives. Front Pharmacol 13:989934. https://doi.org/10.3389/fphar.2022.989934

Boudreau MD, Beland FA (2006) An evaluation of the biological and toxicological properties of Aloe barbadensis (miller), Aloe vera. J Environ Sci Health C Environ Carcinog Ecotoxicol Rev 24(1):103. https://doi.org/10.1080/10590500600614303

Chang HH et al (2021) A system for reporting and evaluating adverse drug reactions of herbal medicine in Taiwan from 1998 to 2016. Sci Rep 11(1):21416. https://doi.org/10.1038/s41598-021-00704-w

Choudhury A, Singh PA, Bajwa N, Dash S, Bisht P (2023) Pharmacovigilance of herbal medicines: concerns and future prospects. J Ethnopharmacol 309:116383. https://doi.org/10.1016/j.jep.2023.116383

Costache II, Miron A, Hăncianu M, Aursulesei V, Costache AD, Aprotosoaie AC (2019) Pharmacokinetic interactions between cardiovascular medicines and plant products. Cardiovasc Ther 2019:1. https://doi.org/10.1155/2019/9402781

Dent J, El-Serag HB, Wallander MA, Johansson S (2005) Epidemiology of gastro-oesophageal reflux disease: a systematic review. Gut 54(5):710. https://doi.org/10.1136/gut.2004.051821

Divakar MC (2022) The need for Herbovigilance. Int J Adv Res (Indore) 10(11):34–44. https://doi.org/10.21474/IJAR01/15639

Ekor M (2014) The growing use of herbal medicines: issues relating to adverse reactions and challenges in monitoring safety. Front Neurol 4:177. https://doi.org/10.3389/fphar.2013.00177

El-Serag HB (2007) Time trends of gastroesophageal reflux disease: a systematic review. Clin Gastroenterol Hepatol 5(1):17. https://doi.org/10.1016/j.cgh.2006.09.016

Ernst E (2003) Serious psychiatric and neurological adverse effects of herbal medicines - a systematic review. Acta Psychiatr Scand 108(2):83. https://doi.org/10.1034/j.1600-0447.2003.00158.x

Felix T, Jordan JB, Akers C, Patel B, Drago D (2019) Current state of biologic pharmacovigilance in the European Union: improvements are needed. Expert Opin Drug Saf 18(3):231. https://doi.org/10.1080/14740338.2019.1577818

Fornasier G, Francescon S, Leone R, Baldo P (2018) An historical overview over pharmacovigilance. Int J Clin Pharm 40(4):744. https://doi.org/10.1007/s11096-018-0657-1

Gowri BS, Platel K, Prakash J, Srinivasan K (2001) Influence of amla fruits (Emblica officinalis) on the bio-availability of iron from staple cereals and pulses. Nutr Res 21(12):1483. https://doi.org/10.1016/S0271-5317(01)00362-1

Gruszycki Kisiel MR, Tauguinas Pérez AL, Baez Carrizo M, Alba Díaz DA, Gruszycki Kisiel AE (2017) Importance of pharmacovigilance in herbal medicine. Rev Cub de Plantas Med 22(1):1

Hadi MA, Neoh CF, Zin RM, Elrggal M, Cheema E (2017) Pharmacovigilance: pharmacists' perspective on spontaneous adverse drug reaction reporting. Integr Pharm Res Pract Volume 6:91. https://doi.org/10.2147/iprp.s105881

Hassan MAG (2014) Need to incorporate pharmacovigilance of herbal medicine to the curriculum. Natl J Physiol Pharm Pharmacol 4(2):99. https://doi.org/10.5455/njppp.2014.4.080620141

Houghton PJ (1988) The biological activity of valerian and related plants. J Ethnopharmacol 22(2):121. https://doi.org/10.1016/0378-8741(88)90123-7

Hugman B, Skalli S (2022) Pharmacovigilance and risk communication for the safe use of herbal and traditional medicines: how to promote evidence and keep people safe. In: Pharmacovigilance for herbal and traditional medicines: advances, challenges and international perspectives. Springer, Cham. https://doi.org/10.1007/978-3-031-07275-8_15

Kalaiselvan V, Srivastava S, Singh A, Gupta S (2019) Pharmacovigilance in India: present scenario and future challenges. Drug Saf 42(3):339. https://doi.org/10.1007/s40264-018-0730-7

Kim JH, Stansbury KH, Walker NJ, Trush MA, Strickland PT, Sutter TR (1998) Metabolism of benzo[α]pyrene and benzo[α]pyrene-7,8-diol by human cytochrome P450 1B1. Carcinogenesis 19(10):1847. https://doi.org/10.1093/carcin/19.10.1847

Kuhn MA (1999) Complementary therapies for health care. Lippincott Williams & Wilkins, Philadelphia, PA. https://books.google.co.in/books/about/Complementary_Therapies_for_Health_Care.html?id=XrK3zQEACAAJ&redir_esc=y. Accessed 21 Sep 2023.

Mamindla S, Kvsrg P, Koganti B (2016) Herb-drug interactions: an overview of mechanisms and clinical aspects. Int J Pharm Sci Res 7(9):3576

Markowitz JS, DeVane CL, Boulton DW, Carson SW, Nahas Z, Risch SC (2000) Effect of St. John's wort (Hypericum perforatum) on cytochrome P-450 2D6 and 3A4 activity in healthy volunteers. Life Sci 66(9):PL133. https://doi.org/10.1016/s0024-3205(99)00659-1

Martin JH, Lucas C (2021) Reporting adverse drug events to the therapeutic goods administration. Aust Prescr 44(1):2. https://doi.org/10.18773/austprescr.2020.077

Nagaraj B, Veeresham C (2018) Effect of ashwagandha on pharmacokinetic and pharmacodynamic parameters of glimepiride in streptozotocin-induced diabetic rats. Asian J Pharm Clin Res 11(4):207. https://doi.org/10.22159/ajpcr.2018.v11i4.23960

Nutescu EA, Shapiro NL, Ibrahim S, West P (2006) Warfarin and its interactions with foods, herbs and other dietary supplements. Expert Opin Drug Saf 5(3):433. https://doi.org/10.1517/14740338.5.3.433

Pansare K, Sonawane G, Tapadiya P, Tapadiya R, Patil C, Vaghela JS, Kokate S (2021) History, current status and future aspects of pharmacovigilance in India. NVEO 8:1558–1565

Parveen A, Parveen B, Parveen R, Ahmad S (2015) Challenges and guidelines for clinical trial of herbal drugs. J Pharm Bioallied Sci 7:329. https://doi.org/10.4103/0975-7406.168035

Penninkilampi R, Eslick EM, Eslick GD (2017) The association between consistent licorice ingestion, hypertension and hypokalaemia: a systematic review and meta-analysis. J Hum Hypertens 31(11):699. https://doi.org/10.1038/jhh.2017.45

Piscitelli SC, Burstein AH, Welden N, Gallicano KD, Falloon J (2002) The effect of garlic supplements on the pharmacokinetics of saquinavir. Clin Infect Dis 34(2):234. https://doi.org/10.1086/324351

Pubrica-Academy (2021)"Recent trends, challenges and future prospects in literature surveillance of pharmacovigilance." *Pubrica*

Rahman S, Rashid S (2020) Pharmacovigilance approach to tropical natural drugs, fruits and supplement. Int J Curr Adv Res 9:22112–22116. https://doi.org/10.24327/ijcar.2020.22116.4357

Rahman S, Ruknuddin G (2022) History of Pharmacovigilance in India (1983–2022). J Pharmacovigil Drug Saf 19:6–17. https://doi.org/10.21276/jpds.2021.19.01.02

Rasmussen P (2022) Pharmacovigilance for herbal medicines: a perspective from the herbal medicines industry. In: Pharmacovigilance for herbal and traditional medicines: advances, challenges and international perspectives. Springer, Cham, pp 249–259. https://doi.org/10.1007/978-3-031-07275-8_14

Robertson SM, Davey RT, Voell J, Formentini E, Alfaro RM, Penzak SR (2008) Effect of Ginkgo biloba extract on lopinavir, midazolam and fexofenadine pharmacokinetics in healthy subjects. Curr Med Res Opin 24(2):591. https://doi.org/10.1185/030079908X260871

Rousseaux CG, Schachter H (2003) Regulatory issues concerning the safety, efficacy and quality of herbal remedies. Birth Defects Res B Dev Reprod Toxicol 68(6):505. https://doi.org/10.1002/bdrb.10053

Shaikh AS, Thomas AB, Chitlange SS (2020) Herb–drug interaction studies of herbs used in treatment of cardiovascular disorders—a narrative review of preclinical and clinical studies. Phytother Res 34(5):1008. https://doi.org/10.1002/ptr.6585

Sharma S (2015) Current status of herbal product: regulatory overview. J Pharm Bioallied Sci 7:293. https://doi.org/10.4103/0975-7406.168030

Sharma AK, Kapoor VK, Kaur G (2022) Herb–drug interactions: a mechanistic approach. Drug Chem Toxicol 45(2):594. https://doi.org/10.1080/01480545.2020.1738454

Sharma R, Kellarai A (2014) Pharmacovigilance and adverse drug reaction reporting perspectives among interns and postgraduates of a teaching hospital. J Pharmacol Pharmacother 5(4):248. https://doi.org/10.4103/0976-500X.142436

Sharma AK, Pundarikakshudu K (2019) Regulatory aspects of traditional Indian medicines (TIM) in India and in international purview. J AOAC Int 102(4):993. https://doi.org/10.5740/jaoacint.18-0379

Shetti S, Kumar CD, Sriwastava NK, Sharma IP (2011) Pharmacovigilance of herbal medicines: current state and future directions. Pharmacogn Mag 7(25):69. https://doi.org/10.4103/0973-1296.75905

Skalli S, Wang JB, Hugman B (2022) Pharmacovigilance of herbal medicines: the vigilance of tomorrow. In: Evidence-based validation of herbal medicine: translational research on botanicals. Elsevier, Amsterdam. https://doi.org/10.1016/B978-0-323-85542-6.00001-9

Sollers Edu (2021) Future prospects of pharmacovigilance. Sollers College, Piscataway, NJ

Thakkar S et al (2020) Regulatory landscape of dietary supplements and herbal medicines from a global perspective. Regul Toxicol Pharmacol 114:104647. https://doi.org/10.1016/j.yrtph.2020.104647

Thillaivanan S (2014) Challenges, constraints and opportunities in herbal medicines-a review. Int J Herb Med 2(1):2321

Toklu HZ (2016) Pharmacovigilance of herbal medicine: Herbovigilance. Adv Pharmacoepidemiol Drug Saf 5(4):1–3. https://doi.org/10.4172/2167-1052.1000208

Tsutani K, Takuma H (2008) Regulatory sciences in herbal medicines and dietary supplements. Yakugaku Zasshi 128(6):867. https://doi.org/10.1248/yakushi.128.867

Uma Devi P (2001) Radioprotective, anticarcinogenic and antioxidant properties of the Indian holy basil, Ocimum sanctum (Tulasi). Indian J Exp Biol 39(3):185

Verma P and Shah M (2018) "Herbal pharmacovigilance"

Wal P, Wal A, Gupta S, Sharma G, Rai AK (2011) Pharmacovigilance of herbal products in India. J Young Pharm 3(3):256. https://doi.org/10.4103/0975-1483.83780

Walji R, Boon H, Barnes J, Austin Z, Baker GR, Welsh S (2009) Adverse event reporting for herbal medicines: a result of market forces. Healthc Policy 4(4):77. https://doi.org/10.12927/hcpol.2009.20820

WHO (2004) WHO guidelines on safety monitoring of herbal medicines in pharmacovigilance systems. World Health Organization, Geneva

World Health Organization (2002) WHO collaborating Centre for International Drug Monitoring. In: The importance of pharmacovigilance. World Health Organization, Geneva

World Health Organization (2012) Safety monitoring of medicinal products. WHO, Geneva. https://www.who.int/publications/i/item/9789241503198. Accessed 21 Sep 2023

Zhang J, Onakpoya IJ, Posadzki P, Eddouks M (2015) The safety of herbal medicine: from prejudice to evidence. Evid Based Complement Alternat Med 2015:316706. https://doi.org/10.1155/2015/316706

Zhang J, Wider B, Shang H, Li X, Ernst E (2012) Quality of herbal medicines: challenges and solutions. Complement Ther Med 20(1–2):100. https://doi.org/10.1016/j.ctim.2011.09.004

Materiovigilance

13

Maneesh Soni, Mukesh Nandave, and Anoop Kumar

Abstract

Materiovigilance is a coordinated system for identifying, gathering, reporting, and analysing any untoward incidents associated with the use of medical devices, the goal of protecting patients' health by reducing the likelihood that they will occur again. Medical device post-marketing surveillance has been started in many nations, but it is still not as advanced and reliable as that for medicines. The current state of Materiovigilance is examined, along with comparisons to developed nations, gaps are noted, and specific actions are suggested to strengthen the programme. The meaning of Materiovigilance (Mv) is safeguarding the use of medical devices must be made clear to consumers and health professionals, who should also become aware regarding the reporting processes and emergency preparations of medical device-related adverse event. This chapter contains the brief information regarding post-marketing surveillance system of medical devices and regulation of medical devices in India and in other countries.

Keywords

Medical device · Adverse events · Medical device adverse events (MDAEs) · Materiovigilance Programme of India (MvPI) · Patient safety · Post-marketing surveillance

---

M. Soni (✉) · M. Nandave·A. Kumar
Department of Pharmacology, Delhi Pharmaceutical Sciences and Research University, New Delhi, India
e-mail: mukeshnandave@gmail.com; anoopdpsru@dpsru.edu.in

M. Nandave, A. Kumar (eds.), *Pharmacovigilance Essentials*,
https://doi.org/10.1007/978-981-99-8949-2_13

13.1 Introduction

The International Medical Device Regulators Forum (IMDRF) was established in 2011 with the aim of introducing the Materiovigilance (Mv) programme, implementing it to track medical device adverse events (MDAEs) and harmonizing international medical device regulation through Materiovigilance. The group members include representatives from the EU (European Commission and EU Member States), Australia, Brazil, Canada, China, Japan, Singapore, South Korea, and the USA (Sapkota et al. 2023). Materiovigilance is the close observation of any unfavourable changes in a medical device's performance or characteristics using a system that can detect, gather, report, and respond to them with a field safety corrective action or device recall during the post-marketing phase of a medical device. Materiovigilance only refers to medical devices, whereas pharmacovigilance refers to medicines (Saifuddin et al. 2022). Keeping a close eye out for potential threats or issues is the act or state of vigilance, according to the Oxford Dictionary. There is some risk associated with every medical device. Materiovigilance is the practice of closely monitoring any unfavourable alterations in the functionality or properties of a medical device. This is accomplished by using a system that, during the post-marketing phase of a medical device, can identify, collect, track, report, and estimate unfavourable occurrences and respond to them with device recalls or field safety corrective actions (Meher et al. 2022).

13.2 Post-Marketing Safety Surveillance System for Medical Devices in Some Other Countries

13.2.1 Safety Surveillance System for Medical Devices in United State (US)

The USFDA maintains the Manufacturer and User Facility Device Experience (MAUDE) database, which collects and analyses adverse event reports and product problems related to medical devices that are used in the US. The MAUDE database is used by manufacturers, importers, and user facilities to report adverse events and device malfunctions to the FDA as soon as they become known. This database enables the FDA to monitor safety incidents and take corrective action to ensure public health (FDA 2023).

13.2.2 Safety Surveillance System for Medical Devices in European Union (EU)

The European Union has established the European Database on Medical Devices (EUDAMED) which serves as a comprehensive repository for data related to post-market monitoring of medical devices. EUDAMED is intended to facilitate the collection and storage of data related to medical devices available on the EU market, including occurrences, field safety remedial measures, and regular safety update reports provided by manufacturers. It aims to enhance transparency and ensure timely actions in response to safety concerns (Europa 2023).

13.2.3 Safety Surveillance System for Medical Devices in Australia

The Therapeutic Good Administration (TGA) is responsible for the oversight and regulation of medical devices within Australia. The TGA administers the Database of Adverse Event Notification (DAEN) in which healthcare professionals, consumers, and manufacturers can submit reports of adverse events related to medical devices. This data is utilized by the TGA to monitor the health and safety of medical devices on the Australian market and to take appropriate action in the event of safety issues (TGA 2023).

13.2.4 Safety Surveillance System for Medical Devices in Japan

In Japan, The Pharmaceuticals and Medical Devices Agency (PMDA) is answerable for monitoring the safety of medical devices after they have been placed on the market. AERS-MD is a system that enables manufacturers and marketing authorisation holders to report any adverse events associated with medical devices. This data is then analysed by PMDA to identify potential safety issues and to make regulatory decisions (PMDA 2023).

13.2.5 Safety Surveillance System for Medical Devices in Canada

In Canada, post-marketing safety surveillance (PMS) for medical devices is the responsibility of the Health Canada. PMS is the collection and analysis of reports of suspected ADRs after a product has been approved for sale. ADRs are adverse reactions that may be caused by a health product. PMS assesses the potential risks and recommends appropriate actions. These actions may include informing the general public or health care professionals about new product safety data, suggesting labelling modifications and taking a product off the market (Health Canada 2023).

13.2.6 Safety Surveillance System for Medical Devices in China

The CFDA distributes medical device regulation responsibilities between the Center for Medical Device Evaluation (CMDE) and the NDRM. What sets the Chinese system apart is the presence of provincial and local agencies that act as the first responders to reports of adverse events and help the CFDA monitor and take action at the local level (Kramer et al. 2014).

13.3 Materiovigilance System in India [Materiovigilance Programme of India (MvPI)]

In the aftermath of serious adverse incidents due to medical device malfunction, such as short circuit in incubators leading to infant charring and hip implants causing blood poisoning, the Ministry of Health and Family Welfare (MoHFW), Government of India, felt the need to institutionalize the Materiovigilance Programme of India (MvPI). In succession, the MvPI was approved with an objective of generating data on post-marketing safety profiles of medical devices and ensuring the confidence of the general public in the availability of safe and effective medical devices across the country. The Drugs Controller General of India (DCGI) on July 6th, 2015, launched the MvPI at the Indian Pharmacopoeia Commission, Ghaziabad. At that time, Sree Chitra Tirunal Institute for Medical Sciences and Technology (SCTIMST) served as the National Coordinating Centre for this programme. The programme was recasted at the Indian Pharmacopoeia Commission (IPC), Ghaziabad, as the National Coordination Centre (NCC) in January in 2018 by a notification issued by MoHFW-GoI with the mission to ensure the health of the Indian population by balancing the advantages of medical devices against the potential risks associated with their use. The vision is to monitor adverse events associated with medical devices, which is essential to reduce the risk of patient safety and improve the well-being of the Indian population (Meher 2018; MvPI 2023). Table 13.1 demonstrates the regulation of globally stabilized Materiovigilance systems (Kramer et al. 2014; Joshi et al. 2021).

13.3.1 Objectives of MvPI

- Developing a national strategy for patient safety monitoring.
- Examine the balance of benefits and risks associated with a medical device.
- Develop evidence-based information for medical equipment related to adverse events.
- Help the CDSCO (Central Drugs Standard Control Organisation) in decision-making regarding medical device regulation in India.
- Share safety-related information with industry stakeholders.
- Collaborate with other health care organizations and global agencies for exchange and data management (Meher 2018; MvPI 2023).

13.3.2 Medical Device Adverse Event (MDAE) Reporting Process and Management Under MvPI

Any healthcare provider, including physicians, nurses, chemists, biomedical engineers, pharmacists, and patients, can report MDAE nationwide by submitting an electronic online available reporting form for medical devices, i.e. MDAE reporting form for healthcare professionals and for consumer (Annexure 9-A & 9-B, respectively), also available at IPC website; www.ipc.gov.in to either the IPC network of 994 (currently established) healthcare facilities, which includes district/government/private/trust hospitals and medical colleges, or directly to NCC-MvPI, IPC. Any reporter who is not a member of MDMC/AMC may also submit the completed MDAE reporting form to the National Collaborating Centre or to the MDMC/AMC that is closest to them. The scanned form can also be mailed to mvpi-ipc@gov.in by the reporter. There are 994 healthcare facilities in total; 293 of them serve as medical device adverse event monitoring centres (MDMCs) under the MvPI and 701 as adverse drug reaction monitoring centres (AMCs) under the Pharmacovigilance Programme of India (PvPI) (List of centres available on www.ipc.gov.in). The NCC-MvPI also regularly receives MDAE reports from specific Marketing Authorization Holders (MAHs) of medical devices in addition to these monitoring centres. Table 13.2 describes the list for the stakeholders who must provide specific minimum essential information of suspected adverse events (AEs) in order to validate and evaluate the report. Additionally, the NCC-MvP, IPC encourages consumers and healthcare professionals to submit any adverse events associated with medical devices through the PvPI ADR Android app or the toll-free helpline number (18001803024). The helpline is operational between 09:00 a.m. and 05:00 p.m. on weekdays, from Monday to Friday. Flow diagram of MDAE reporting and management system under MvPI and process of recognizing a center (Medical Institution/ Hospital/ Clinical Establishments etc.) as an MDMCs under MvPI, represented in Figs. 13.1 and 13.2, respectively (Kalaiselvan et al. 2020; Kalaiselvan and Saxena 2020).

13.3.3 Who Can Report MDAE

Healthcare professionals, like biomedical engineers and clinical engineers, as well as hospital techies like pharmacists and nurses, as well as patients can report any medical device-related adverse events. Manufacturers/importer/distributors of medical devices could also voluntarily report any specific adverse events related to their product (MvPI 2023; Kalaiselvan et al. 2015).

13.3.4 Why to Report MDAE

It is the ethical duty of a healthcare professional or an ethical medical device manufacturer to report any adverse events associated with the utilization of medical devices in order to protect the health of the public (MvPI 2023; Kalaiselvan et al. 2015).

13.3.5 What to Report in MDAE

Although Materiovigilance is primarily concerned with adverse events connected with medical devices used in India, MvPI encourages reporting of all types of

Table 13.1 Regulation of globally stabilize Materiovigilance system (Kramer et al. 2014; Joshi et al. 2021)

Sr. No.	Country	Regulatory authority	Guideline	Reporting mechanism	Penalties to the violators	Reporting timeline	Database name and link
1	India	CDSCO	Guidance document of MvPI version 1.2	MDAE reporting form to MvPI	Rs. 5,00000/– fine or for 1 year imprisonment or both for the manufacture, importer, and seller	Serious adverse events—Within 15 calendar days and nonserious adverse events within 30 calendar days	MvPI database www.ipc.gov.in CDSCO www.cdscomdonline.gov.in
2	USA	USFDA	21CFR803A	Form 3500A, Form 3419 for user facilities	If the Federal Food, drug, and cosmetic act (FFDCA) is violated, the FDA may recall products, seize them, and refuse to import them. When a case is brought before the court, the judge may order criminal penalties, such as prison terms, depending on the circumstances	Manufacturers have 30 days to report fatalities, serious injuries, and product malfunctions, and only 5 days to report an occurrence that necessitates taking corrective action to reduce risks. Ten days to report a user facility's death or serious injury	MAUDE—Manufacturer and User facility device experience www.accessdata.fda.gov
3	Canada	Health Canada	Regulation for Canadian medical devices, section 60 and 61 Canadian medical devices regulations, section 60 and 61	For industries: Mandatory medical device problem reporting form	Warning to manufacturer, importer, or distributor to recall or fix the issues	Within 10 calendar days for serious adverse events and within 30 for nonserious adverse events	Canada vigilance adverse reaction online database www.canada.ca

4	Australia	TGA	Guideline for Australian medical devices; guidance document number 11, version 1.7	Medical device incident reporting (MDIR) system	Up to $15,000 in fines for manufacturers or suppliers	A serious injury or death must be reported within 10 days, a significant public health threat must be reported within 2 days, and a near event must be reported within 30 days	Database of adverse event notifications (DAEN) for medical devices https://www.tga.gov.au
5	EU	European medicines agency (EMA)	Medical device regulation (EU) 2017/745	Reporting and recording system for incidents and corrective action	In Germany, France, and the UK, repeat offenders and serious first-time offenders face hefty fines and prison terms	Serious public health threats must be reported in two days. Report serious injury or death within ten days. Any incident that could lead to death or significant deterioration must be reported promptly, with a deadline of no more than 30 days thereafter	EUDAMED—European database on medical devices https://ec.europa.eu
6	Japan	Ministry of health, labour and welfare (MHLW)	Pharmaceutical affairs law article 77–4-2	Reports collected in the PMDA safety database	Being informed of recalls, labelling changes, or package inserts	For serious adverse events, 15 days	Pharmaceuticals and medical device agency (PMDA) https://www.pmda.go.jp/english
7	China	China FDA (CFDA)	Provisions for monitoring and reevaluating adverse event reporting for medical devices	National Medical Product Administration (NMPA)	Device permit is denied, and within 5 years, no application for the relevant licence or permit has been accepted	Serious adverse events (SAEs) must be reported within 15 days of the event, deaths must be reported within 5 days, and normal MDAEs must be reported within 30 days	China FDA (CFDA) http://www.sfdachina.com/ NMPA Database (nmpa.gov.cn)

Table 13.2 Essential information for MDAE reporting

Information	Details
General information	Reporting date, report type (initial/follow-up/trend)
Details of reporter	Reporter type (manufacturer/importer/distributors/ HCPs/others) and contact information
Category of device	Medical device/in vitro diagnostics/medical equipment/machines and their details
Details of device	Device name/trade name/brand name; MAHs details; licence no. batch/model no.; mfg. and exp. dates
Description of events	Event date, implant/explant date, serious/nonserious, event description, etc.
Information of patient	Patient's initial, age, gender, weight. Relevant medical history and patient outcome
Assessment of causality	Information of investigation action taken; information of root cause of problem
Manufacturer/authorized representative investigation and action taken	Report of device risk analysis, corrective/preventive and device history review

adverse events related to medical devices, regardless of whether they are known or unknown, serious or nonserious, frequent or rare (MvPI 2023; Kalaiselvan et al. 2015).

13.3.6 Role of Regulatory Authority of India (CDSCO) in MvPI

The National Regulatory Authority (NRA) is responsible for safeguarding the public's health and safety in India. As NRA, CDSCO is responsible for the smooth conduct of MvPI all over the country. IPC serves as the National Coordination Center (NCC). The Sree Chitra Tirunal Institute for Medical Sciences and Technology (SCTIMST) Thiruvananthapuram acts as National Collaborating Centre; National Health System Resource Centre (NHSRC), New Delhi, serves as the technical support partner and CDSCO continues to serve as the regulator for this programme (MvPI 2023; Kalaiselvan et al. 2020).

13.4 Medical Device Rule-2017: Regulation of Medical Devices in India

The National Regulatory Authority (NRA)-CDSCO is responsible for approving the manufacturing, import, conduct of clinical trials, setting standards, sale, and distribution of medical devices in the country. CDSCO has the onus of enforcing and implementing the Medical Devices Rules, 2017, which were published in the Gazette of India notification G.S.R. 78 (E), Dated January 31st, 2017 by the MoH&FW, GoI. MDR-2017 is effective from January 1st, 2018 under the Drugs and Cosmetic Act 1940.

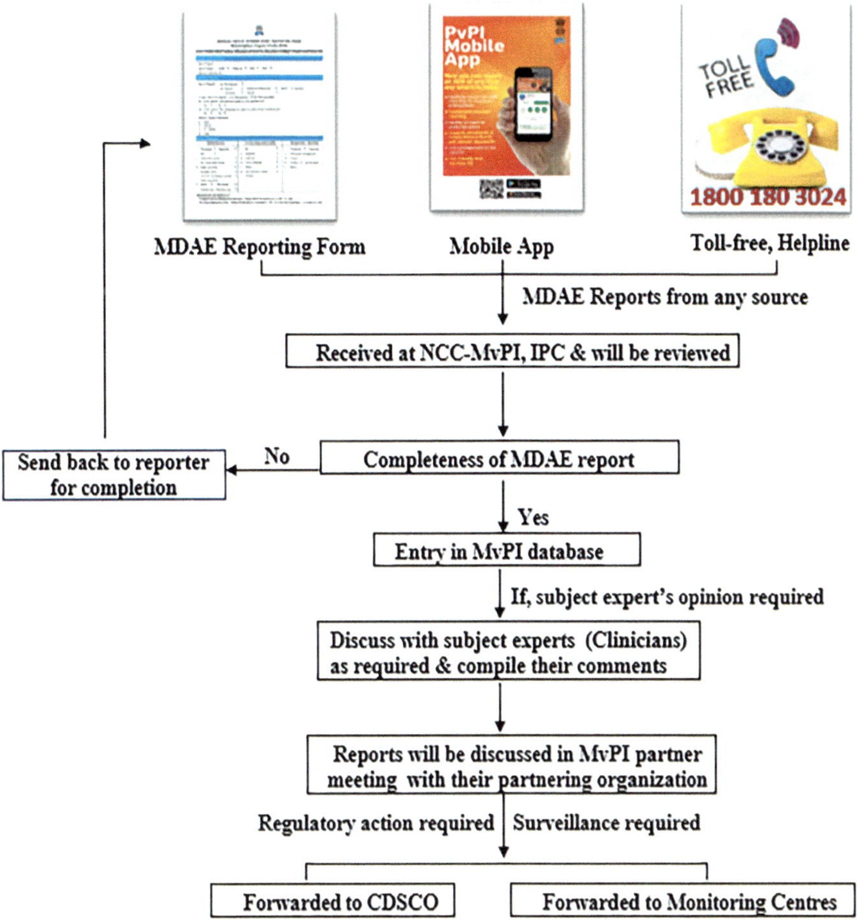

Fig. 13.1 Flow diagram of MDAE reporting and management system under MvPI

The MDR- 2017 provides comprehensive legislation for the regulation of medical devices and are in line with international regulatory best practices, which will support Make in India. Regulation of medical devices in India for their import, manufacturing, clinical investigation permission is provided in Table 13.3.

The MDR-2017 contains 12 chapters (Table 13.4), 8 schedules (Table 13.5), and 40 forms for medical devices (Table 13.6) to assistance for manufactures of MDs, modernizers in adopting MDR- 2017 (THE MEDICAL DEVICES RULES 2017).

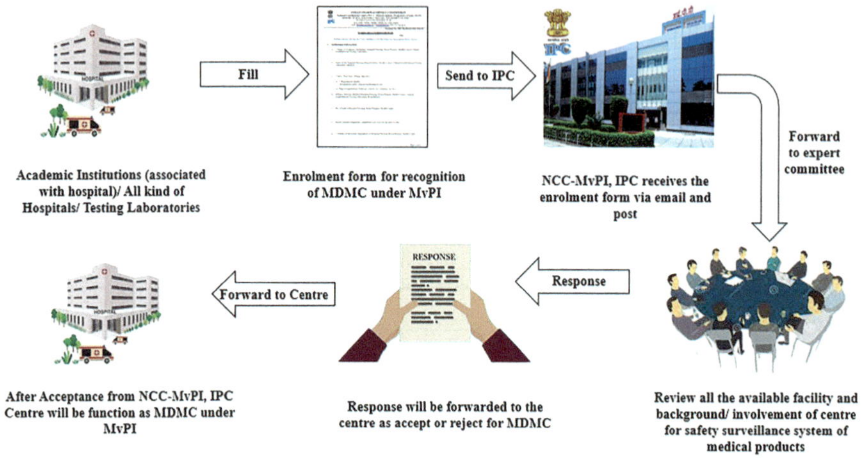

Fig. 13.2 Flow diagram of process to recognition of MDMC

13.4.1 Medical Device

Any device that is intended by its manufacturer to be used specifically for humans or animals, whether used alone or in combination, including software or an accessory, but which does not achieve the primary intended action in or on humans or animals through pharmacological, immunological, or metabolic means but which may assist in performing its intended function by such means for one or more of the specific purposes of:

- For any disease or disorder: Diagnosis/prevention/monitoring/treatment/alleviation;
- For any injury or disability: Diagnosis/monitoring/treatment/alleviation/assistance;
- For support of the anatomy or of a physiological process: Investigation/replacement/modification;
- For supporting/sustaining life;
- For disinfection of medical devices; and
- For control of conception (The Gazette of India; [F. No. X.11035/281/2018-DRS]) (THE MEDICAL DEVICES RULES 2017).

13.4.2 Medical Devices Classification

According to the MDR 2017, MDs are categorized into four classes on the basis of their risk; they are as represented in Table 13.7 (THE MEDICAL DEVICES RULES 2017).

Table 13.3 Medical devices regulation in India

Action	Class A	Class B	Class C	Class D
Importing	CLA			
Manufacturing	SLA		CLA	
QMS verification by	Notified body		CLA	
Sale	SLA			
Permission to conduct clinical investigation	CLA			

CLA central licencing authority, *SLA* state licencing authority

Table 13.4 Chapters of MDR-2017

Chapter with title	Description of chapter
Chapter I Preliminary	This chapter contains the detailed information regarding **short title, commencement, and application** of MDR rule. This chapter also contains some **definitions** which are used in this rule, i.e. medical device, notified body, sponsor, state licencing authority, etc.
Chapter II Medical devices regulation	This chapter contains the detailed information regarding the regulation of medical devices in terms of: • Medical device classification • Grouping of medical devices • Medical device manufacturing essential principles • Medical devices product standards
Chapter III Authorities, officers, and bodies	This chapter contains the detailed information regarding the licencing authorities. Delegation of power of licencing authorities and their controlling officer. National accreditation body and their functions. Notified body, their duties and procedure to be adopted. Fees charges by notified body. Registration certificates suspension and cancellation of notified body. Officers for medical device and medical device testing. And central testing laboratories for medical devices
Chapter IV Medical devices manufacturer for sale or distribution	This chapter contains the detailed information regarding the application for manufacturer for sale or distribution of medical devices comes under the class A or class B. Application for class C or class D medical devices manufacturing. Requirements of granting the licence for manufacturing or loan. Inspection of granting the licence or loan licence for medical devices comes under class C or class D. Report of inspection. Granting of licence or loan licence to manufacturer for sale or distribution. Manufacturing licence or loan licence conditions. State licencing authority unannounced inspection. Cancellation of test licence to manufacturer for test, evaluation, clinical investigations, etc.
Chapter V Importing of medical devices	This chapter contains the detailed information regarding import of medical devices, in terms of application for import licence Grant. Inspection of a manufacturing facility abroad. Import licence grant. Validity of licence. The licence holder must adhere to the terms of the licence. A new application in the event of a constitutional amendment. Import test licence for testing, evaluating, conducting clinical research, etc. grant of import licence. Issuing import test licences for testing, evaluating, conducting clinical research, etc. importation of an experimental medical device for use in patient care by a government hospital or other statutory medical facility. Import of medical equipment for individual use

(continued)

Table 13.4 (continued)

Chapter with title	Description of chapter
Chapter VI Medical devices labelling	This chapter contains the detailed information regarding the medical device labelling. Exemption of medical device export labelling requirements. The medical device's unique device identification. Medical device longevity. Labelling a new in vitro diagnostic medical device or a medical device for testing, evaluating, conducting clinical research, etc.
Chapter VII Medical device clinical investigation and new in vitro diagnostic medical device clinical performance evaluation	This chapter contains the detailed information regarding conducting clinical research. The use of rule 122DD of the 1945 drugs and cosmetics rules in relation to the ethics committee. Request for authorization to carry out clinical research. Permission to carry out clinical research. Requirements for authorization. Permission suspension, cancellation, etc. medical management and reimbursement for clinical research. Search and seizure authority, etc. record keeping 9. Disclosure of the names, addresses, etc., of those taking part in clinical research or clinical performance evaluation. Permitting the use of a new in vitro diagnostic medical device in clinical performance evaluation. Requirements for conducting clinical performance evaluations. Revocation or suspension of permission. Medical supervision
Chapter VIII Medical devices import or manufacture which does not have reference/devices	This chapter contains the detailed information regarding permission to manufacture or import a medical device without a predicate device. Authorization to manufacture or import a new in vitro diagnostic medical device. Requirements for importing or manufacturing new in vitro diagnostic medical devices and medical devices without a predicate device
Chapter IX Duties of the officer of medical devices, officers of medical device testing and notified body	This chapter contains the detailed information regarding a medical device testing officer's obligations. Sample evaluation or testing in accordance with subsection (4) of section 25 of the act. The steps the medical device testing officer must take after receiving a sample. Request for testing or assessment of a medical device. A medical device officer's obligation. Information that cannot be disclosed is prohibited, and the stock disposal order form is number seven. Forbidden sales. The type of receipt for medical equipment, records, registers, documents, or other tangible objects seized. How to certify copies of documents that have been seized. The reason samples were collected. Sample medical device receipt form when fair price offer is rejected. Procedure for dispatch of sample to medical device testing officer. Confiscation of medical devices, implements, machinery, etc. procedure for disposal of confiscated medical device
Chapter X Laboratory registration for carrying out test or evaluation	This chapter contains the detailed information regarding a medical device testing laboratory registration application. Requirements for medical device testing lab registration. Registration of a laboratory for testing medical devices. Registration validity. Registration requirements. Registration suspension and cancellation
Chapter XI Medical devices sale	This chapter contains the detailed information regarding arrangements for the sale of medical equipment. Medical device supply to hospitals in exchange for a delivery challan. Medical device recall
Chapter XII Miscellaneous	This chapter contains the detailed information regarding exemption from provisions related to medical devices. Export of medical devices. Rejection of application. Debarment of applicant. Mode of payment of fee. Digitalisation of form. Overriding effect. Savings

Table 13.5 Schedules of MDR-2017

Schedule with title	Description
Schedule first Medical devices and in vitro diagnostic devices classification criteria	**Part I** classification criteria for medical devices other than in vitro diagnostic **Part II** classification criteria for in vitro diagnostic medical devices
Schedule second Licence, permission, and registration certificates are subject to fees	This schedule has the details about the fees which is payable for licence, permission, and certificate registration. Subjects are, i.e. notified body's registration. Notified body's registration retention fee. A manufacturing permit or a loan permit for the production of class A or class B medical devices. In order to produce class C or class D medical devices. Manufacturers must have a manufacturing licence or loan licence and pay a retention fee, etc.
Schedule third Documents needed for the notified body's registration, as well as its obligations and functions	**Part I** documents to be provided with form MD-1 application for certificate of registration **Part II** notified body duties and functions
Schedule fourth Documents necessary for granting a licence to manufacture for distribution, sale, or import	**Part I** attorney power **Part II** (1) documents required to be submitted with an application for an import licence or a licence to produce a class A medical device for sale or distribution (2) documents needed to support the application for a licence to import or manufacture class B, class C, or class D medical devices **Part III** appendix I: Site or plant master file contents Appendix II other than in vitro diagnostic medical devices, device master files for medical devices are available Appendix III in vitro medical devices master file **Part IV** information needed to be submitted along with the application form for the manufacture or import of medical devices without a base device
Schedule fifth Medical device and in vitro diagnostic device quality management system	This schedule has the details about medical device and in vitro diagnostic device quality management system in terms of general requirements, applicability, quality management system, responsibility of management, management resource, realization of product, improvement, measurement, and analysis
Schedule sixth Changes after approval	(a) Changes to the following will be regarded as significant changes in: Construction material, design that will impact the medical device's performance, stability, performance according to specifications, and indication for use, sterilization methods, self-life approved, a manufacturing procedure, piece of equipment, or testing that could impact the device's quality, etc. (b) the following changes will be regarded as minor changes in: Design that will not compromise the medical device's performance, stability, performance criteria, or specifications, in the equipment, testing, or manufacturing process that should not have an impact on the device's quality, Packaging specifications excluding the main substance used in packaging

(continued)

Table 13.5 (continued)

Schedule with title	Description
Schedule seventh Conditions for obtaining authorization to manufacture or import an investigational medical device for use in conducting clinical research	This schedule has the details about: Application for permission. Investigation of clinical, sponsor responsibilities, investigator responsibilities, ethics committee responsibility, informed consent, clinical investigation (Pillot), clinical investigation (pivotal), clinical investigation of post-marketing, post-marketing surveillance, etc.
Schedule eighth Exemptions	This schedule has the details about medical devices class: • Custom medical devices • Medical bandages and dressings for first aid • Medical equipment provided by a licenced physician to a patient who is also that physician's own patient or any medical equipment provided by a licenced physician at the request of another • Medical equipment provided by a hospital or pharmacy that is supported or maintained by the government or a local organization • Mechanical contraceptives • Importation of a modest amount of medical equipment donated to a nonprofit hospital for use in providing free care to patients

Table 13.6 List of forms under MDR-2017

Form no.	Description
MD 1	Request for a notified Body's certificate of registration
MD 2	Medical Devices Rules, 2017: Certificate of Registration for a Notified Body
MD 3	Application for licence to produce class A or class B medical devices for sale and distribution
MD 4	Application for loan licencing to manufacture class A or class B medical devices for sale or distribution
MD5	Licence to produce class A or class B medical devices for distribution or sale
MD 6	Loan licence to manufacture class A or class B medical device for sale or distribution
MD 7	Application for licence to manufacture class C or class D for sale or distribution
MD 8	Application for loan licencing to manufacture class C or class D goods for sale or distribution
MD 9	Licence to manufacture class C or class D for sale or distribution
MD 10	Loan licence to manufacture class C or class D medical device for sale or distribution
MD 11	The audit or inspection book must be maintained in this format
MD 12	Requesting a licence to produce medical devices for clinical research, testing, evaluation, examination, demonstration, or training
MD 13	Authorization to produce medical devices for clinical investigations, testing, evaluation, demonstration, or training
MD 14	Request for issuance of import permit for medical device
MD 15	Medical device import licence

(continued)

Table 13.6 (continued)

Form no.	Description
MD 16	Obtaining a licence to import medical equipment for clinical research, testing, evaluation, demonstration, or training
MD 17	Obtaining a licence to import medical equipment for clinical research, testing, evaluation, demonstration, or training
MD 18	A government hospital or statutory medical institution's request for a licence to import experimental medical equipment for the purpose of treating patients
MD 19	A government hospital or statutory medical institution's authorization to import a medical device under investigation for the purpose of treating patients
MD 20	Request for authorization to import a limited number of medical devices for personal use
MD 21	Obtaining authorization to import a small number of medical devices for personal use
MD 22	Request for permission to conduct clinical research on an experimental medical device
MD 23	Conduct permission for clinical investigation
MD 24	Requesting authorization to test the clinical effectiveness of a new in vitro diagnostic medical device
MD 25	Getting authorization to test a new in vitro diagnostic medical device's clinical performance
MD 26	Application for granting permission to import or manufacture a medical device without a predicate medical device for sale or distribution
MD 27	Permission to import or produce a medical device without a predicate medical device for the purpose of selling or distributing
MD 28	Application for authorization to import or produce new in vitro diagnostic medical device for sale or distribution
MD 29	A licence to manufacture or import new in vitro diagnostic medical devices
MD 30	Central medical device testing laboratory memorandum
MD 31	Central medical device testing laboratory certificate of testing or evaluation
MD 32	Report of medical device testing officer's test or evaluation of medical devices
MD 33	Request for testing or evaluation of a medical device from a purchaser made pursuant to section 26 of the drugs and cosmetics act of 1940 (23 of 1940)
MD 34	A person to refrain from disposing of stock in his possession pursuant to an order made under clause (c) of subsection (1) of section of the Drugs and Cosmetics Act, 1940 (23 of 1940)
MD 35	Receipt for medical device stock for a record, register, document, or tangible object seized in accordance with subsection (1) of section 22 of the drugs and cosmetics act (23 of 1940) clauses (c) or (cc)
MD 36	Intimation for that person from whom sample booked
MD 37	Receiving a sample of a medical device when the fair price offered under section 23's subsection (1) of the 1940 drugs and cosmetics act is rejected
MD 38	Medical device testing officer memorandum
MD 39	For the purpose of testing or evaluating a medical device on behalf of the manufacturer, a medical device testing laboratory has requested registration
MD 40	For the purpose of testing or evaluating a medical device on behalf of the manufacturer, a certificate of registration to medical device testing laboratory is required

Table 13.7 Classification of medical devices

Class	Risk	Device examples
Class A	Lower	Thermometer, surgical taps, swaps, bandages, ice bag, etc.
Class B	Lower moderate	Hypodermic syringes/needles, ENT chair, general disinfectant, etc.
Class C	Moderate high	Incubator, intraocular lens, dry heat sterilizer, orthopaedic fixation plate, etc.
Class D	High	Cardiac stent, cardiac monitor, aneurysm clip Cochlear implant, etc.

13.5 Recall of Medical Devices

Recall refers to any action taken by a medical device's manufacturer, an authorized representative, or a supplier to remove the medical device from circulation or to recover the medical device from anyone to whom it has been distributed. (a) is harmful to one's health; or (b) fails to meet any quality, safety, or effectiveness claim made by the product's manufacturer; or (c) does not adhere to the act's and these rules' requirements. Recalled medical devices (last 3 years) in India are presented in Table 13.8 (CDSCO 2023).

13.6 Conclusion

The use of medical devices has increased significantly over the past few years, according to healthcare professionals around the world. Materiovigilance programmes are effective measures taken by different nations to ensure the security of medical devices being used. Medical device regulation is essential for ensuring the performance, efficacy, and availability of the device in the market to improve community health. Customers' trust and confidence in a product will automatically increase if it is safer and more efficient. Devices are categorized according to their risks, as was discussed in the review, so reporting and regulation must be done in accordance.

The worldwide market size of medical devices is projected to $612.7 billion in value by the year 2025, with approx. 5% compound annual growth rate. Due to growing consumer demand and technological advancement, we might see significant growth in product categories like wearable health technology, robotics nanotechnology, and extended reality gadgets. Additionally, the development in increasingly sophisticated data-driven algorithms, like autonomous diagnostics, is made possible by artificial intelligence. Medical equipment's companies of all extents have sufficient of opportunities despite recent setbacks. By establishing connections with patients and customers, medical devices will actively contribute to value creation on a global scale by 2030. This will probably call for a shift away from cure and treatment towards prevention through clever solutions and services that will lower costs and improve outcomes. This chapter may help to understand the safety surveillance system and regulatory aspect of medical devices.

Table 13.8 Recalled medical devices (last 3 years) in India

Sr. No.	Medical device	Recalled date	Reason for recall
1.	HOYA Vivinex Toric IOLs (certain model no.)	08th May 2023	Customers in Australia and Japan have complained about damage (such as scratches) and fragment adhesion on the IOL optic surface, IOLs from the specified manufacturing period (June 2022 to January 2023)
2	Adsorba Hemoperfusion cartridge 300 C	21st July 2022	Due to the potential presence of particular matter within the cartridge, there was a recall. If particles are not detected before use, they may enter the patient's vascular system and have a serious negative impact on their health
3	Peripheral stent on OPTA.035 delivery system, Palmaz genesis	21st June 2022	Cordis has observed an increase in complaints for stent dislodgment and associated failure modes, specifically produced during a particular time (October 2019–April 2021)
4	EEA auto suture circular stapler/ loading unit with DST series technology (staple)	14th June 2022	The component could become disengaged if a staple guide is not attached to the instrument, which would allow the tool to transect tissue without creating staples Treatment delays, prolonged hospital stays, unknown tissue injuries, unintended radiation exposure, unforeseen medical interventions, foreign bodies in patients, failure to anastomose, and haemorrhage could all result from this
5	Remote controller MMT 500 and MMT 503, Used in conjunction with ambulatory insulin infusion pumps as an optional accessory	8th November 2021	These particular remote controllers from Medtronic have been recalled due to possible cybersecurity risks. The wireless communication between the remote and MiniMed insulin pump could potentially be recorded and replayed by an unauthorized person (someone other than a patient, patient carer, or healthcare professional). An unauthorized person could use specialized equipment to instruct the insulin pump to either over-deliver insulin to a patient, causing hypoglycaemia, or stop insulin delivery, causing high blood sugar, diabetic ketoacidosis, and even death

(continued)

Table 13.8 (continued)

Sr. No.	Medical device	Recalled date	Reason for recall
6	MiniMed 600 series insulin pumps (MiniMed 620 G and 640 G insulin pump/pump kits)	11th October 2021	Any insulin pump with a clear retainer ring should be exchanged for one with the updated black retainer ring free of charge after Medtronic recalled the relevant insulin pumps. Even if the clear retainer ring is undamaged and regardless of the pump's warranty status, a replacement insulin pump will be given The clear retainer ring of the MinMed 630G and 670G insulin pumps was missing or broken, and Medtronic had previously discovered this and informed customers. The insulin cartridge is secured in the pump reservoir compartment with the aid of the retainer ring. Low blood sugar (hyperglycaemia or high blood sugar) may result from under- or over-delivery of insulin if the cartridge is not locked firmly into place. Extreme hyperglycaemia and hypoglycaemia can be fatal or have life-threatening consequences
7	HeartWare™ HVAD system	17th September 2021	The internal pump was linked to an increased risk of neurological adverse events and mortality. If the internal pump breaks down, it might take a while to restart or not at all. Both issues have the potential to cause serious patient harm or death, such as stroke, heart attack, worsening heart failure, the requirement for further procedures, and hospitalizations A growing body of observational clinical studies compares patients who receive the HVAD system to those who receive other commercially available durable left ventricular assist devices (LVAD), and they reveal a higher frequency of neurological adverse events and mortality. According to Medtronic, there were over 100 complaints about the HVAD internal pump taking too long or failing to restart, which resulted in a total of 14 fatalities and 13 pump removals

References

CDSCO (2023) Central Drugs Standard Control Organization, Directorate General of Health Services Ministry of Health & Family Welfare Government of India. https://cdsco.gov.in/opencms/opencms/en/Medical-Device-Diagnostics/Medical-Device-Diagnostics/. Accessed 3 Oct 2023

Europa (2023) European Commission—EUDAMED. https://ec.europa.eu/health/md_eudamed/

FDA (2023) U.S. Food and Drug Administration (FDA)—postmarket requirements and commitments. https://www.fda.gov/medical-devices/postmarket-requirements-and-commitments

Health Canada (2023). Drug and medical device post market surveillance - Canada.ca. Accessed 2 Oct 2023

Joshi D, Sharma I, Gupta S, Singh TG, Dhiman S, Prashar A, Gulati M, Kumar B, Vishwas S, Chellappan DK, Gupta G (2021) A global comparison of implementation and effectiveness of materiovigilance program: overview of regulations. Environ Sci Pollut Res 28:1–22

Kalaiselvan V, Saxena R (2020) Intraocular devices associated adverse events reporting system in India. Indian J Ophthalmol 68(11):2343

Kalaiselvan V, Kumar P, Mishra P, Singh G (2015) System of adverse drug reactions reporting: what, where, how, and whom to report? Indian J Crit Care Med 19(9):564

Kalaiselvan V, Tripathi SK, Prakash J (2020) Materiovigilance programme of India: a scheme to assure cardiovascular devices safety surveillance. Indian Heart J 72(4):316–318

Kramer DB, Tan YT, Sato C, Kesselheim AS (2014) Ensuring medical device effectiveness and safety: a cross-national comparison of approaches to regulation. Food Drug Law J 69(1):1

Meher BR (2018) Materiovigilance: an Indian perspective. Perspect Clin Res 9(4):175

Meher BR, Padhy BM, Srinivasan A, Mohanty RR (2022) Awareness, attitude, and practice of materiovigilance among medical professionals at a tertiary care institute of national importance: a cross-sectional study. Perspect Clin Res 13(2):94

MvPI (2023) Guidance document, Materiovigilance Programme of India (MvPI), version 1.2. Guidance_Document_MvPI.pdf (ipc.gov.in). Accessed 3 Oct 2023

PMDA (2023) Pharmaceuticals and Medical Devices Agency (PMDA)—adverse event reporting system for medical devices. https://www.pmda.go.jp/english/safety/safety.html

Saifuddin PK, Tandon M, Kalaiselvan V, Suroy B, Pattanshetti V, Prakash A, Medhi B (2022) Materiovigilance programme of India: current status and way forward. Indian J Pharmacol 54(3):221

Sapkota B, Palaian S, Shrestha S, Ibrahim MI (2023) Materiovigilance in perspective: understanding its concept and practice in the global healthcare system. Ther Innov Regul Sci 57:1–3

TGA (2023) Therapeutic Goods Administration (TGA)—medical devices. https://www.tga.gov.au/medical-devices

THE MEDICAL DEVICES RULES (2017) [GSR 78(E), dt. 31-1-2017, w.e.f. 1-1-2018] (As amended vide GSR 777(E) dt. 14-10-2022(w.e.f. 14-10-2022). https://cdsco.gov.in/opencms/resources/UploadCDSCOWeb/2022/m_device/Medical%20Devices%20Rules,%202017.pdf

Haemovigilance

14

Mohammad Hamid, Mukesh Nandave, and Anoop Kumar

Abstract

Haemovigilance is a vital process encompassing safe blood collection, processing, and transfusion for donors and recipients. Originating in France, it has evolved globally to mitigate reactions, infections, and quality issues tied to blood transfusion. This chapter explores the evolution of haemovigilance, its scope, significance, limitations, and recommendations. Donor and recipient viewpoints on blood transfusion and related reporting are provided. This chapter also showcases the ISTARE database's role in international haemovigilance collaboration, the Indian National Haemovigilance Programme, and other countries' initiatives. A discussion on the challenges of implementing a haemovigilance system, such as inconsistent reporting and funding, and recommendations for a better haemovigilance system are reported. Throughout the chapter, emerging trends and global initiatives outlining the prospects of haemovigilance in ensuring safe blood transfusion practices are provided.

Keywords

Blood safety · Adverse reaction · Imputability

M. Hamid (✉) · M. Nandave · A. Kumar
Department of Pharmacology, Delhi Pharmaceutical Sciences and Research University, New Delhi, India
e-mail: mukeshnandave@gmail.com; anoopdpsru@dpsru.edu.in

M. Nandave, A. Kumar (eds.), *Pharmacovigilance Essentials*,
https://doi.org/10.1007/978-981-99-8949-2_14

14.1 Introduction

The administration of blood and its constituents via transfusion is a crucial medical procedure that can potentially rescue lives. Nevertheless, inherent risks accompany blood collection, processing, and transfusion, leading to a broad spectrum of unfavorable occurrences. These events encompass reactions, incidents narrowly averted, mistakes, deviations from established protocols, and accidents that may arise throughout the blood donation and transfusion process. Therefore, it is crucial to improve the standard of care for blood donors and recipients, as well as the efficacy, safety, and cost-effectiveness of the blood and its constituent parts.

In this context, "haemovigilance," a term derived from the Greek word "haema," signifying blood, and the Latin term "vigil," indicating watchful, plays a central role. According to the World Health Organization (WHO), "haemovigilance is a collection of monitoring procedures encompassing the entire transfusion continuum, spanning from blood and its components' donation and processing to their delivery and transfusion to patients, followed by subsequent monitoring. This encompasses the tracking, reporting, investigating, and analyzing unfavorable events linked to blood donation, processing, and transfusion, along with implementing measures to prevent their occurrence or recurrence."

Haemovigilance must be seamlessly included in the quality systems of all organizations involved in the supply chain for blood and blood products to guarantee the safety of both donors and recipients at every stage. This integration spans crucial domains like clinical transfusion, inventory management, testing, processing, storage, and distribution (World Health Organization 2016). The classification of blood products is shown in Table 14.1.

14.2 History of Haemovigilance

The pioneering efforts in haemovigilance began in France in 1994, as shown in Fig. 14.1, with the establishment of monitoring systems and a national haemovigilance system. Shortly after that, in 1995, the European Council issued a resolution

Table 14.1 Classification of blood products

Category/components	Blood products
Cellular components	Red cell concentrates
	Platelet concentrates
	Granulocyte concentrates
Plasma components	Fresh frozen plasma
	Cryoprecipitates
	Cryo-poor plasma
	Stored plasma
Plasma derivatives	Albumin
	Immunoglobulin
	Coagulation factors

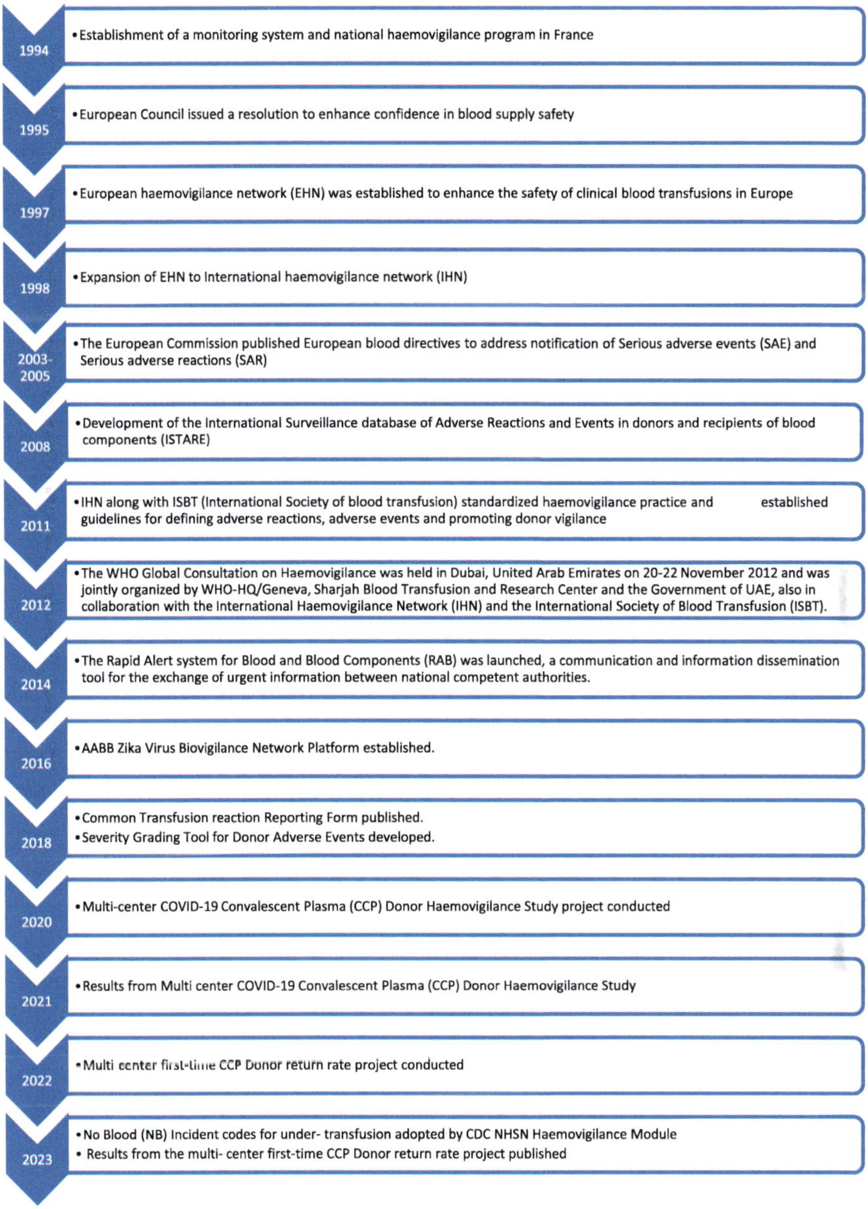

Fig. 14.1 History of haemovigilance

to bolster public confidence in blood supply safety. This initiative led to the establishment of legal oversight over haemovigilance systems (Watson 2005; Faber 2004). Valuable lessons in enhancing blood safety have been drawn from well-established haemovigilance systems in countries such as the UK (Serious Hazards of Transfusion [SHOT]), Canada (Transfusion Transmitted Injuries Surveillance System [TTISS]), the Netherlands (Transfusion Reactions in Patients [TRIP]), Japan, Russia, Switzerland, and the USA.

The European Haemovigilance Network (EHN) was established in 1997 to increase the safety of clinical blood transfusion services in Europe. Starting with just five members, the network steadily expanded to include 28 members. The International Haemovigilance Network (IHN) was established in 1998 as the International Haemovigilance Network (EHN)'s scope grew over time. Collaborating with the working party on Haemovigilance of the International Society of Blood Transfusion (ISBT), the IHN strives to establish a unified framework for ensuring the safety of blood and blood components on a global scale while also promoting haemovigilance. Through activities such as digital information exchange, meetings, and seminars, the IHN has made substantial contributions to advancing the quality of haemovigilance in Europe. In 2011, the IHN, in partnership with ISBT, played a pivotal role in standardizing haemovigilance practices. They provided definitions for adverse reactions and adverse events in patients. They laid out guidelines for promoting and managing donor vigilance, including uniform definitions for donor complications and adverse events.

Additionally, the European Commission published European Blood Directives between 2003 and 2005, imposing binding rules controlling the collection, testing, processing, storage, and distribution of human blood and blood components. These guidelines notably addressed the need for haemovigilance and emphasized the significance of comprehensive donor-to-receiver blood product traceability as well as the reporting of serious adverse events (SAE) and severe adverse reactions (SAR) that can endanger recipient safety. By strengthening haemovigilance networks, these directives enhanced the support and services provided more stringently (Mukherjee 2016).

The International Surveillance of Transfusion-Associated Reactions and Events (ISTARE) database was created further to improve the safety of blood donors and receivers. This international database, accessible at http://www.ihn-org.com/haemovigilance-databases/istare-2/, facilitates the global sharing of haemovigilance data. ISTARE's primary objective is to capture adverse reactions, incidents, and events related to blood transfusion, categorized as certain, probable, or possible. It also records adverse events occurring in blood donors. Utilizing ISTARE aims to maximize the safety and well-being of donors and recipients in blood transfusion practices.

14.3 Scope

The scope of haemovigilance systems can vary due to differences in reporting practices, including distinctions between reporting adverse reactions and adverse events, deciding whether to include all or serious events and considering incidents in both recipients and donors. An ideal haemovigilance system would cover blood donation, processing, and transfusion to patients as part of the entire transfusion chain. It should make it possible to keep track of, report, and look into any negative blood transfusion-related incidents, reactions, or near-misses. The blood transfusion service, hospital staff, transfusion laboratories, transfusion committees, regulatory agencies, and national health authorities must all work together effectively (Jain and Kaur 2012).

Haemovigilance systems play a critical role in enhancing donor and patient safety through various means:

- Identify trends in adverse events and reactions in blood transfusion practices.
- Determine the root causes of these issues and raise awareness to prevent similar incidents in the future.
- Providing valuable evidence for developing and modifying policies and practices to enhance transfusion safety.
- Guiding research efforts to address knowledge gaps and improve transfusion outcomes.
- Acting as an immediate alarm system and early warning system for dangers in transfusion procedures.
- Demonstrating a commitment to continuous improvement in transfusion safety by implementing haemovigilance measures (World Health Organization 2016).

By fulfilling these functions, haemovigilance systems substantially enhance the safety and quality of blood transfusion processes.

14.4 Benefits

Haemovigilance plays a pivotal role in ensuring the safety and well-being of various stakeholders within the blood transfusion ecosystem:

14.4.1 Blood Donors

Haemovigilance measures are instrumental in enhancing the safety of blood donors. They minimize complications and issues that may arise during the blood transfusion process, thus ensuring the well-being of voluntary blood donors. Furthermore, haemovigilance encourages their continued participation and support by instilling trust among donors.

14.4.2 Blood Transfusion Services

Haemovigilance is an early warning system that promptly identifies flaws or issues within the blood transfusion process. This enables swift reporting and resolution of safety concerns, facilitating the development and improvement of transfusion procedures. Continuous monitoring and evaluation through haemovigilance empower healthcare professionals to enhance the safety and efficiency of blood transfusion services.

14.4.3 Hospital Blood Banks and Healthcare Facilities

Haemovigilance systems integrated into hospital blood banks and healthcare facilities are pivotal in detecting and reducing errors and system faults. These systems enable timely intervention and the implementation of corrective measures by ensuring accurate and ongoing reporting of adverse events. Haemovigilance data also serves as the foundation for comprehensive strategies to improve blood banks' and healthcare facilities' safety and overall functioning.

14.4.4 Patient Safety

Haemovigilance is critical in safeguarding patient safety by identifying concerns and potential risks affecting individual patients. Through data analysis and root cause investigations, haemovigilance provides valuable insights that inform corrective actions and improvements. Evidence-based policy recommendations derived from haemovigilance data contribute to policy changes to enhance patient safety and ensure optimal healthcare outcomes.

14.4.5 Physicians and Healthcare Professionals

Haemovigilance actively supports healthcare professionals in monitoring transfusion-related adverse events and complications. It facilitates continuous learning and improvement by providing feedback and keeping healthcare professionals updated on the latest transfusion safety measures. This leads to improved patient care and better transfusion outcomes.

14.4.6 Regional and National Health Authorities, Regulatory and Health Agencies

Haemovigilance programs are invaluable to regional and national health authorities, regulatory bodies, and health agencies in safeguarding public health. They enable the early diagnosis of new diseases and the adoption of risk-reduction strategies for related dangers, such as infections transferred through blood transfusions. Haemovigilance also helps identify and mitigate non-infective risks, allowing proactive measures to be taken. By monitoring adverse event trends, haemovigilance facilitates timely corrective actions, improving overall transfusion safety and healthcare practices.

14.4.7 Community

The community benefits from haemovigilance efforts through improved care and responsible stewardship of the gift of blood donation. By promoting awareness of the importance of haemovigilance, the community contributes to the safety and effectiveness of the blood system. This support fosters greater confidence and trust among blood donors and patients, ensuring the transfusion meets the highest safety standards.

These collective efforts, as outlined, demonstrate how haemovigilance plays a central role in safeguarding the interests and well-being of all stakeholders involved in blood transfusion (World Health Organization 2016; Sadique Hussain 2022).

14.5 Characteristics of a Successful Haemovigilance System

Though varying from one country to another, national haemovigilance systems exhibit shared characteristics that contribute to their success. These characteristics can be grouped into organizational and operational perspectives:

Organizational Perspective:

- Efficiency, Resources, and Sustainability: A successful national haemovigilance system operates efficiently, is adequately resourced, and is designed for long-term sustainability. It actively involves all relevant stakeholders, ensuring a collaborative approach.
- Non-punitive Environment and Learning Culture: Such a system promotes a non-punitive culture where reporting adverse events is encouraged rather than discouraged. This environment fosters a culture of learning from incidents.
- Confidentiality: Ensuring the confidentiality of submitted data is a priority in this system. Protecting the identity of the source encourages transparency and openness in reporting adverse events.
- Integration with Quality Systems: Haemovigilance is seamlessly integrated into the quality systems of healthcare establishments, covering the entire transfusion process. This comprehensive approach helps identify potential risks and implement necessary measures to enhance patient safety.
- Traceability: The system enables traceability from the blood donor blood unit to the recipient and vice versa. This allows for the tracking and investigation adverse events, facilitating the implementation of corrective actions when needed.
- Adherence to International Standards and Definitions: The system adheres to international recommendations, utilizing standardized standards and definitions for consistency and compatibility with global best practices.
- Education and Training: Adequate education and training programs are in place to equip healthcare professionals with the necessary knowledge and skills for

haemovigilance. This promotes awareness and understanding of adverse events and reporting procedures.

- Feedback Reporting: The system provides feedback reports to the stakeholder community, offering insights into trends, analyses, and recommendations. This fosters a culture of continuous improvement and collaboration among stakeholders.

Operational Perspective:

- Simplicity: The system is designed to be user-friendly and easy to navigate, ensuring straightforward reporting of adverse events.
- Clear and Standardized Reporting Forms: Standardized reporting forms are employed to collect essential information that enables effective analysis of adverse events.
- Standard Procedures: Written standard procedures are established for initiating, investigating, and coordinating reports. This ensures a systematic approach to handling adverse events.
- Timely Reporting and Analysis: Adverse events are reported promptly, and trends are identified in a timely manner. Expert analysis is conducted to provide recommendations for improvement, minimizing the occurrence or recurrence of adverse events.
- Monitoring of Corrective Actions: Mechanisms are in place to monitor the implementation of corrective actions, ensuring they are executed promptly. This helps track the progress of improvement efforts and demonstrates enhanced clinical outcomes (World Health Organization 2016).

Incorporating these characteristics into national haemovigilance systems helps optimize their effectiveness in enhancing the safety and quality of blood transfusion processes.

14.6 Need for Haemovigilance

The need for haemovigilance emerged during the twentieth century, driven by significant advancements in understanding blood groups, cross-matching techniques, and anticoagulation methods. These developments led to the widespread acceptance of blood transfusion as a therapeutic intervention. However, in the 1970s and 1980s, concerns about infection transmission through blood transfusion brought to light the critical importance of prioritizing the safety of blood-related procedures. During this period, a significant public health crisis occurred when it was discovered that up to 4689 people with hemophilia and other bleeding disorders were infected with HIV and hepatitis viruses due to contaminated clotting factors derived from infected blood products. This tragic event served as a stark reminder of the potential risks of blood transfusion and the urgent need for enhanced safety measures. In response to these challenges, France took a pioneering step in 1991 by establishing monitoring systems through blood transfusion committees. This initiative culminated in the creation of a national hemovigilance network in 1994. France's leadership in this regard served as a model for other nations and prompted the formation of the International Haemovigilance Network (IHN). The IHN is dedicated to promoting global collaboration in haemovigilance practices, sharing knowledge, and developing common standards to ensure the safety and quality of blood transfusion practices worldwide. While many developed countries have successfully implemented robust haemovigilance systems overseen by regulatory authorities, adopting comprehensive haemovigilance programs in Asian countries and other regions has been limited. This gap has resulted in a scarcity of haemovigilance data in these areas.

Therefore, it is imperative to underscore the global significance of haemovigilance and advocate for establishing robust systems in all regions. These systems are crucial for ensuring the continued safety and quality of blood transfusion practices and preventing the transmission of infectious diseases through blood products. By fostering international collaboration and knowledge sharing, we can collectively enhance the safety of blood transfusion worldwide and prevent the tragic events of the past from recurring (Khobragade et al. 2022).

14.7 Haemovigilance for Recipient

Implementing haemovigilance is paramount in ensuring the safety and well-being of patients who undergo blood transfusions. In the context of haemovigilance for recipients, an internationally accepted scale is utilized to assess the severity of adverse reactions that occur following blood transfusion. This assessment is crucial in determining the likelihood of attributing the adverse reaction to the specific blood component or blood product received. To promote consistency in reporting and facilitate meaningful data comparison, the International Haemovigilance Network (IHN) and the International Society of Blood Transfusion (ISBT) have collaborated to establish standardized definitions for adverse reactions in recipients. These standardized definitions provide a common language and framework for describing and categorizing adverse reactions, ensuring that data collected from different regions and healthcare systems can be effectively compared and analyzed. Furthermore, the criteria for assessing the severity and imputability (the extent to which the adverse reaction can be attributed to the transfused blood component) have been defined by ISBT. These criteria help healthcare professionals accurately evaluate the seriousness of adverse reactions and determine their connection to the transfusion, which is essential for appropriate management and follow-up care.

In summary, the collaboration between IHN and ISBT in establishing standardized definitions and criteria for assessing adverse reactions in recipients is a crucial step in enhancing the consistency and quality of haemovigilance practices worldwide. It ensures that adverse events following blood transfusion are accurately documented, analyzed, and addressed to improve patient safety in the context of transfusion medicine (Mukherjee 2016).

The severity of recipients has been graded by 4 levels and shown in Table 14.2.

Indeed, by utilizing imputability levels and severity criteria, the haemovigilance system for recipients significantly improves our comprehension of adverse events and their connection to transfusion. This, in turn, plays a pivotal role in enhancing patient safety and enables continuous efforts to improve the quality of transfusion practices.

The standardized definitions and reporting framework established through the collaboration of the International Haemovigilance Network (IHN) and the International Society of Blood Transfusion (ISBT) working committee group are instrumental in achieving these goals. They provide a common language and structured approach for describing adverse events following transfusions. This standardized approach facilitates consistent reporting within individual haemovigilance systems and promotes information sharing and comparative analysis of data across different systems. By sharing data and insights across borders and healthcare settings, the global medical community can identify trends, patterns, and best practices related to transfusion safety. This collaborative effort empowers healthcare professionals to make informed decisions, implement preventive measures, and continuously enhance the quality of care provided to patients undergoing blood transfusions. Harmonizing definitions and reporting practices through the IHN-ISBT partnership contributes to a safer and more effective transfusion medicine landscape (NIB 2019).

14.8 Haemovigilance for Donor

The haemovigilance system also assumes a critical role in safeguarding the safety and well-being of blood donors throughout the entire transfusion process. In the context of haemovigilance for donors, the focus is on monitoring and addressing adverse reactions or events that may occur during whole blood or component donation. These complications can arise from various factors related to the donation

Table 14.2 Imputability levels to grade severity of recipient's reaction

Definite (certain)	When there is conclusive evidence beyond reasonable doubt that the adverse event can be attributed to the transfusion
Probable (likely)	When the evidence is clearly in favor of attributing the adverse event to the transfusion
Possible	When the evidence is indeterminate for attributing the adverse event to the transfusion or an alternate cause
Unlikely (doubtful)	When the evidence is clearly in favor of attributing the adverse event to causes other than the transfusion
Excluded	When there is conclusive evidence beyond reasonable doubt that the adverse event can be attributed to causes other than the transfusion

process, donor selection, and donor management, and they have the potential to directly impact the health of the donor, the quality of the collected blood product, and the health of the recipient.

To systematically classify and define these donor-related complications, a collaborative working group from the International Society of Blood Transfusion (ISBT) and the European Haemovigilance Network (EHN) has put forward a classification system (Mukherjee 2016), as shown in Table 14.3. This system provides a structured framework for categorizing and describing adverse events or reactions that may occur during the donation process, facilitating accurate reporting and analysis to ensure donor safety and the quality of donated blood products.

The severity and imputability of these complications experienced by blood donors are assessed using a scale that is comparable to the one utilized for grading adverse reactions in recipients. This internationally accepted scale provides a standardized framework for evaluating and reporting adverse events that occur during the process of blood donation. It ensures consistency in assessing and reporting adverse events affecting blood donors.

Through the systematic classification and categorization of these donor-related adverse events or reactions, haemovigilance systems can efficiently monitor and address potential risks to donors, thereby enhancing their safety and well-being throughout the entire donation process. This structured approach ensures that donor complications are appropriately assessed, reported, and managed, contributing to a safer and more reliable blood donation system (NIB 2022a).

14.9 National Haemovigilance Programme of India

The Haemovigilance Programme of India (HvPI), launched on December 10, 2012, is a joint initiative run by the Indian Pharmacopoeia Commission in collaboration with the National Institute of Biologicals, working under the Ministry of Health and Family Welfare, Government of India. HvPI is a centralized program with a primary objective of monitoring, facilitating the reporting of adverse reactions associated with blood transfusion, and the administration of blood products throughout India, as shown in Fig. 14.2. This program plays a crucial role in enhancing the safety and quality of blood transfusion practices in the country by systematically collecting and analyzing data on adverse events, thereby promoting patient and donor well-being. HvPI's centralized approach ensures that adverse reactions are consistently monitored and reported nationwide, contributing to improved transfusion safety standards in India.

The proper functioning of the Haemovigilance Programme of India involves various centers and entities working collaboratively:

Table 14.3 Classification and characterization of donor adverse events/reactions

A	Local symptoms 1. Blood outside vessel (a) Hematoma (bruise) (b) Arterial puncture (c) Delayed (bleeding/re-bleeding) 2. Arm pain (a) Nerve injury/irritation (b) Other arm pain 3. Localized infection/inflammation along the course of a vein (a) Thrombophlebitis (b) Cellulitis 4. Other major blood vessel injury: Serious conditions needing specialist medical diagnosis and attention (a) Deep venous thrombosis (DVT) (b) Arteriovenous fistula (c) Compartmental syndrome (d) Brachial artery pseudoaneurysm
B	Complications mainly with generalized symptoms: Vasovagal reactions • Without loss of consciousness (LOC) • With LOC (loss of consciousness) < 60 s • With LOC (loss of consciousness) > 60 s • With injury • Without injury • Within the blood collection facility • Outside blood collection facility
C	Complications related to apheresis • Citrate reactions • Hemolysis • Air embolism • Infiltration • Infiltration of IV fluids
D	Allergic reactions • Local allergic reactions • Generalized allergic reactions (anaphylactic reactions)
E	Serious complications • Acute cardiac symptoms • Myocardial infarction (MI) • cardiac arrest • Transient ischemic attack (TIA) • Cerebrovascular accident • Death
F	Other reactions

Core Group and Advisory Committee: These entities play a pivotal role in the program by finalizing guidance documents and actively participating in developing reporting forms. Their expertise and input contribute to the effective operation of haemovigilance activities.

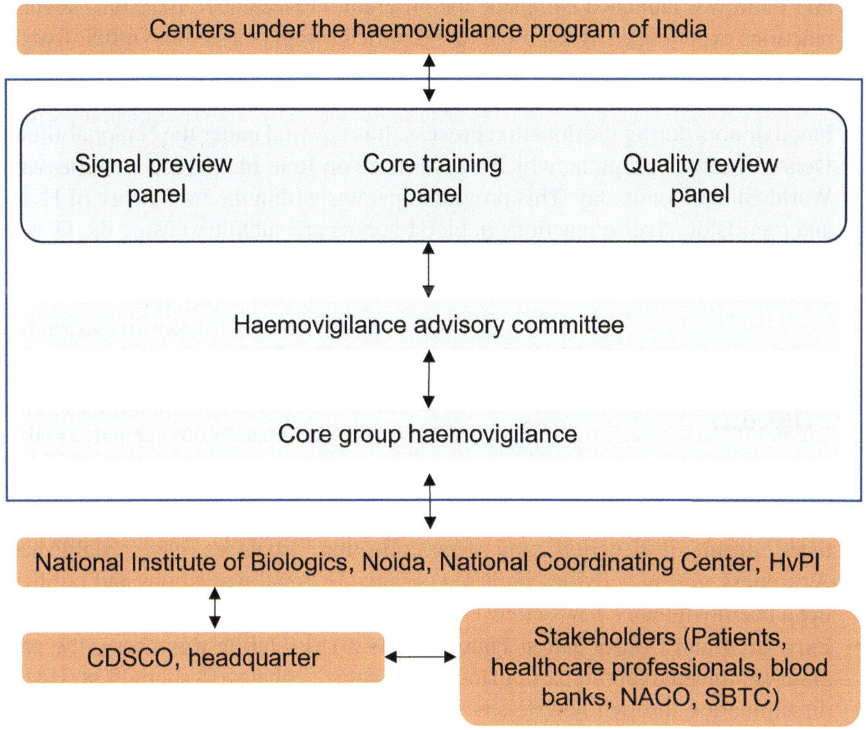

Fig. 14.2 Haemovigilance Programme of India

National Institute of Biologicals: This institution is the coordinating center for the Haemovigilance Programme of India. It is responsible for collecting, collating, and analyzing data related to biologicals and haemovigilance. Their efforts are central to the program's success in monitoring and responding to adverse events.

ADR Monitoring Centers: These centers are distributed across medical colleges, hospitals, and blood banks registered with the Pharmacovigilance National Coordinating Center. They serve as the frontline reporting entities for adverse reactions related to blood transfusion and blood product administration. Their participation is essential in identifying and reporting adverse events, contributing to the overall safety of blood-related procedures.

The collaboration among these various centers and committees ensures a comprehensive and organized approach to Haemovigilance in India. It allows for collecting, analyzing, and responding to data regarding adverse reactions associated with blood transfusions and blood products, ultimately promoting the safety and quality of these critical medical interventions.

The Haemovigilance Programme of India (HvPI) operates through two distinct arms, each focused on different aspects of monitoring and reporting adverse events:

- Recipient's Arm: This arm is dedicated to reporting adverse reactions related to blood transfusions and their impact on the patient. It falls under the purview of

HvPI and was launched alongside the program on December 10, 2012. Adverse reactions experienced by recipients are reported using the Haemo-Vigil Software, which employs the Transfusion Reactions Reporting Form (TRRF).
- Donor's Arm: The Donor's Arm deals with adverse reactions experienced by blood donors during the donation process. It is covered under the National Blood Donor Vigilance program, which was initiated on June 14, 2015, coinciding with World Blood Donor Day. This program operates within the framework of HvPI, and reports of adverse reactions in blood donors are submitted using the Donor-Vigil Software, along with the Adverse Blood Donor Reaction Reporting Form (NIB 2022b).

HvPI was established with dedicated funding of Rs 29.36 crore during the 12th Five Year Plan (2012–2017), and it unfolded in three distinct phases, each with specific objectives:

- Initiation Phase (2012–2013): This phase focused on setting up the necessary systems, procedures, and software development. Participant enrollment was initiated during this period, and data collection processes were established. Awareness-raising activities included organizing zonal workshops and publishing a haemovigilance newsletter.
- Expansion and Consolidation Phase (2013–2015): During this phase, the program continued to enroll participants and organize zonal workshops. Knowledge dissemination through newsletters was prioritized, and staff training was conducted. Efforts were made to secure International Haemovigilance Network (IHN) membership to enhance global collaboration.
- Expansion and Maintenance Phase (2015–2017): The primary objective of this phase was to maintain and optimize the haemovigilance system and its associated procedures. The focus included identifying gaps and planning appropriate training programs. Enhancements were made to donor vigilance, and the development of a rapid alert system was prioritized. Plans for developing epidemiological surveillance for transfusion-transmissible infections (TTI) were also initiated (Mukherjee 2016; Sreekumar et al. 2016).

The HvPI program aims to track and analyze adverse reaction incidents across the blood transfusion chain. By doing so, it seeks to identify patterns, assess trends, and recommend best practices, policies, and interventions to enhance patient care and safety in the context of blood transfusion. To facilitate efficient data collection and analysis, HvPI has developed a specialized software called "Haemo-Vigil." The program operates through close collaboration and communication among haemovigilance units, each having specific roles and responsibilities as shown in Table 14.4.

The objectives of the Haemovigilance Programme of India (HvPI) are comprehensive and essential for enhancing the safety and quality of blood transfusion practices in the country. These objectives can be summarized as follows:

1. Collect, Consolidate, and Evaluate Data: HvPI aims to systematically collect, consolidate, and evaluate data on adverse reactions and events associated with

Table 14.4 Roles and responsibilities of various haemovigilance units

S. no	Haemovigilance unit	Roles and responsibilities
1	CDSCO-DCGI	• Formulate safety-related regulatory decisions • Communication of blood and blood products transfusion-safety-related decisions to stakeholders • To monitor compliance
2	National coordinating center—HvPI	• Review the quality and completeness of the data • Collation and analysis • Preparation of guidance documents • Training and awareness programs • Feedback to reporting units • Recommendations for blood safety to NCC-PvPI at IPC
3	National coordinating center—PvPI	• Forward recommendations of HV—National Advisory Committee to CDSCO
4	Reporting units	• Generate transfusion reaction reports • Causality assessment • Submit a report through HV software

blood transfusion and its components. This data serves as a valuable resource for monitoring and improving transfusion safety.

2. Raise Awareness Among Healthcare Professionals: HvPI strives to raise awareness among healthcare professionals about the importance of actively participating in the haemovigilance initiative. Engaging healthcare providers is crucial for successfully monitoring and reporting adverse events.
3. Generate Evidence-Based Recommendations: The program is committed to generating evidence-based recommendations. It provides valuable insights and data to support the Central Drugs Standard Control Organisation (CDSCO) in making regulatory decisions related to transfusion safety. Evidence-based decision-making is fundamental to enhancing patient and donor safety.
4. Transmit Essential Information: HvPI serves as a communication platform for transmitting essential information related to transfusion safety to stakeholders. This includes sharing recommendations, best practices, and safety guidelines with healthcare institutions, blood banks, and other entities involved in the blood transfusion process.
5. Establish National and International Relationships: The program actively establishes and fosters national and international relationships. Collaborative efforts with other haemovigilance programs and organizations enhance knowledge sharing, collaboration, and the exchange of best practices in transfusion safety.

The joint efforts of the Indian Pharmacopoeia Commission and the National Institute of Biologicals have resulted in a well-structured haemovigilance Programme with clearly defined functions and responsibilities. Through HvPI, India aims to build a robust system for monitoring and addressing adverse reactions, ultimately contributing to the improvement of transfusion practices and the overall quality of patient care in the country. This initiative aligns with global efforts to ensure the safety and efficacy of blood transfusions. The flow chart for reporting adverse reactions associated with blood transfusion is shown in Fig. 14.3.

ANNEXURE IX

FLOW CHART FOR REPORTING ADVERSE REACTIONS ASSOCIATED WITH BLOOD TRANSFUSION

Clinical Transfusion site: Adverse Reaction noted by the Physician / Nurse/Bedside staff

↓

Clinical site: Documentation in Form No.1 **(Annexure II)**

↓

Clinical site: Fill up Form No.2 **(Annexure III)**. Along with Form No.2 send Blood Bag, Transfusion Set, and Post-transfusion Sample to Department of Transfusion Medicine/ Blood Centre for further investigation including Repeat ABO & Rh (D) Grouping, Repeat Antibody Screen and Cross Match, Direct Antiglobulin Test.

↓

Clinical site: Send Post Transfusion Blood in special Blood Culture Bottles to Microbiology Lab.

↓

Clinical site: Send EDTA and Citrated Blood Sample and Urine Sample of the patient to Haematology Lab for Complete blood count (CBC), Plasma haemoglobin, Urine haemoglobin, Coagulation screen.

↓

Clinical site: Send clotted Blood Sample to Biochemistry Lab. for Renal Function Test (Urea, Creatinine and Electrolytes), Liver Function Tests (Bilirubin, ALT and AST).

↓

Department of Transfusion Medicine/ Blood Centre to further investigate the Transfusion Reaction as per the Transfusion Reaction Work up Form, document the findings, compilation of the reports from other departments and reporting results and inferences to the respective Medical Ward.

↓

Department of Transfusion Medicine/ Blood Centre: Assess the Imputability Level of the Transfusion Reaction in coordination with the attending Physician of the respective Medical Ward.

↓

Department of Transfusion Medicine/ Blood Centre: Enter the details in the Transfusion Reaction-Traceability Document (TR-TD). **(Annexure VII)**

↓

Haemo-Vigil Software: Enter the information as per the Transfusion Reaction Reporting Form for Blood & Plasma Products for onward transmission of data to NCC, NIB.

Fig. 14.3 Flow chart for reporting adverse reactions associated with blood transfusion

14.10 Haemovigilance Program of Various Countries

14.10.1 United States of America

In the USA, it is a requirement to notify the Food and Drug Administration (FDA) of any fatal transfusion reactions. However, it took until 2009 to establish a formal national haemovigilance system. The US Department of Health and Human Services, including the Centers for Disease Control and Prevention, and organizations involved in blood donation, transfusion, tissue donation, and organ transplantation came together to launch the US Biovigilance Network in 2006. The AABB Donor Haemovigilance Program is used to track and minimize the incidence of unfavorable outcomes related to blood donation. The American Red Cross, America's Blood Centers, Blood Systems, Inc., the United States Department of Health and Human Services, and hospital blood collection facilities all worked together to design this initiative. It enables participating facilities to enter information into a web-based electronic data collection system and use it for trend and donor data analysis.

According to the most recent FDA annual report on transfusion fatalities, the blood supply is safer now than ever. This improvement is credited to developments in donor screening, improved testing methods, automated data systems, and modifications to transfusion medicine practices. There were 190 transfusion-related fatalities reported in the USA between the fiscal years 2009 and 2013. 74 deaths were attributed to transfusion-related acute lung injury (TRALI), followed by 45 deaths from transfusion-associated circulatory overload (TACO) and 19 deaths from bacterial infections.

14.10.2 United Kingdom (UK)

The Serious Hazards of Transfusion (SHOT) program was launched in the United Kingdom (UK) in 1996 to facilitate reporting adverse events in patients receiving blood transfusions. The National Blood Service (NBS) in England, the Scottish National Blood Transfusion Service, the Northern Ireland Blood Transfusion Service, and the Welsh Blood Service are the four blood transfusion services in the United Kingdom. The SHOT program, which is entirely voluntary, includes all labile blood components offered by these services, and it guarantees strict confidentiality for donors, recipients, and those reporting incidents. The SHOT program introduced an evidence-based approach to enhance patient safety through a robust reporting system. An increase in the reporting of adverse reactions would contribute to raising the standards of transfusion practices in hospitals, the development of clinical transfusion guidelines, and the education of clinicians on the judicious use of blood products (Mani et al. n.d.)

14.10.3 Australia

Australia's "National Safety and Quality Health Service Standards" incorporate a specific standard focused on blood and blood products. This standard outlines the procedures and methods required for the healthcare system's safe, appropriate, and effective management of blood and blood products. Within the Australian National Haemovigilance System, hospitals play a pivotal role in identifying, reviewing, and reporting incidents related to blood and blood products to their respective regional haemovigilance programs. These regional programs are responsible for reviewing, validating, assessing the severity, and determining the imputability of reported events. These similar incidents are subsequently reported to the national framework and data dictionary. The National Haemovigilance Advisory Committee then analyzes this data and generates comprehensive reports and recommendations. It is important to note that different regions in Australia assign responsibility for jurisdictional practice improvement and haemovigilance activities to various organizations. In South Australia, this responsibility falls under the purview of "Blood Safe." In New South Wales, it is managed by "Blood Watch." In the Australian Capital Territory (ACT), the "Appropriate Use of Blood Reference Group" oversees these activities. In the Northern Territory, it is the "Transfusion Safety Program." In Queensland, the "Blood Management Program" is responsible. In Victoria and Tasmania, "Blood Matters" takes the lead, and In Western Australia, it is managed by the "Patient Blood Management Program" (WHO 2013).

14.10.4 France

The "Agence Française du Sang" (AFS) took on overseeing the haemovigilance system starting in 1994. The primary objective of the AFS was to identify and thoroughly analyze any adverse effects associated with blood transfusions to prevent their recurrence. Transfusion incident reports (TIR) were centralized at the AFS level, and the reporting is mandatory. Within the French Haemovigilance System, blood center physicians at each hospital conducting transfusions were designated as responsible for gathering reports on transfusion reactions and subsequently reporting them to the local health authorities. These local authorities, in turn, were obligated to transmit these reports to the AFS's centralized haemovigilance cell (Mani et al. n.d.).

14.10.5 Japan

In Japan, a haemovigilance system was started in 1993 by the Japanese Red Cross Society (JRCS). The JRCS holds the exclusive responsibility for providing labile blood products, overseeing the entire process from blood product collection and processing to distribution, and managing adverse reactions and infectious disease concerns. The information collected through reported cases is then shared with medical institutions, aiming to assist treating physicians in making precise diagnoses. This collaborative effort enhances the quality and safety of blood products (Mani et al. n.d.).

14.11 Problems Concerned with the Implementation of Haemovigilance

The implementation of haemovigilance indeed faces various challenges and potential errors throughout the blood transfusion process, which can have severe consequences if not addressed effectively. Here is a summary of some of the critical challenges and potential solutions:

1. Deficiencies in Standard Definitions and Reporting Protocols: Standardized definitions and uniform reporting protocols are essential to ensure consistent reporting and analysis of adverse events. Efforts should be made to harmonize definitions and protocols at both national and international levels to address this challenge. Collaboration with organizations like the International Haemovigilance Network (IHN) can help establish common standards.
2. Organizational Problems: Issues such as inadequate funding, ambiguous mandates, and unclear responsibilities can hinder the effectiveness of haemovigilance programs. Governments and healthcare authorities should provide sufficient resources and support to ensure the proper functioning of these programs. Clear mandates and responsibilities should be defined, and staff should receive adequate training.
3. Underreporting of Adverse Reactions: Concerns about underreporting of adverse reactions to blood and blood products are valid. Encouraging a culture of reporting adverse events is crucial. Healthcare professionals should be educated about the importance of reporting, and reporting mechanisms should be made user-friendly and accessible. Whistleblower protections can also help in addressing underreporting.
4. Errors in Transfusion Process: Blood or blood component distribution, testing, processing, storage, and storage errors can be fatal. Strict adherence to established protocols and procedures is critical. Training of healthcare staff involved in transfusion, including thorough verification processes, can significantly reduce the risk of errors. Implementing technologies like barcoding and electronic matching systems can enhance patient safety.
5. Disparities in Haemovigilance Practices: Disparities in haemovigilance practices between countries can lead to variations in the quality and safety of blood transfusion. International collaboration and knowledge sharing can help countries with less developed haemovigilance systems learn from those with more established programs. The exchange of best practices and expertise can contribute to global improvements in haemovigilance.

Addressing these challenges requires a multi-faceted approach involving standardization, education, funding, and a safety culture. By improving haemovigilance practices and promoting strict adherence to established procedures, the safety and effectiveness of blood transfusion processes can be enhanced, ultimately leading to better patient outcomes and reduced risks associated with transfusion-related adverse events.

14.12 WHO's Recommendations and Priorities for Action on Haemovigilance

The World Health Organization (WHO) has put forth numerous recommendations and action priorities in a report following a global consultation on haemovigilance events. This consultation was a collaborative effort between WHO HQ/Geneva, the Sharjah Blood Transfusion Research Center, and the government of the United Arab Emirates. It involved partnerships with the International Haemovigilance Network and the International Society of Blood Transfusion. These recommendations and priorities aim to enhance the safety and effectiveness of blood transfusion practices worldwide.

14.12.1 Recommendations to Hospital/Institutional Level

For the successful implementation of haemovigilance in hospitals and other healthcare facilities, hospital administrators and clinical staff should consider the following key actions and recommendations:

1. Implement Clinical Guidelines: Follow clinical guidelines for blood and blood product transfusions based on national standards. These guidelines should cover:
   (a) positive patient identification before transfusion,
   (b) transfusion triggers (criteria for when transfusions are necessary),
   (c) accurate transfusion process documentation,
   (d) continual evaluation of clinical transfusion procedures, and,
   (e) compliance with traceability requirements.
2. Establish Policies and Procedures: Create Comprehensive Policies and Procedures for Each Step in the Blood Transfusion Process, including those related to haemovigilance. Ensure that these policies align with local, national, or international standards. They are non-punitive to encourage reporting and are regularly reviewed and updated.
3. Define Quality Indicators: Identify quality indicators that serve as measures of clinical practice and traceability. These indicators should include confirmation of transfusion and indicator data should be regularly collected and analyzed to drive continuous quality improvement efforts.
4. Reporting Mechanisms: Create mechanisms for reporting adverse transfusion events, reactions, and incidents. This should include:

   (a) using standardized incident reporting forms and adverse transfusion reaction forms,
   (b) creating procedures for examining transfusion responses,
   (c) clearly outlining reporting and follow-up duties and responsibilities, and,
   (d) consistently reviewing events and adverse responses via the hospital transfusion committee.
5. Resource Allocation: Establish and maintain an efficient haemovigilance system at the hospital level by allocating enough human and financial resources.
6. Training and Education: Create systems to assure the competency and knowledge of all staff members involved in the transfusion chain by educating and training them on haemovigilance and transfusion safety.
7. Transfusion Committees: Establish, activate, and maintain hospital transfusion committees to oversee and coordinate haemovigilance activities within the facility.
8. Transfusion Nurse or Haemovigilance Officer: Designate or appoint a Transfusion Nurse or Haemovigilance Officer within the hospital. This individual should be responsible for:
   (a) following up on all reports of adverse transfusion events,
   (b) reporting incidents to the hospital transfusion committee, and,
   (c) reporting incidents to the National Haemovigilance Office, if applicable.

By following these recommendations, healthcare facilities can enhance the safety, quality, and effectiveness of blood transfusion practices and contribute to improved patient outcomes.

14.12.2 Recommendations at National Level

For the successful implementation of haemovigilance at the national level, Ministries of Health and state/local health authorities should consider the following key actions and recommendations:

1. Recognition of Importance: Acknowledge the critical importance of haemovigilance for ensuring the quality and safety of blood donation and transfusion.
2. Incorporate into National Blood Policy: Include surveillance of the entire blood cold chain within the framework of the national blood policy.
3. Establish National Haemovigilance System: Create and maintain a national haemovigilance system that covers all aspects of the blood chain, including donors and recipients, processes, and products.
4. Strategic Planning: Develop strategic plans for gradually developing the haemovigilance system, evolving from basic to more complex stages.
5. Leadership and Governance: Provide effective leadership, direction, and governance to drive the development and operation of the national haemovigilance system.

6. Stakeholder Coordination: Establish mechanisms for coordination and collaboration among all stakeholders, including institutions and organizations involved in the blood chain.
7. Organizational Structure: Create an efficient organizational structure that monitors the entire blood chain, including donors, recipients, products, and processes.
8. Non-Punitive Environment: Ensure a non-punitive environment when developing the haemovigilance system to encourage reporting and transparency.
9. Data Management: Implement methods and channels for data collection, monitoring, analysis, reporting, evaluation, assessment, rapid alerting, and early warning.
10. Policy Integration: Ensure that haemovigilance is effectively integrated into policy formulation and quality management, ultimately improving the quality and safety of the entire blood chain.
11. Resource Allocation: Allocate the necessary financial and human resources to implement the haemovigilance system effectively.
12. Access to Expertise: Facilitate access to current medical and scientific expertise to enhance the haemovigilance system's capabilities.

Similarly, for the implementation of haemovigilance at the national level, all blood centers and transfusion services should consider the following actions and recommendations:

1. Define Roles and Responsibilities: Clearly define the roles and responsibilities of blood centers concerning their involvement in the haemovigilance system.
2. Reporting Systems: Develop comprehensive systems for reporting adverse donor reactions and errors, covering data collection, notification, reporting, monitoring, analysis, and evaluation.
3. Liaison Mechanism: Establish a mechanism for effective liaison and communication with hospitals, blood banks/blood transfusion laboratories, and hospital transfusion committees (HTC).
4. Traceability: Ensure bidirectional tracking from donor to transfused patient and vice versa (vein to vein) using appropriate information technology and communication tools to guarantee traceability.
5. Integration with Quality Management: Integrate haemovigilance into the existing quality management system to harmonize quality and safety efforts.

By following these recommendations, Ministries of Health, state/local health authorities, blood centers, and transfusion services can collectively contribute to a robust and effective national haemovigilance system, enhancing blood transfusion safety and quality across the healthcare system.

14.12.3 Recommendations at International Level

International organizations, such as the World Health Organization (WHO), the International Haemovigilance Network (IHN), and the International Society of Blood Transfusion (ISBT), are essential to the advancement of haemovigilance initiatives worldwide. These are the recommended actions and responsibilities for these organizations:

1. Advocacy and Support: Promote and offer high-level advocacy to national health authorities, imploring them to set up, carry out, assess, and continuously enhance haemovigilance systems within their respective nations.
2. Guidelines and Standardization: Create global technical standards, educational materials, uniform/standardized reporting systems, and definitions. These resources should make establishing, implementing, assessing, and enhancing national haemovigilance systems easier.
3. Technical Assistance: Offer technical support to countries by:
   (a) determining the particular requirements they have for the creation of a national haemovigilance system,
   (b) conducting evaluations to find gaps and create plans for implementing the system, and,
   (c) enabling the creation and execution of haemovigilance plans.
4. Networking and Partnerships: Facilitate networking opportunities and support establishing partnerships or twinning mechanisms for haemovigilance within and between Member States. This collaborative approach can foster knowledge exchange and capacity building.
5. Building Capacity: To increase capacity and assist the development of haemovigilance skills in nations, organize educational and training initiatives in haemovigilance at the regional and national levels.
6. Sharing of Information: Develop or strengthen channels for global networking through consultation and discussion. Promote international exchange of knowledge regarding haemovigilance, including ideas, best practices, statistics, information, experiences, and reports.
7. Establish an online forum or electronic forum where nations may easily share publications and information on haemovigilance, fostering cooperative study and information exchange.
8. Information Dissemination: Disseminate information, website addresses, and links related to different haemovigilance systems, making it easier for stakeholders to access relevant resources and information.
9. Publication and Communication: Encourage and support the publication and communication of haemovigilance findings and reports at international forums, including WHO, IHN, ISBT, and other international conferences and meetings. This sharing of knowledge helps raise awareness and promotes best practices.
10. Collaborative Partnerships: Develop collaborative partnerships among international organizations working on Haemovigilance. Cooperation between organizations can amplify the impact of haemovigilance efforts worldwide and ensure a coordinated approach.

By taking on these roles and responsibilities, international organizations can contribute significantly to establishing and enhancing effective haemovigilance systems globally, ultimately improving the safety and quality of blood transfusion practices across countries.

14.12.4 Priorities for Action

1. Advocacy for Establishment: Provide high-level advocacy to decision-makers in the Ministry of Health and National Health Authorities, emphasizing the importance of establishing national haemovigilance systems for blood safety.
2. Expand Networking: Intensify and broaden networking efforts with international organizations already engaged in the field of haemovigilance. Collaboration and information sharing can enhance global efforts.
3. Technical and Managerial Information: Offer technical and managerial guidance and information to assist countries in setting up and developing haemovigilance systems effectively.
4. Protocols and Tools: Facilitate access to or develop standardized protocols and tools for collecting, analyzing, and utilizing national blood donor and transfusion data. These tools should align with international standards.
5. Standardized Case Definitions: Assist in establishing efficient processes for providing standard case definitions, which are essential for consistent data collection in haemovigilance systems.
6. Strengthen Clinical Interface: Strengthen the clinical interface between hospitals and blood banks/supplying blood centers to improve communication and collaboration.
7. Hospital Transfusion Committees (HTC): Advocate for and encourage creating and maintaining functional hospital transfusion committees (HTC) to oversee and enhance transfusion safety within healthcare facilities.
8. Support IT Systems: Provide support for information technology (IT) systems, including:
   (a) developing a system for donor data management,
   (b) enhancing patient record systems in hospitals concerning transfusion,
   (c) establishing a database for traceability, and,
   (d) offering training to staff on IT usage.
9. Capacity Building: Strengthen capacity in haemovigilance through:
   (a) national training programs for various stakeholders, such as clinicians, nurses, midwives, and blood bank workers, focus on best transfusion practices and haemovigilance;
   (b) assisting in establishing haemovigilance systems at the local level, such as hospitals and blood banks (including protocols, forms, reporting systems, and administrative organization);
   (c) providing support and assistance to priority countries in setting up haemovigilance systems; and,
   (d) Implementing a stepwise approach to gradually introduce haemovigilance programs, starting with major medical college hospitals and expanding to other healthcare facilities over time.

By taking on these roles and responsibilities, international organizations can significantly contribute to establishing and strengthening national haemovigilance systems, thereby enhancing the safety and quality of blood transfusion practices worldwide.

14.13 Database Used in Haemovigilance

The International Surveillance of Transfusion-Associated Reactions and Events (ISTARE) database is valuable for improving haemovigilance. Here are some critical points about ISTARE:

- Purpose: ISTARE is designed to collect national haemovigilance data on adverse reactions and events related to blood transfusion practices from around the world. Its primary goal is to enable international comparisons, facilitate information sharing, and provide a platform for benchmarking haemovigilance practices globally.
- Establishment: ISTARE was established in 2008, and since then, it has been instrumental in compiling data on adverse reactions and events, both from blood component donors and recipients, across various countries.
- Comprehensive Approach: The International Haemovigilance Network (IHN), which oversees ISTARE, promotes a holistic haemovigilance approach. This means that ISTARE does not solely focus on serious adverse events but also includes a broader range of reactions and events related to blood transfusions.
- Data Analysis: ISTARE has features that automatically generate rates and ratios of adverse reactions. It also produces charts that allow for the comparison of national data with international data for periods of up to one or more years.
- Covered Areas: ISTARE compiles data on various aspects of haemovigilance, including event rates (both overall and by product type), the type of reaction categorized by severity and imputability, distributions of event types, averages for global regions, and monitoring of trends in adverse reactions and events.

By providing a centralized and standardized platform for haemovigilance data collection and analysis, ISTARE contributes significantly to the global understanding of transfusion-related adverse events and helps identify trends and areas for improvement in transfusion safety practices.

ISTARE is a comprehensive database that captures a wide range of data related to haemovigilance efforts. Types of data it captures:

General Information: This includes information about the structure and coverage of the haemovigilance system in a given region or country. It provides an overview of how haemovigilance is organized and managed.

General Denominators: ISTARE collects data on the numbers of donors and donations and the main categories of blood products. This information provides context and basic statistics about the blood transfusion system.

Specific Denominators: Besides general denominators, the database also captures denominator data for particular types of blood components issued and transfused. This allows for a more detailed analysis of blood product usage.

Donor Complications: ISTARE records events related to donor complications, including those associated with whole blood donations and apheresis donations. This information helps monitor and improve donor safety.

Errors—Incorrect Blood Component Transfused (IBCT): This category includes data on errors related to transfusion, such as ABO-incompatible transfusions, sampling errors, and cases of wrong labeling. These errors can have serious consequences, and tracking them is crucial for patient safety.

Adverse Transfusion Reactions: ISTARE compiles data on adverse transfusion reactions, categorizing them by various factors:

- By blood component: This categorizes adverse reactions based on the specific type of blood component involved.
- By imputability: Adverse reactions are categorized as "possibly," "probably," or "definitely" related to the transfusion. This helps assess the likelihood of the reaction being linked to the transfusion.
- By severity: Adverse reactions are classified based on severity, including non-severe, severe, life-threatening, and fatal reactions. This classification helps in understanding the seriousness of adverse events.

By capturing data across these categories, ISTARE provides:

- a comprehensive view of haemovigilance practices,
- enabling international comparisons,
- trend analysis, and,
- the development of evidence-based recommendations for improving transfusion safety and donor well-being.

14.14 Conclusion

In conclusion, haemovigilance plays a crucial and continuous role in ensuring the safety and quality of the blood transfusion process. By systematically collecting and analyzing data on adverse reactions, haemovigilance serves as a vigilant guardian of patient safety. It helps identify trends, investigates root causes, and enables the implementation of corrective and preventive measures, ultimately minimizing risks and enhancing the entire blood transfusion chain's safety and quality. Moreover, haemovigilance serves as a powerful quality indicator, shedding light on the effectiveness of transfusion practices and highlighting areas where improvements are needed. The knowledge gained from haemovigilance activities informs policy changes, guideline development, and the enhancement of standards and processes, fostering a culture of professionalism and continuous improvement within healthcare systems.

Furthermore, haemovigilance is not confined to national boundaries; it plays a pivotal role in international cooperation. Collaboration among countries facilitates the exchange of best practices, benchmarking, and harmonizing haemovigilance systems worldwide. This global approach strengthens the collective knowledge base and promotes the advancement of haemovigilance efforts on an international scale. In essence, haemovigilance is an indispensable tool that safeguards the well-being of both blood donors and recipients, drives ongoing improvements in transfusion practices, and contributes significantly to the healthcare system's ability to provide optimal care.

References

Faber JC (2004) The European blood directive: a new era of blood regulation has begun. Transfus Med 14(4):257–273. https://doi.org/10.1111/J.0958-7578.2004.00513.X

Jain A, Kaur R (2012) Hemovigilance and blood safety. Asian J Transfus Sci 6(2):137. https://doi.org/10.4103/0973-6247.98911

Khobragade RS, Paranjape SG, Gadhade JB, Premchand A (2022) Hemovigilance: a momentous step to blood safety. Int J Basic Clin Pharmacol 11(3):267. https://doi.org/10.18203/2319-2003.ijbcp20221043

Mani A, Chaitanya Kumar IS, Bodade AG, Khade A (n.d.) Hemovigilance and transfusion safety: a review on the hemovigilance systems across various countries. Eur J Mol Clin Med 1:1

Mukherjee S (2016) Haemovigilance: a current update in Indian perspective. J Clin Diagn Res 10:EE05. https://doi.org/10.7860/JCDR/2016/21029.8868

NIB (2019) Haemovigilance Programme of India, "Guidance document for reporting adverse transfusion reactions in blood transfusion services". Accessed 9 Jul 2023. https://www.nib.gov.in/Haemovigilance/G%20D%20Ver%203%20(2019).pdf. Accessed 20 Aug 2023

NIB (2022a) National blood donor vigilance program, "Guidance document for reporting blood donor adverse reactions". https://nib.gov.in/Haemovigilance/Final%20Guidance%20document%20for%20donor%20haemovigilance.pdf. Accessed 9 Jul 2023

NIB (2022b) Haemovigilance Programme of India, "Haemovigilance newsletter". Accessed 9 Jul 2023. https://nib.gov.in/Haemovigilance/Haemovigilance%20Newsletter%20Vol.%20No.%2010%20Issue%2020,%20July-December,%202022.pdf. Accessed 4 Sept 2023

Sadique Hussain M (2022) Mini-review on haemovigilance: an Indian perspective. Pharm Pharm Res 5(6):01–06. https://doi.org/10.31579/2693-7247/090

Sreekumar P, Pramod Kumar T, Partha Sarathi G, Gupta D (2016) Haemovigilance and its significance in transfusion safety. Int J Drug Res Technol 6(4):245–249; http://www.ijdrt.com

Watson R (2005) EU tightens rules on blood safety. BMJ 331(7520):800. https://doi.org/10.1136/BMJ.331.7520.800-C

WHO (2013) "Haemovigilance-report," Dubai, United Arab Emirates. https://cdn.who.int/media/docs/default-source/biologicals/blood-products/document-migration/haemovigilance-report.pdf?sfvrsn=7a7a74ed_3&download=true. Accessed 26 Aug 2023

World Health Organization (2016) A guide to establishing a national haemovigilance system. WHO, Switzerland, pp 1–44

Role of Pharmacogenetics in Pharmacovigilance

15

Ruchika Sharma, Mukesh Nandave, and Anoop Kumar

Abstract

Pharmacovigilance information is most important and has been involved in the summary of product characteristics (SPC) of medications since the turn of the century. Both newly launched medications and those that have a strong market presence rely on pharmacovigilance to help assure patient safety. Adverse events occur after post-marketing if pharmacovigilance reporting is not implemented or enforced for clinical studies. Precisely, it is estimated that between 90% and 100% of adverse events associated with currently available drugs are not reported. As a result, identifying drug safety issues in people with severe comorbidities and complicated conditions is very difficult. Because conventional doses of pharmacological drugs are utilised to treat each patient in populations without these concerns, a complete awareness of potential difficulties and contraindications associated with genome in the population is inadequate. Therefore, pharmacogenetics is a cutting-edge technology that can help to solve these challenges. This chapter discusses pharmacovigilance science, pharmacogenetics, and the importance of pharmacogenetics in adverse drug reactions (ADRs), patient care, and clinical trials. Furthermore, this chapter discusses current pharmacogenetics issues.

R. Sharma (✉)
Centre for Precision Medicine and Pharmacy, Delhi Pharmaceutical Sciences and Research University DPSRU, New Delhi, India

M. Nandave · A. Kumar
Department of Pharmacology, Delhi Pharmaceutical Sciences and Research University, New Delhi, India
e-mail: mukeshnandave@gmail.com; anoopdpsru@dpsru.edu.in

M. Nandave, A. Kumar (eds.), *Pharmacovigilance Essentials*,
https://doi.org/10.1007/978-981-99-8949-2_15

Keywords

Omics · Genetics · ADRs · Clinical trials · Drug safety

15.1 Introduction

The availability of many new drugs due to improvements in drug development technologies has increased the risk of adverse drug reactions (ADRs) (Coleman and Pontefract 2016). These have supported the establishment of pharmacovigilance systems, which monitor the safety of medications. The primary pharmacovigilance system components are struggling with substantial under-reporting issues. The study of drug-metabolising enzymes, pharmacogenetics of adverse drug reactions (ADRs), the discovery of genetic biomarkers, diagnostic tests for pharmacogenetic decisions, recommendations for gene/drug pairs, and individualised use of medications are the main topics covered by pharmacogenomics, in addition to drug safety and efficacy studies (Ventola 2013). There is a lot of variation in how each person reacts to medications. This may be caused by the heterogeneity of the disease being treated as well as clinical patient factors such as age, sex, nutrition, concurrent drug use, and renal or hepatic functioning (Venter et al. 2018). Additionally, inherited traits of the genome may contribute to some of the heterogeneity in medication response. The pharmacokinetics, pharmacodynamics, or susceptibility of an individual may be affected by these genetic differences (Venter et al. 2018; Roden et al. 2011).

Pharmacogenetics is the study of differences in each person's deoxyribonucleic acid (DNA) sequence that are related to how drugs are disposed of (pharmacokinetics) or how they work (pharmacodynamics), which may have an impact on their therapeutic response (Sharma et al. 2022). For nearly 60 years, the phrase has been in use. The use of genomic technologies (such as next generation sequencing) to comprehend disease susceptibility, conservation, drug discovery, precision medicine, biomarker discover, and treatment response is known as pharmacogenomics, a term that has just recently been coined (Sharma et al. 2022; Crews et al. 2012). Thus, pharmacogenomics illustrates the transition from genetics to genomics by presenting a genome-wide approach to identifying genes that contribute to a certain disease (Ventola 2011).

Pharmacogenetics information has been included in the summary of product characteristics (SPC) of medications since the turn of the century. Pharmacogenetic tests are mainly focused on the P450 cytochromes, which are key players in the metabolism of medicines. Some patients are metabolisers of some medications more slowly than others, leading to overdoses and ADRs (Forster et al. 2021). The most well-known examples are clopidogrel and CYP2C19 or AVK and VKORC1-CYP2C9. Testing for HLA-B*1502 and HLA-B*5801 before commencing carbamazepine and allopurinol, respectively, and only administering the medication to non-carriers, is another illustration of the value of pharmacogenomic biomarkers in reducing adverse drug responses through the selection of patients (Brown and Pereira 2018; Pereira et al. 2019). As a result, there is now a lower likelihood of these medications causing severe cutaneous side effects such as Stevens-Johnson syndrome and toxic epidermal necrolysis. It should be remembered that ethnicity matters and that the biomarkers HLA-B*1502 and HLA-B*5801 are particularly common in some Asian groups (Pereira et al. 2019).

To avoid the occurrence of ADRs, testing is advised in the USA prior to the administration of these medications. To assess the toxicity of specific anticancer medications (such as UGT1A1-irinotecan and TPMT 6-mercaptopurine), additional tests are frequently conducted (Varughese et al. 2020; Franczyk et al. 2022). Many affluent nations have adopted pharmacogenomics-based practises; nonetheless, this development has presented difficulties for medical professionals acting as suppliers of health care services. This chapter's primary goal is to examine pharmacovigilance concerns connected to pharmacogenomic and to connect pharmacogenetics to pharmacovigilance for improved drug safety and efficacy. The International Society of Pharmacovigilance (ISoP) is a non-profit international scientific organisation that promotes pharmacovigilance through science and education and works to improve all facets of the safe use of medications worldwide (Yue 2021).

15.1.1 Pharmacogenetics

Pharmacogenetics is a subfield of pharmacology that examines how individual differences in DNA sequence relate to how well and how badly people respond to medications. These variations could be found in both the pharmacodynamics and the pharmacokinetics (Abdullah-Koolmees et al. 2021). Any kind of polymorphism in the genome can change a drug's function, causing it to either not produce a clinical response to a given treatment or to produce unfavourable responses.

15.1.2 Pharmacogenomics

The term "pharmacogenomics" refers to a group of techniques used to identify new therapeutic targets by using knowledge of the genome and its byproducts. These techniques include rational pharmacology, the discovery and use of drugs, and research into the effects of those drugs on human genetic variability (Abdullah-Koolmees et al. 2021). As a result, it should be feasible to develop customised therapy procedures that are safer and more logical, as well as targeted drugs.

15.2 Pharmacogenovigilance

Generally talking, "pharmacogenovigilance" refers to pharmacovigilance operations that are influenced by pharmacogenomics studies and analyses. It includes the investigation and understanding of genetic variants in all facets of patient care and healthcare delivery. To explain individual and inter-population variation in medication pharmacokinetics and pharmacodynamics, pharmacovigilance and pharmacogenomics share this goal. Pharmacogenomics is crucial for maximising drug safety, even while pharmacovigilance enhances patient care and safety (Suke et al. 2015; Bhimaneni et al. 2021).

Pharmacogenovigilance, which incorporates pharmacogenomics, has a more mechanistic surveillance strategy than conventional pharmacovigilance. This is very helpful for determining causation. Furthermore, if the global polymorphism distribution associated with a specific pharmacological reaction is known, it enables extrapolation from one population to another. It also aids in understanding how medications behave pharmacokinetically and pharmacodynamically in diverse genetic subpopulations (Jeetu and Anusha 2010).

As a result, pharmacovigilance in the modern era of pharmacogenomics cannot disregard this idea. Future pharmacovigilance efforts may even be unethical if pharmacogenomic tests are not taken into account. Thus, it is necessary to build a national pharmacovigilance system that takes pharmacogenomics into account. This will make it easier to combine various data sources and evaluate the causal links between genetic markers, medications, and ADRs (Jeetu and Anusha 2010). Pharmacogenovigilance is still not frequently used in clinical practise, nevertheless. The fact that pharmacogenomics is still a young field is one of the causes. Despite recent developments, it has taken time for its integration into healthcare services. The lack of knowledge among healthcare professionals is another significant hurdle.

15.3 Drug Safety Challenges

ADRs are a significant issue for all stakeholders globally. According to the WHO, an adverse drug reaction is any reaction to a drug that is harmful and unexpected and that takes place at levels given to humans for prevention, diagnosis, or therapy, excluding failure to achieve the intended goal (Coleman et al. 2006). After the thalidomide crisis in the 1960s, an international drug monitoring program was established in response to the issues that ADRs presented to medical practitioners (Coleman et al. 2006; Davies et al. 2009). Between 0.3% and 11% of hospital admissions are ADRs, which is a sizable percentage (Davies et al. 2009; Aronson and Ferner 2003). In the United States of America (USA), adverse medication reactions are the fourth greatest cause of death, and the cost of treating drug problems has increased by up to 20%. Short-term hospitalisation, long-term hospitalisation, and even mortality are potential outcomes of ADRs. ADRs to medications cause over 100,000 American deaths annually, and about two million people are hospitalised (Aronson and Ferner 2003; Sultana et al. 2013; Mejía et al. 2020). ADRs and medication errors are thought to be the cause of 2.3% of hospital stays in the United Kingdom (UK), 4.8% in Germany, and 7.3% in the USA. According to studies, 20–25% of deaths are related to prescription medicines, and in the vast majority of cases, the deaths might have been avoided (Mejía et al. 2020). It has been determined that up to 50% of recently approved medicines have major ADRs that were discovered at the post-marketing stage, but sadly only 5% were reported. Therefore, structural and functional pharmacogenomics play a vital role in drug discover as presented in Fig. 15.1.

Genetic factors that cause genetic polymorphism, individual variations in an enzyme's capacity to metabolise drugs, and variations in drug receptors and transporters are thought to determine ethnic background. ADRs occurrence varies from patient population to patient population due to genetic variations. African-Americans are more sensitive to ACE-related angioedema than other ethnic groups, according to a cohort study that used 2225 participants to look into characteristics that predispose patients to ADRs with angiotensin-converting enzyme (ACE) inhibitors. According to studies, black people had a 3.0 relative risk of angioedema and a higher risk of cerebral haemorrhage than non-black people. People from East Asia are three times more likely than white people to develop cough while using ACE inhibitors (Mathey et al. 2022). Parkinson disease patients with the UDP-glucuronosyltransferase 1A9 genotype are more likely to experience adverse drug reactions (ADRs) when taking catechol-O-methyltransferase inhibitors. According to recent studies, patients who acquired ADRs had higher levels of CYP1A2, low allele combinations (8/12; 67%), and lower levels of CYP1A2-mRNA than patients

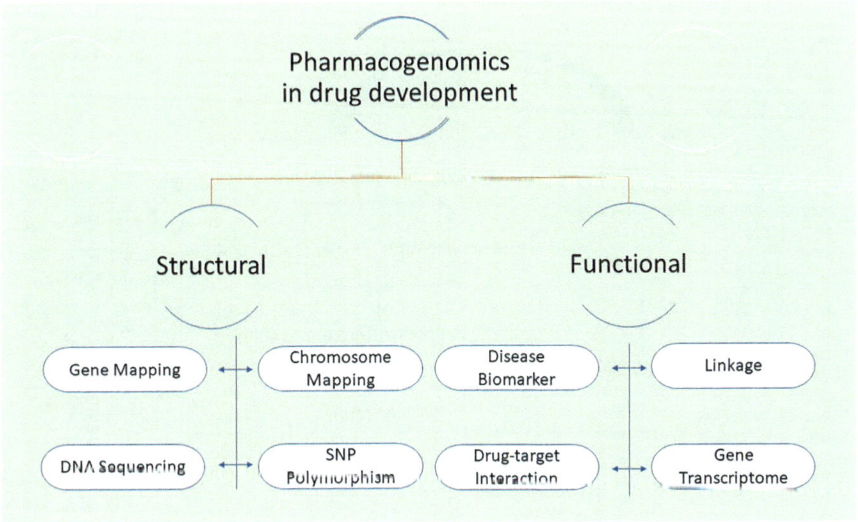

Fig. 15.1 Role of pharmacogenomics in drug development and safety

who did not (6/22; 27%, $p = 0.019$) (Ferrari et al. 2012; Sheng et al. 2021; Babayeva and Loewy 2023).

15.4 Pharmacogenetics: A Potential Tool in Pharmacovigilance

15.4.1 Role of Pharmacogenetics in Adverse Drug Reactions

ADRs play a major role in poor medication adherence, hospitalisation, and even mortality. In the USA, it is estimated that ADRs alone cause 100,000 fatalities per year. The fourth most frequent cause of death is this. As a result, identifying those who are highly susceptible to idiosyncratic ADRs may aid in reducing their occurrence and associated expenses (Davies et al. 2009; Aronson and Ferner 2003). Depending on an individual's variations in the genes that code for the drugs' receptors and the proteins that transport or metabolise them, drug efficacy and toxicity may differ. Pharmacogenomics therefore has great potential and is currently being investigated for its capacity to lower ADRs (Alomar 2014; Mathey et al. 2022) as described in Fig. 15.2.

It is common for the long-term safety of a drug to be unknown at the time of market approval. Furthermore, clinical trial samples are rarely entirely representative of the patient population in practise. In actual clinical practise, patients usually have numerous comorbidities and use multiple medications. Pharmacovigilance is the process of continuing to monitor a drug's effects after it has received approval. The major objectives are to identify, evaluate, comprehend, and stop any short- and long-term ADRs. Additionally, it is essential for establishing a favourable

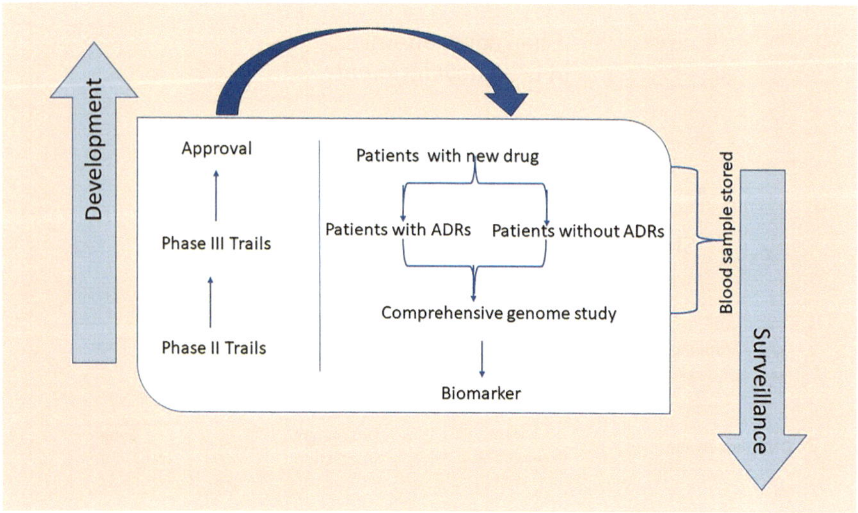

Fig. 15.2 Role of pharmacogenetics in adverse drug reactions

risk–benefit ratio. In light of this, pharmacovigilance is essential for quality control in all areas of healthcare delivery (Hamid et al. 2022; Lucas et al. 2022).

Currently, the pharmacovigilance system is heavily reliant on adverse event reports that are submitted voluntarily. This system, however, confronts many difficulties. ADRs can affect any organ or device and be caused by a wide range of therapeutics, including anticonvulsants, antibiotics, antiretrovirals, and antiarrhythmics (Coleman et al. 2006). Because of the clinical complexity and variability of ADRs, their causes are still poorly understood. In this scenario, genetic predisposition to ADRs is emerging, not only in anticancer chemotherapy but also in many other medical specialties such as anaemia, malignant hyperthermia, necrosis, epilepsy, thyroid disorders, diabetes, etc. The involvement of genetic changes in the development of ADRs has been revealed for both dose-dependent and dose-independent reactions (Wilke et al. 2007; Osanlou et al. 2018; Micaglio et al. 2021). Thus, the expanded use of pharmacogenetic testing in the investigation of ADRs will result in new clinical diagnoses of diseases that were not previously recognised as well as enhanced therapeutic safety and effectiveness. Future advancements in genotype–phenotype correlation through the use of artificial intelligence and improved lab techniques may result in personalised medicine that can predict ADR and, as a result, select the best chemical and dosage for each patient.

15.4.2 Role of Pharmacogenetics in Clinical Trails

Pharmaceutical corporations have demonstrated a great deal of caution in the relatively recent area of pharmacogenomics in clinical trials. There are many benefits to including pharmacogenomic testing in clinical studies. Safety and efficacy are the two main issues to be addressed in the creation of new medications. Both of these characteristics had very little prediction prior to the development of pharmacogenetic techniques. This resulted in significant financial loss as a result of drug compound attrition during clinical trials. Currently, the situation has changed, and the attrition rate can be greatly decreased, thanks to the availability of powerful pharmacogenetic methods. This results in less money being lost that could be used to create new drugs. With the aid of in vitro techniques, it is possible to determine whether the drug is metabolised by polymorphic enzymes during preclinical investigations and then decide whether to continue the study.

Additionally, choosing appropriate individuals for phase I clinical trials with normal metabolising enzymes and preventing adverse events can both benefit from this information (Rioux 2000; Burt and Dhillon 2013; Harper and Topol 2012; Sukumar et al. 2002). It should be highlighted that only when the drug's metabolic pathway is identified can pharmacogenetic principles be utilised as inclusion or exclusion criteria (Fig. 15.3).

In the early stages of research, when knowledge regarding the drug's metabolism is unknown, pharmacogenetic concepts cannot be employed for subject selection. However, as demonstrated in Table 15.1 (Surendiran et al. 2008), obtaining pharmacogenetic data in the early stages of a clinical study can be beneficial later on.

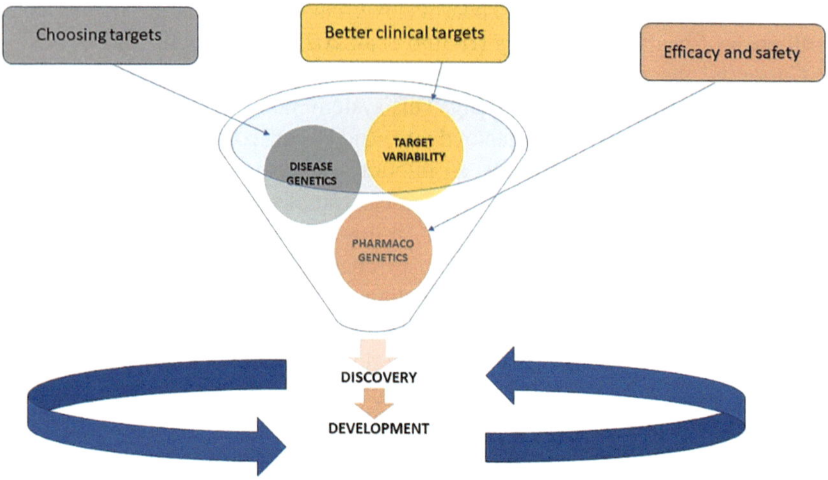

Fig. 15.3 Role of pharmacogenetics in clinical trials

Table 15.1 Application of pharmacogenetic/pharmacogenomic techniques at different phases of drug development

Stage	Technique	Application of pharmacogenetics/pharmacogenomics
	Drug target identification	Identification and characterisation of the gene coding for the drug target and to assess the variability
Phase I	Clinical trial	Patient selection—inclusion/exclusion criteria
		Dose range selection
Phase II	Clinical trial	Dose modification
Phase III	Clinical trial	Interpretation of trial results based on pharmacogenetic test results
Phase IV	Clinical trial	Analysis of reported adverse events with pharmacogenetic tests
	Regulatory issues	Requirements for submission of pharmacogenetic data during development by FDA
	Patient therapeutics	Personalisation of drug therapy
		Pharmacogenetic data in drug labelling
		Identification of responders and nonresponders
		Identification of high-risk groups of adverse events

15.4.3 Pharmacogenetics in Patient Care

The most often used pharmacogenetic testing for patient care involves finding polymorphisms in the genes that code for drug metabolising enzymes and helping to choose or modify the dosage. According to a recent study, polymorphic enzymes are involved in the metabolism of 59% of medications that result in negative side effects. For example, at regular doses, warfarin has been proven to have an improved effect in patients with elevated INR (International Normalised Ratio). Following pharmacogenetic testing, it was shown that these patients had *3/*4 and *1/*3 CYP2C9 polymorphisms, indicating that they were poor metabolisers. The FDA has approved the inclusion of pharmacogenetic data in the warfarin product label, and the warfarin product label now includes genetic data as a result of the significant association between CYP2C9 polymorphisms and warfarin toxicity. As a result, starting and sustaining warfarin treatment is safer (Kapoor et al. 2016; Rigter et al. 2020; O'Shea et al. 2022; Lee et al. 2007; Higashi et al. 2002).

Identification of populations with risk characteristics not directly related to the medicine is a further possible application of pharmacogenetics. In another example, patients with single nucleotide polymorphism have been discovered to be at increased risk for cerebral vein thrombosis, and this risk increases when these patients are taking oral contraceptives. When made available, this knowledge could shield high-risk patients with a genetic predisposition from experiencing negative side effects from oral contraceptives (O'Shea et al. 2022; Higashi et al. 2002). The decrease in side effects has an impact on both the drug's marketing value and safety profile. Pharmaceutical companies are consistently hesitant to base their drug offerings on pharmacogenetic testing (Fig. 15.4).

This is brought on by a number of variables, including market segmentation based on genetic profile and rising product and healthcare prices. Due to these circumstances, the pharmaceutical industry continues to take a "wait and see" approach when it comes to producing pharmacogenetic data for their medicines.

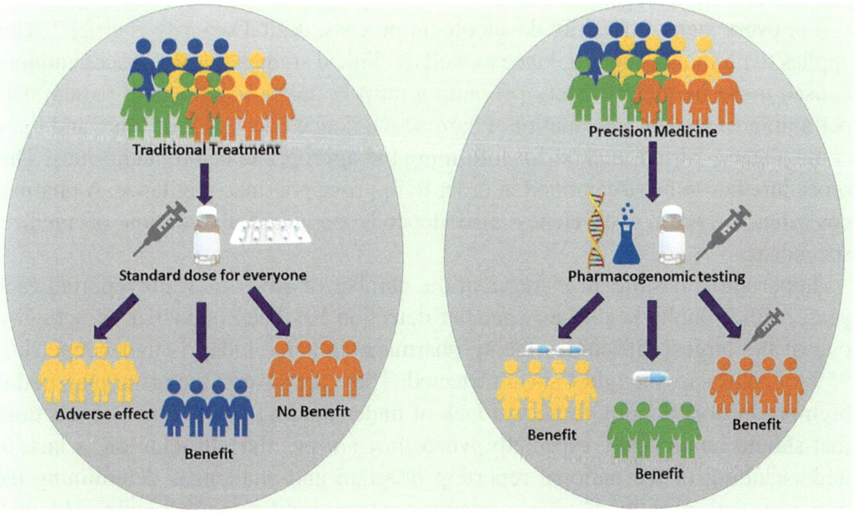

Fig. 15.4 Role of pharmacogenetics in patient care

15.5 Challenges of Current Pharmacogenovigilance

One of the main barriers preventing the use of pharmacogenomic in pharmacovigilance reporting is the lack of prospective clinical trials demonstrating the value of pharmacogenomic biomarkers in aiding in the drug selection and dose for the specific patient to achieve an optimal therapeutic response. The extent to which genetic factors influence drug response or toxicity phenotype is determined by the size of the gene effect—whether massive, moderate, or minor—as well as non-genetic components such as drug–drug interactions. The pharmacogenomic biomarker test's poor predictability prevents it from advising genotype-guided dose, such as for the drug (Dal Pan 2014; Giacomini et al. 2007). Randomised clinical trials, however, have not conclusively demonstrated the benefits of preventative genetic testing. Combining data from all of the genes that contribute to a medication response is anticipated to increase the prediction power of pharmacogenomic testing (Wilke et al. 2007; Kapoor et al. 2016; Lee et al. 2007).

Additional obstacles to the widespread application of pharmacogenovigilance result from moral and legal concerns about data security and privacy. Healthcare delivery uses technology more and more. Researchers and developers now have unprecedented access to enormous amounts of patient data because of technological and digital advancements. The majority of pharmaceutical businesses currently claim employing digital technologies for data collection, archiving, and sharing. In the future, researchers may freely exchange genetic information in order to work together on clinical trials, create more effective targeted treatments, and more readily incorporate new technologies (Dal Pan 2014). Drugs that are safer and more effective can be created as a result. The risk of cybercrime is rising, meanwhile, as stakeholders utilise digital technologies to share data more frequently, digital security is therefore essential.

For every step of the drug development process, digital security is crucial. This applies to pharmacogenovigilance as well as clinical studies. As pharmacogenomics is used more frequently, every precaution must be taken to safeguard patient data pertaining to genetic information. Pharmacovigilance takes a lot of time, and there is not a standardised method for informing the appropriate health authorities. This procedure has to be streamlined in order to improve pharmacovigilance. A pharmacovigilance system's efficiency also depends on the collaboration of medical specialists.

Importantly, despite an increase in the number of adverse events reported each year, neither public health nor speedier detection has been impacted. In actuality, one of the largest difficulties facing pharmacovigilance today is under-reporting. 95% of ADRs are thought to be undetected. There are several factors at play in this high proportion. Among these is a lack of understanding of the kinds of reactions that should be reported, especially when they are peculiar. In addition, a lack of understanding of the national reporting program and challenges determining the processes and causality of adverse occurrences are significant roadblocks. Although taking into account pharmacogenomic data can help to overcome some of these obstacles, the pharmacogenomic era also presents new difficulties (Sienkiewicz et al. 2021; Pérez García and Figueras 2011).

15.6 Pharmacogenovigilance: Considerations for the Present and the Future

One of the most important difficulties for the proper administration of patients is inter-individual heterogeneity in drug response clinical trials. The potential unanticipated differences in how each patient reacts to medications that might lead to therapeutic failures and adverse reactions are clinically important (Lavertu et al. 2021). A problem that has always been noted but is now magnified due to the increased use of polytherapy is the finding that the same medication administered at the same dose may be effective in the majority of the subjects treated but have poor effectiveness and/or cause side effects, sometimes serious ones also represented in Fig. 15.4 (Choudhury et al. 2023; Kalaiselvan et al. 2019). Although non-genetic variables (such as age, gender, nutritional status, other diseases, and the presence of comorbidities) used to dominate pharmacokinetic and pharmacodynamic variability (Castillo-Carniglia et al. 2019; Bonevski et al. 2014). Around the 1950s, scientists noticed a significant component of diversity in individual response to drugs in hereditary factors. Studies on pharmacogenetic features, or allelic changes in genes connected with drug absorption, distribution, metabolism, excretion, and biological activity that can affect drug action, have grown as a result over time (Pecoits-Filho et al. 2016).

15.7 Therapeutic Promise of the Human Genome Project

After the Human Genome Project was finished, there was a lot of hope that genetic information would significantly advance medicine, make side effects more predictable, and allow for the screening of individuals for potential medication reactions. However, despite the early excitement, progress has been far slower than expected. The fact that a person's reaction to medications is multifactorial and the product of numerous gene and environmental interactions accounts for a large portion of this delay. Despite the fact that the body of information is constantly growing, scientists are aware that before treatment can be tailored to a patient's genotype, empirical evidence must first be generated for a certain disease and drug combination.

15.8 Conclusion

It is crucial to identify and evaluate ADRs as soon as possible in order to best protect patients. Drug safety and efficacy have been considerably enhanced by discoveries in the field of pharmacogenomics. Individual genetic makeup has a significant impact in the variety of drug reactions. The identification of genetic biomarkers is proof that the need for pharmacogenovigilance research inclusion in clinical practise is further validated. Pharmacogenomics is crucial for maximising medication safety, whereas pharmacovigilance improves patient care, safety, and supports public health initiatives. Despite the fact that pharmacovigilance centres are well-established and play a critical role in assuring medication safety, pharmacogenomics has received inadequate financing from governments, particularly in developing nations. The existing pharmacovigilance system does not take into account the genetic diversity in drug response when healthcare practitioners notice and report adverse reactions to medications that have been on the market for a long time. Since it has been determined that no pharmaceutical is suitable for everyone, it is now required to analyse and track medications using unique genetic indicators. Pharmacogenomics is not generally regarded as a crucial tool in medication safety; hence it has not yet been incorporated into pharmacovigilance. This is a result of healthcare workers' lack of knowledge and awareness, as well as misunderstandings of the purpose and goals of the two disciplines. Finally, pharmacogenomics advancements have the potential to significantly improve drug-related issues if properly investigated. Since 134 countries participated in the WHO pharmacovigilance program as of the end of 2010, connecting pharmacogenomics with pharmacovigilance research would be the quickest and easiest way to close the knowledge and awareness gap currently present.

References

Abdullah-Koolmees H, van Keulen AM, Nijenhuis M, Deneer VHM (2021) Pharmacogenetics guidelines: overview and comparison of the DPWG, CPIC, CPNDS, and RNPGx guidelines. Front Pharmacol 11:595219. https://doi.org/10.3389/fphar.2020.595219

Alomar MJ (2014) Factors affecting the development of adverse drug reactions (review article). Saudi Pharm J 22(2):83–94. https://doi.org/10.1016/j.jsps.2013.02.003

Aronson JK, Ferner RE (2003) Joining the DoTS: new approach to classifying adverse drug reactions. BMJ 327(7425):1222–1225. https://doi.org/10.1136/bmj.327.7425.1222

Babayeva M, Loewy ZG (2023) Cannabis pharmacogenomics: a path to personalized medicine. Curr Issues Mol Biol 45(4):3479–3514. https://doi.org/10.3390/cimb45040228

Bhimaneni S, Sharma R, Dey P, Kumar A (2021) Pharmacovigilance of herbal medicines: an overview. In: Mandal SC, Chakraborty R, Sen S (eds) Evidence based validation of traditional medicines. Springer, Singapore. https://doi.org/10.1007/978-981-15-8127-4_25

Bonevski B, Regan T, Paul C, Baker AL, Bisquera A (2014) Associations between alcohol, smoking, socioeconomic status and comorbidities: evidence from the 45 and up study. Drug Alcohol Rev 33(2):169–176. https://doi.org/10.1111/dar.12104

Brown SA, Pereira N (2018) Pharmacogenomic impact of CYP2C19 variation on clopidogrel therapy in precision cardiovascular medicine. J Pers Med 8(1):8. https://doi.org/10.3390/jpm8010008

Burt T, Dhillon S (2013) Pharmacogenomics in early-phase clinical development. Pharmacogenomics 14(9):1085–1097. https://doi.org/10.2217/pgs.13.81

Castillo-Carniglia A, Keyes KM, Hasin DS, Cerdá M (2019) Psychiatric comorbidities in alcohol use disorder. Lancet Psychiatry 6(12):1068–1080. https://doi.org/10.1016/S2215-0366(19)30222-6

Choudhury A, Singh PA, Bajwa N, Dash S, Bisht P (2023) Pharmacovigilance of herbal medicines: concerns and future prospects. J Ethnopharmacol 309:116383. https://doi.org/10.1016/j.jep.2023.116383

Coleman JJ, Pontefract SK (2016) Adverse drug reactions. Clin Med (Lond) 16(5):481–485. https://doi.org/10.7861/clinmedicine.16-5-481
Coleman JJ, Ferner RE, Evans SJ (2006) Monitoring for adverse drug reactions. Br J Clin Pharmacol 61(4):371–378. https://doi.org/10.1111/j.1365-2125.2006.02596.x
Crews KR, Hicks JK, Pui CH, Relling MV, Evans WE (2012) Pharmacogenomics and individualized medicine: translating science into practice. Clin Pharmacol Ther 92(4):467–475. https://doi.org/10.1038/clpt.2012.120
Dal Pan GJ (2014) Ongoing challenges in pharmacovigilance. Drug Saf 37(1):1–8. https://doi.org/10.1007/s40264-013-0123-x
Davies EC, Green CF, Taylor S, Williamson PR, Mottram DR, Pirmohamed M (2009) Adverse drug reactions in hospital in-patients: a prospective analysis of 3695 patient-episodes. PLoS One 4(2):e4439. https://doi.org/10.1371/journal.pone.0004439
Ferrari M, Martignoni E, Blandini F, Riboldazzi G, Bono G, Marino F, Cosentino M (2012) Association of UDP-glucuronosyltransferase 1A9 polymorphisms with adverse reactions to catechol-O-methyltransferase inhibitors in Parkinson's disease patients. Eur J Clin Pharmacol 68(11):1493–1499. https://doi.org/10.1007/s00228-012-1281-y
Forster J, Duis J, Butler MG (2021) Pharmacogenetic testing of cytochrome P450 drug metabolizing enzymes in a case series of patients with Prader-Willi syndrome. Genes 12(2):152. https://doi.org/10.3390/genes12020152
Franczyk B, Rysz J, Gluba-Brzózka A (2022) Pharmacogenetics of drugs used in the treatment of cancers. Genes 13(2):311. https://doi.org/10.3390/genes13020311
Giacomini KM, Krauss RM, Roden DM, Eichelbaum M, Hayden MR, Nakamura Y (2007) When good drugs go bad. Nature 446(7139):975–977. https://doi.org/10.1038/446975a
Hamid AAA, Rahim R, Teo SP (2022) Pharmacovigilance and its importance for primary health care professionals. Korean J Fam Med 43(5):290–295. https://doi.org/10.4082/kjfm.21.0193
Harper AR, Topol EJ (2012) Pharmacogenomics in clinical practice and drug development. Nat Biotechnol 30(11):1117–1124. https://doi.org/10.1038/nbt.2424
Higashi MK, Veenstra DL, Kondo LM, Wittkowsky AK, Srinouanprachanh SL, Farin FM, Rettie AE (2002) Association between CYP2C9 genetic variants and anticoagulation-related outcomes during warfarin therapy. JAMA 287(13):1690–1698. https://doi.org/10.1001/jama.287.13.1690
Jeetu G, Anusha G (2010) Pharmacovigilance: a worldwide master key for drug safety monitoring. J Young Pharm 2(3):315–320. https://doi.org/10.4103/0975-1483.66802
Kalaiselvan V, Srivastava S, Singh A, Gupta SK (2019) Pharmacovigilance in India: present scenario and future challenges. Drug Saf 42(3):339–346. https://doi.org/10.1007/s40264-018-0730-7
Kapoor R, Tan-Koi WC, Teo YY (2016) Role of pharmacogenetics in public health and clinical health care: a SWOT analysis. Eur J Hum Genet 24(12):1651–1657. https://doi.org/10.1038/ejhg.2016.114
Lavertu A, Vora B, Giacomini KM, Altman R, Rensi S (2021) A new era in pharmacovigilance: toward real-world data and digital monitoring. Clin Pharmacol Ther 109(5):1197–1202. https://doi.org/10.1002/cpt.2172
Lee SY, Nam MH, Kim JS, Kim JW (2007) A case report of a patient carrying CYP2C9*3/4 genotype with extremely low warfarin dose requirement. J Korean Med Sci 22(3):557–559. https://doi.org/10.3346/jkms.2007.22.3.557
Lucas S, Ailani J, Smith TR, Abdrabboh A, Xue F, Navetta MS (2022) Pharmacovigilance: reporting requirements throughout a product's lifecycle. Ther Adv Drug Saf 13:20420986221125006. https://doi.org/10.1177/20420986221125006
Mathey CM, Maj C, Scheer AB, Fazaal J, Wedi B, Wieczorek D, Amann PM, Löffler H, Koch L, Schöffl C, Dickel H, Ganjuur N, Hornung T, Forkel S, Greve J, Wurpts G, Hallberg P, Bygum A, Von Buchwald C, Karawajczyk M, Forstner AJ (2022) Molecular genetic screening in patients with ACE inhibitor/angiotensin receptor blocker-induced angioedema to explore the role of hereditary angioedema genes. Front Genet 13:914376. https://doi.org/10.3389/fgene.2022.914376

Mejía G, Saiz-Rodríguez M, Gómez de Olea B, Ochoa D, Abad-Santos F (2020) Urgent hospital admissions caused by adverse drug reactions and medication errors-a population-based study in Spain. Front Pharmacol 11:734. https://doi.org/10.3389/fphar.2020.00734

Micaglio E, Locati ET, Monasky MM, Romani F, Heilbron F, Pappone C (2021) Role of pharmacogenetics in adverse drug reactions: an update towards personalized medicine. Front Pharmacol 12:651720. https://doi.org/10.3389/fphar.2021.651720

Osanlou O, Pirmohamed M, Daly AK (2018) Pharmacogenetics of adverse drug reactions. Adv Pharmacol 83:155–190. https://doi.org/10.1016/bs.apha.2018.03.002

O'Shea J, Ledwidge M, Gallagher J, Keenan C, Ryan C (2022) Pharmacogenetic interventions to improve outcomes in patients with multimorbidity or prescribed polypharmacy: a systematic review. Pharmacogenomics J 22(2):89–99. https://doi.org/10.1038/s41397-021-00260-6

Pecoits-Filho R, Abensur H, Betônico CC, Machado AD, Parente EB, Queiroz M, Salles JE, Titan S, Vencio S (2016) Interactions between kidney disease and diabetes: dangerous liaisons. Diabetol Metab Syndr 8:50. https://doi.org/10.1186/s13098-016-0159-z

Pereira NL, Rihal CS, So DYF, Rosenberg Y, Lennon RJ, Mathew V, Goodman SG, Weinshilboum RM, Wang L, Baudhuin LM, Lerman A, Hasan A, Iturriaga E, Fu YP, Geller N, Bailey K, Farkouh ME (2019) Clopidogrel pharmacogenetics. Circ Cardiovasc Interv 12(4):e007811. https://doi.org/10.1161/CIRCINTERVENTIONS.119.007811

Pérez García M, Figueras A (2011) The lack of knowledge about the voluntary reporting system of adverse drug reactions as a major cause of underreporting: direct survey among health professionals. Pharmacoepidemiol Drug Saf 20(12):1295–1302. https://doi.org/10.1002/pds.2193

Rigter T, Jansen ME, de Groot JM, Janssen SWJ, Rodenburg W, Cornel MC (2020) Implementation of pharmacogenetics in primary care: a multi-stakeholder perspective. Front Genet 11:10. https://doi.org/10.3389/fgene.2020.00010

Rioux PP (2000) Clinical trials in pharmacogenetics and pharmacogenomics: methods and applications. Am J Health Syst Pharm 57(9):887–901. https://doi.org/10.1093/ajhp/57.9.887

Roden DM, Wilke RA, Kroemer HK, Stein CM (2011) Pharmacogenomics: the genetics of variable drug responses. Circulation 123(15):1661–1670. https://doi.org/10.1161/CIRCULATIONAHA.109.914820

Sharma R, Patil C, Majeed J, Kumar S, Aggarwal G (2022) Next-generation sequencing in the biodiversity conservation of endangered medicinal plants. Environ Sci Pollut Res Int 29(49):73795–73808. https://doi.org/10.1007/s11356-022-22842-y

Sheng Y, Yang H, Wu T, Zhu L, Liu L, Liu X (2021) Alterations of cytochrome P450s and UDP-glucuronosyltransferases in brain under diseases and their clinical significances. Front Pharmacol 12:650027. https://doi.org/10.3389/fphar.2021.650027

Sienkiewicz K, Burzyńska M, Rydlewska-Liszkowska I, Sienkiewicz J, Gaszyńska E (2021) The importance of direct patient reporting of adverse drug reactions in the safety monitoring process. Int J Environ Res Public Health 19(1):413. https://doi.org/10.3390/ijerph19010413

Suke SG, Kosta P, Negi H (2015) Role of pharmacovigilance in India: an overview. Online J Public Health Inform 7(2):e223. https://doi.org/10.5210/ojphi.v7i2.5595

Sukumar S, Colah R, Mohanty D (2002) G6PD gene mutations in India producing drug-induced haemolytic anaemia. Br J Haematol 116(3):671–672. https://doi.org/10.1046/j.0007-1048.2001.03328.x

Sultana J, Cutroneo P, Trifirò G (2013) Clinical and economic burden of adverse drug reactions. J Pharmacol Pharmacother 4(Suppl 1):S73–S77. https://doi.org/10.4103/0976-500X.120957

Surendiran A, Pradhan SC, Adithan C (2008) Role of pharmacogenomics in drug discovery and development. Indian J Pharmacol 40(4):137–143. https://doi.org/10.4103/0253-7613.43158

Varughese LA, Lau-Min KS, Cambareri C, Damjanov N, Massa R, Reddy N, Oyer R, Teitelbaum U, Tuteja S (2020) DPYD and UGT1A1 pharmacogenetic testing in patients with gastrointestinal malignancies: an overview of the evidence and considerations for clinical implementation. Pharmacotherapy 40(11):1108–1129. https://doi.org/10.1002/phar.2463

Venter WDF, Fabian J, Feldman C (2018) An overview of tenofovir and renal disease for the HIV-treating clinician. South Afr J HIV Med 19(1):817. https://doi.org/10.4102/sajhivmed.v19i1.817

Ventola CL (2011) Pharmacogenomics in clinical practice: reality and expectations. P T 36(7):412–450
Ventola CL (2013) Role of pharmacogenomic biomarkers in predicting and improving drug response: part 1: the clinical significance of pharmacogenetic variants. P T 38(9):545–560
Wilke RA, Lin DW, Roden DM, Watkins PB, Flockhart D, Zineh I, Giacomini KM, Krauss RM (2007) Identifying genetic risk factors for serious adverse drug reactions: current progress and challenges. Nat Rev Drug Discov 6(11):904–916. https://doi.org/10.1038/nrd2423
Yue QY (2021) The International Society of Pharmacovigilance (ISoP) pharmacogenomic special interest group: pharmacogenomics in pharmacovigilance. Drug Saf 44(6):615–617. https://doi.org/10.1007/s40264-021-01068-w

Introduction to Signal Detection in Pharmacovigilance

16

Ruchika Sharma, Mukesh Nandave, and Anoop Kumar

Abstract

Signal detection and evaluation are the most important aspects of pharmacovigilance to generate the hypothesis regarding drug and adverse event which should be tested further. The signal can be detected using qualitative and quantitative methods. This chapter starts with introduction to signal followed by sources of signals and qualitative and quantitative methods. The various databases which are being used widely for the detection of signals are also discussed. Finally, the recent methodological developments and future perspectives are also briefly discussed.

Keywords

Adverse drug reactions · Pharmacovigilance · Spontaneous reporting system

16.1 Introduction

Signal is one of the most important parts of pharmacovigilance which generate hypothesis regarding drugs and adverse events. In simpler terms, a health-related safety signal is simply a risk-adjusted hypothesis based on data and supporting

R. Sharma
Centre for Precision Medicine and Pharmacy, Delhi Pharmaceutical Sciences and Research University DPSRU, New Delhi, India

M. Nandave · A. Kumar (✉)
Department of Pharmacology, Delhi Pharmaceutical Sciences and Research University, New Delhi, India
e-mail: mukeshnandave@gmail.com; anoopdpsru@dpsru.edu.in

M. Nandave, A. Kumar (eds.), *Pharmacovigilance Essentials*,
https://doi.org/10.1007/978-981-99-8949-2_16

documentation. Drug safety signal detection technologies and databases, as a result, are critical components of public health monitoring systems (Suke et al. 2015). It is merely a preliminary signal that must be evaluated, validated, and confirmed. The investigation operations progress from evidence gathering through information analysis and, finally, signal recognition and management. To dismiss or formulate a drug safety issue, a collective "qualitative" case-by-case clinical analysis of safety reports combined with a "quantitative" assessment employing data mining technologies has been ideal. Serious signals are prioritised for assessment and validation because they are caused by a novel medical product, pose a potential risk to public health, and have high-quality evidence for a causal association. Traditional PV signal detection practises employ both qualitative and quantitative methodologies (Ventola 2018).

A signal, according to the WHO, is "reported information on a possible causal relationship between an adverse event and a drug, of which the relationship was previously unknown or incompletely documented". A small number of reports can frequently indicate a signal. These signals are transmitted to regional pharmacovigilance centres, which are then passed on to zonal centres. Finally, all case reports are submitted in the National Centres' databases and sent to the WHO Collaborating Centre for International Drug Monitoring (the Uppsala Monitoring Centre) (Imran et al. 2022). To study the cause-and-effect relationship, the signal is assessed using the Uppsala Monitoring Scale (UMC) and the Naranjo Scale of likelihood. Signal identification and evaluation is a critical and complex process. With a rising volume of safety reports and complicated data, it is critical to gather, organise, assemble, and analyse data in a timely and relevant manner to maintain patient safety and locate "needle from haystack" (Suke et al. 2015).

The Council for International Organizations of Medical Sciences (CIOMS) defines signal as "information that arises from one or more sources that suggest a new potentially causal association, or a new aspect of a known association, between an intervention and an event or set of related events, either adverse or beneficial, that is judged to be of sufficient likelihood to justify verifying action" (Ventola 2018; Sartori et al. 2020). According to both definitions, a causal relationship between AE and drug must be established.

Early identification of safety signals is becoming increasingly crucial and is of significant interest to the pharmaceutical business, regulators, and the general public. Signals contain both qualitative and quantitative information. Different types of adverse events necessitate different detection methods (Sartori et al. 2020). Early detection of signals is the core function of pharmacovigilance. The thalidomide disaster occurred in the 1960s as a result of late signal detection. However, spontaneous reporting systems have now been designed and implemented worldwide. The number of case reports received by the World Health Organization Collaborating Centre for International Drug Monitoring in Uppsala, Sweden, is steadily increasing, reaching about 200,000 each year.

16.2 Source of Signals

The primary goal of pharmacovigilance is to discover early warning signs. However, processes for reporting unexpected events have been developed and are now used globally. Only a few of the sources that generate safety signals are case-control, cohort, and spontaneous reporting. Safety signals are provided by a variety of sources, including spontaneous reporting, case-control and cohort studies, and pre-clinical research (Jacob et al. 2013; Wisniewski et al. 2016). The various sources of signals are explained in below sections.

16.2.1 Spontaneous Reporting System

The majority of contemporary pharmacovigilance is based on a spontaneous reporting mechanism. Case reports and case series are frequently included in the spontaneous reporting system. The fundamental goal of spontaneous reporting system is to detect signals from novel, unusual, and severe ADRs as soon as possible. A medically qualified individual voluntarily reports an occurrence to a drug information centre, where the reports are analysed. Spontaneous reports are used to keep track of adverse pharmaceutical reactions and quality deviations that are underreported. The main reason for the public's lack of understanding among health professionals and the general public is underreporting. Another problem with this method is selective reporting, which might provide the impression of a risk when there is not one (Salvador et al. 2022). As a result, while spontaneous reporting is affordable, it is not the best approach for post-marketing drug surveillance. Nonetheless, we cannot deny that spontaneous reporting has been and continues to be the major technique of finding early medication safety warnings. Most pharmaceutical goods are withdrawn from the market on the basis of spontaneous reporting effectiveness in spotting new safety signals.

16.2.2 Electronic Health Records (EHRs)

This includes patient medical records, discharge summaries, laboratory findings, administrative files, insurance and reimbursement claims, and so on. EHRs can undoubtedly solve spontaneous reporting limitations such as underreporting and selective reporting; nevertheless, because the data is unstructured, poorly maintained medical records, their quality, completeness, and retrieval may be difficult. Furthermore, there may be privacy and ethical concerns, as well as ownership issues when accessing the data. Disease-specific registries based on facts and evidence can be a good source of quality data if they are effectively maintained and organised with predetermined scientific and therapeutic objectives (Menachemi and Collum 2011).

16.2.3 Biomedical Literature

This includes a thorough screening and assessment of available medical literature for critical PV data, such as case reports, case series, pharmacoepidemiologic studies, clinical trials, and observational studies. Furthermore, monthly safety update reports given to regulatory authorities by marketing authorisation holders have been assessed for the benefit and risk associated with medication use. Nonetheless, a lack of critical information for ICSR reporting, unstructured data for meaningful assessment, a proper search technique, and duplicate publications may be difficult. Unbiased effective information-extraction strategies, as well as significant time and effort, are required for effectively and efficiently monitoring medical literature (Samara et al. 2023). As a result, it has been found that a significant proportion of published literatures are not retrieved and are chosen for signal detection.

16.2.4 Registries

Both illness and drug registries have the capacity to produce safety signals. A registry mostly consists of a list of patients who share similar characteristics. A particular exposure (drug registry) or an illness may be characteristics. The sole difference between the two types of registries is the kind of patient data that is of interest, but both can gather a lot of data using standardised questionnaires. A case report study comparing the drug exposure of cases found in a disease registry and controls chosen from either patients with another ailment inside the registry or patients outside the registry may also be built on the foundation of a disease registry (Gliklich et al. 2014).

16.2.5 Periodic Safety Update Report (PSUR)

The PSUR can be a valuable resource for locating fresh safety signals. A PSUR is designed to give the Competent Authorities an update on the global safety experience of a medical product at specific post-authorisation time points. For all registered items, regardless of whether they are currently on the market, PSURs must be submitted. One report may cover all goods authorised by one marketing authorisation (MA) holder that contains the same active substance(s) (Detela and Lodge 2019). The recurrent safety update report is used to provide the appropriate authorities with updates on the overall safety experience of a medical product at predetermined intervals following authorisation. Signals are evaluated using a variety of criteria. High-quality report facts must be present before a report of a brand-new adverse drug response may be taken into consideration (Ebbers et al. 2013).

16.3 Data Collection

Data collecting is gathering pertinent information about the drug's safety profile from a variety of sources, including incident reports, clinical trials, post-marketing studies, and scholarly publications (Yao et al. 2013; Lucas et al. 2022).

16.4 Databases

The Argus Safety 3.0.1 database is one of the most crucial parts of the pharmacovigilance software system. Employers can assist pharmacovigilance and other pertinent operations using the digital database while assuring compliance with global legislation. As a comprehensive pharmaceutical software solution, it offers a pharmacovigilance business process that takes place during the drug's pre- and post-marketing phases. The Argus database is kept in a data centre with ISO 9001 accreditation and conforms with all FDA safety requirements. The Oracle Argus Safety products Oracle Argus Insight, Oracle Argus Perceptive, Oracle Argus Affiliate, Oracle Argus Dossier, Oracle Argus Interchange, Oracle Argus Reconciliation, and Oracle Argus Unblinding are all connected to Oracle Argus Safety (Hauben and Zhou 2003).

16.4.1 VigiFlow (India)

A web-based system for managing Individual Case Safety Reports (ICSRs) called VigiFlow was created specifically for national centres participating in the WHO Programme for International Drug Monitoring. Pharmaceutical firms or clinical research organisations may also use it to track their ICSR. VigiFlow is a trademark of the UMC and is managed by the UMC in Uppsala, Sweden. It is based on the ICH E2B standard and complies with it. The WHO's worldwide ICSR database measure (IC value), which has important filtering features, is known by the moniker VigiBase. For more than three decades, it has been in use. Since 1978, it has been in Uppsala and is run by the UMC; it is intended for spontaneous reports (Vogler et al. 2020; Khaleel et al. 2022).

16.4.2 AERS (USA) (Adverse Event Reporting System)

As can be seen in Table 16.1, the FDA's Adverse Event Reporting System (AERS) is a database that holds details on reports of drug errors and adverse events. The FDA's post-marketing safety surveillance programme for pharmaceutical and therapeutic biologic products is supported by the database. The AERS database's informatics design complies with the international safety reporting recommendations

Table 16.1 Sources of individual case reports

Sources of individual case reports	Description of the source
Unsolicited sources	Informal reports; literature; the internet; and other sources (including the lay press or other media)
Solicited sources	Organised data collection systems (such as clinical trials, registries, post-approval named patient use programmes, other patient support and disease management programmes, surveys of patients or healthcare professionals, information gathering on effectiveness or patient outcome; some of these may involve record-linkage, i.e. finding entries that refer to the same entity in two or more files) are a type of data collection method
Contractual agreements	Exchange of safety data between companies
Regulatory authority sources	Suspected unexpected serious adverse reactions (SUSARs), which come from regulatory authorities, are one type of individual case safety report

provided by the International Conference on Harmonisation (ICH E2B) (Khaleel et al. 2022). The Med DRA language is used to code adverse events and drug mistakes.

The FDA can use AERS to do tasks like searching for fresh safety issues that might be connected to marketed products, assessing a manufacturer's adherence to reporting requirements, and responding to information requests from third parties. Clinical reviewers at the Center for Drug Evaluation and Research (CDER) and the Center for Biologics Evaluation and Research (CBER) assess the reports in AERS to keep track of the safety of drugs following FDA approval. Further analysis is done if an AERS possible safety concern is found.

16.4.3 EudraVigilance (Europe)

The European data processing network and management system for reporting and evaluating suspected adverse reactions during the development of new drugs and for monitoring the marketing authorisation of medicinal products in the European Economic Area is called EudraVigilance (European Union Drug Regulating Authorities Pharmacovigilance). The electronic exchange of individual case safety reports is dealt with via the European EudraVigilance System (Khaleel et al. 2022).

16.4.4 Canada Vigilance (Canada)

Information about adverse reactions that have happened in Canada can be found in the Canada Vigilance Adverse Reaction Online Database. Each quarter, the database is updated to include fresh data that Health Canada has received. The Canada Vigilance Adverse Reaction Online Database only employs general wording that does not include any patient- or reporter-specific identification. The Canada Vigilance Adverse Reaction Online Database has a variety of features, such as the ability to search by brand name, active ingredient name, adverse reaction phrases, or system organ class, background information and help material, and the ability to print, save, and export search results (Vogler et al. 2020; Osborne 2010).

16.4.5 Argus Safety Database

A crucial component of the pharmacovigilance software system Argus safety 3.0.1 is the Argus safety database. With regard to pharmacovigilance and other relevant activities, the corporations use the digital database to assure compliance with international rules. It provides a pharmacovigilance business process that occurs during both the pre- and post-marketing phases of the medicine as a full pharmaceutical software solution. The Argus database is housed in an ISO-9001-certified data centre that is run in accordance with the security standard established by FDA regulations. Oracle Argus Safety, Oracle Argus Safety Japan, Oracle Argus Insight, Oracle Argus Perceptive, Oracle Argus Affiliate, Oracle Argus Dossier, Oracle Argus Interchange, Oracle Argus Reconciliation, and Oracle Argus Unblinding are all related products (Hauben and Zhou 2003).

16.4.6 ARISg Software

More than 300 firms globally retain their crucial medication safety data in ARISg, which is the top pharmacovigilance and clinical safety system in the world. From case input through the automatic generation of submission-ready adverse event (AE) reports, including CIOMS I, Med Watch 3500A, and many more, ARISg offers all the capability needed to manage adverse event reporting and adverse reaction requirements of various authorities around the world (Khaleel et al. 2022; Osborne 2010).

16.4.7 Gate Patni

Sponsors can track the status and development of the clinical study in terms of the safety and efficacy of the investigational medicine using the Clinical Trials Dashboard provided by iGATE (Khaleel et al. 2022).

16.5 Approaches for the Detection of Signals

Various approaches regarding detection of signals are described in below sections.

16.5.1 Traditional Approaches

Traditional signal detection techniques can be divided into qualitative and straightforward quantitative methods. The traditional qualitative technique entails reviewing individual case reports and/or case series that may be present in pharmacovigilance databases or in the medical literature in order to analyse spontaneously reported adverse occurrences. When using simply traditional methods, the sheer amount and complexity of data in these enormous datasets can make it more likely that some drug-induced adverse drug reactions (ADRs) will not be detected early, which could have a significant impact on public health (Harpaz et al. 2012). The aggregate analysis through individual case count, assessing simple reporting rates or exposure adjusted reporting rates is a straightforward quantitative approach of signal discovery (Ibrahim et al. 2021).

16.5.2 Qualitative Approach

16.5.2.1 Review of Individual Cases or Case Series

Signals are discovered while qualified specialists analyse cases that have been reported. The "index case" or "striking case" strategy, in which the first well-reported example of an adverse event following the administration of a vaccine may be viewed as a signal, is the method utilised here most frequently for signal discovery. Clinically, however, a collection of related reported cases (referred to as clustering) is necessary to firmly suspect a connection between the administration of the vaccination and the emergence of an adverse event.

Special attention is given during the review process to "designated medical events" (rare, serious events with a high vaccine-related risk), "events of special interest" (which can vary from region to region and organisation to organisation), "targeted medical events" (whose classification is based on vaccine), and "hyper-acute events". In these circumstances, one to three identically reported cases are typically thought to be enough to produce a signal.

Signal detection uses analysis of information from periodic safety reviews, such as periodic safety update reports (PSUR, in India and Europe) (Hauben and Zhou 2003; Ibrahim et al. 2021).

16.5.2.2 Cross-Sectional Study (Survey)

Regardless of exposure or disease condition, data is gathered from a population of patients in cross-sectional studies at a specific point in time or interval of time. When examining the prevalence of an illness at a certain time, these studies work well. Additionally, these investigations are utilised to investigate the basic relationship between exposure and result in ecological analysis. It is ideal to do cross-sectional research when exposure does not alter over time. The primary drawback of these research is that the time link between exposure and result is only indirectly assessed (Capili 2021).

16.5.2.3 Case-Control Study

In order to ascertain the kind and degree of exposure, a case-control study is a retrospective, descriptive, observational study of a person, disease, or result. These studies frequently compare participants with the condition or disease (the "cases") to patients who do not have the condition or disease (the "controls") in order to uncover characteristics that may contribute to the ailment or disease (Capili 2021).

The odds ratio, an estimation of the relative risk of disease in two groups, is used to examine case-control studies. These studies are helpful in determining risk factors for adverse events and determining whether there is a connection between a medicine and a particular unusual adverse event. These studies' findings could be complicated by additional factors.

16.5.2.4 Cohort Study

In a prospective, observational study known as a cohort study, a group of individuals with comparable features are monitored in order to ascertain the kind and degree of exposure. A population that is at risk for the disease (or event) is monitored throughout time to determine when the condition may manifest. The comparator cohorts of interest are often chosen based on drug use and followed throughout time in cohort studies incorporating drug exposure.

When it is necessary to understand the incidence rates of adverse events in addition to the relative risks of adverse events, cohort studies can be helpful. The utilisation of cohort studies to assess safety concerns in certain populations (the elderly, children, patients, and pregnant women) is also common. The relative risk (disease rate in exposed group/disease rate in unexposed group) is used to analyse these research. These research' biggest flaws are their reliance on time (interesting outcomes might not materialise right away) and the influence of confounding variables (Capili 2021).

16.5.2.5 Anecdotal Reporting

Most initial reports of adverse medication responses come from individual doctors through anecdotal reporting. The occurrence of an incident connected to the usage of a specific medicine is described. Such instances need to be confirmed because they are anecdotal, but it might not be possible to do so.

16.5.2.6 Meta-Analysis

Meta-analysis is a quantitative, formal, epidemiological study design that uses statistical techniques to systematically evaluate earlier research works in order to draw conclusions about the body of work. Results from a meta-analysis may be more accurate estimates of the impact of a treatment, a disease risk factor, or other outcomes than those from any one study that contributed to the pooled analysis. In pharmacovigilance, this analysis seeks to determine the link between medications and adverse events, to estimate how frequently ADRs occur, and to pinpoint subgroups that are more likely to have ADRs (Sharma et al. 2022; Khouri et al. 2021; Kumar 2023).

16.5.3 Statistical Approaches

The majority of these techniques (disproportionality analysis) rely on the relative reporting (of adverse events) frequencies. Traditional signal detection techniques should not be replaced by statistical approaches, often known as data mining algorithms; rather, they should be supported so that they may analyse huge amounts of datasets more effectively and methodically.

Finding statistically significant reporting connections between a certain drug and adverse event pair within spontaneous reporting database(s) is the goal of disproportionality analysis. A statistic known as the "statistic of disproportionate reporting" (SDR) is computed using statistical methods. Because pharmacovigilance data contains inherent biases and artefacts, finding an SDR (statistically prominent reporting relationship) does not prove causation or prove the existence of a signal. Similarly, the absence of an SDR does not rule out the existence of causation between an adverse event and a drug pair. Because of this, the conclusion regarding the existence of a signal should not just be based on statistical prominence but also requires a thorough clinical evaluation (Ibrahim et al. 2021).

16.5.3.1 Frequentist's Approach

For each drug-adverse event pair, data mining techniques transform information from a vast database into 2 × 2 contingency tables (Table 16.2).

This table can be used to compute the relative reporting, reporting odds ratio (ROR), proportional reporting ratio (PRR), and information component (IC) measures of association strength. Based on Frequentist's idea of repeated sampling, the confidence interval is generated for these measurements. The two most popular frequentist approaches are ROR and PRR. Table 16.3 provides association measures and formulas for calculating them (based on the 2 × 2 table above).

16.5.3.2 Bayesian Methods

In a big data collection, millions of 2 × 2 tables for each drug-event combination may be created, and it may be laborious to calculate the measures of association for each table. Therefore, it was necessary to create more modern signal detection techniques. The World Health Organisation developed the first Bayesian approaches of signal detection in pharmacovigilance in the 1990s. "Bayesian Confidence

Table 16.2 A 2 × 2 contingency table formed based on reports of a particular drug-adverse event pair in a database

	Reports of event of interest	Reports of all other events	Total
Reports for drug of interest	A	B	A + B
Reports for all other drugs	C	D	C + D
Total	A + C	B + D	A + B + C + D

Table 16.3 Measures of association between drug and adverse event

Measures of association	Formulae
ROR	AD/BC
PRR	A × (C + D)/C × (A + B)
RR	A (A + B + C + D)/(A + C) (A + B)
IC	$\log_2$IC = A (A + B + C + D)/(A + C) (A + D)

Propagation Neural network (BCPNN)" and "Multi-item Gamma Poisson Shrinker (MGPS)" are two important Bayesian approaches used for signal detection.

16.6 Signal Validation

The evaluation of the detected signals to determine their applicability, causality, and possible influence on public health constitutes signal validation. Following the detection of the signal through individual or aggregate analysis, it is evaluated through a series of sequential steps, including signal triage, clarification, and early evaluation, and if necessary, formal evaluation using additional data from sources such as mechanistic studies about the adverse event, non-clinical studies, observational studies, registry-based studies, clinical trials, population databases like electronic patient record, background event, the signal may be communicated to the relevant parties, such as regulatory agencies, healthcare providers, and the general public (Hsieh et al. 2023).

16.7 Signal Prioritisation and Risk Assessment

The process of evaluating validated signals according to their potential influence on public health and the availability of funding for additional research is known as signal prioritisation. A drug's potential dangers, including the likelihood and seriousness of side effects, are evaluated throughout the risk assessment process.

16.8 Risk Management

Signal management entails the constant assessment and tracking of drug safety concerns, as well as the application of risk management tactics to reduce any possible risks connected to a drug. Implementing actions to reduce a drug's potential dangers, such as altering the product label or prescribing information, restricting use, or pulling the drug off the market, is known as risk management (Malikova 2020). In order to identify, characterise, prevent, or minimise risk linked to pharmaceutical products, including the assessment of the effectiveness of intervention, risk management plans (RMPs) have recently been established in post-marketing surveillance. During the post-authorisation period, these RMPs can give users a greater grasp of the drug's advantages and disadvantages.

16.9 Signal Evaluation

Signal evaluation is the process of continuously tracking and assessing signals to ascertain their applicability and potential impact on the general public's health, which can help guide future risk management decisions. Pharmacovigilance is essential to maintaining the safety and effectiveness of pharmaceuticals on the market, and signal detection and management play a key role in this process (Malikova 2020).

16.10 Conclusion

The most crucial part of pharmacovigilance is the accurate signal identification and their assessment. Signal detection is accomplished using a variety of techniques. Pharmacovigilance signals come from a variety of sources. Pharmacovigilance requires a plan of complementing actions rather than relying solely on one method. Through effective training and retraining of the staff involved in the pharmacovigilance activity, the quality of the reports can be improved. The use of artificial intelligence tools to supplement and optimise the drug safety signal detection process is gaining popularity. However, such ideas are in their early stages and must be validated before being used in the real world and allowed by regulatory authorities. While advanced technology may supplement and enhance PV efforts, detailed clinical judgement will always be essential for final adjudication of causality and signal detection.

References

Capili B (2021) Cross-sectional studies. Am J Nurs 121(10):59–62. https://doi.org/10.1097/01.NAJ.0000794280.73744.fe

Detela G, Lodge A (2019) EU regulatory pathways for ATMPs: standard, accelerated and adaptive pathways to marketing authorisation. Mol Ther Methods Clin Dev 13:205–232. https://doi.org/10.1016/j.omtm.2019.01.010

Ebbers HC, Mantel-Teeuwisse AK, Sayed-Tabatabaei FA, Moors EH, Schellekens H, Leufkens HG (2013) The role of periodic safety update reports in the safety management of biopharmaceuticals. Eur J Clin Pharmacol 69(2):217–226. https://doi.org/10.1007/s00228-012-1317-3

Gliklich RE, Dreyer NA, Leavy MB (eds) (2014) Registries for evaluating patient outcomes: a user's guide, 3rd edn. Agency for Healthcare Research and Quality (US)

Harpaz R, DuMouchel W, Shah NH, Madigan D, Ryan P, Friedman C (2012) Novel data-mining methodologies for adverse drug event discovery and analysis. Clin Pharmacol Ther 91(6):1010–1021. https://doi.org/10.1038/clpt.2012.50

Hauben M, Zhou X (2003) Quantitative methods in pharmacovigilance: focus on signal detection. Drug Saf 26(3):159–186. https://doi.org/10.2165/00002018-200326030-00003

Hsieh MH, Liang HY, Tsai CY, Tseng YT, Chao PH, Huang WI, Chen WW, Lin SJ, Lai EC (2023) A new drug safety signal detection and triage system integrating sequence symmetry analysis and tree-based scan statistics with longitudinal data. Clin Epidemiol 15:91–107. https://doi.org/10.2147/CLEP.S395922

Ibrahim H, Abdo A, El-Kerdawy AM, Eldin AS (2021) Signal detection in pharmacovigilance: a review of informatics-driven approaches for the discovery of drug-drug interaction signals in different data sources. Artif Int Life Sci 1:100005

Imran M, Bhatti A, King DM, Lerch M, Dietrich J, Doron G, Manlik K (2022) Supervised machine learning-based decision support for signal validation classification. Drug Saf 45(5):583–596. https://doi.org/10.1007/s40264-022-01159-2

Jacob D, Marrón B, Ehrlich J, Rutherford PA (2013) Pharmacovigilance as a tool for safety and monitoring: a review of general issues and the specific challenges with end-stage renal failure patients. Drug Healthc Patient Saf 5:105–112. https://doi.org/10.2147/DHPS.S43104

Khaleel MA, Khan AH, Ghadzi SMS, Adnan AS, Abdallah QM (2022) A standardized dataset of a spontaneous adverse event reporting system. Healthcare (Basel) 10(3):420. https://doi.org/10.3390/healthcare10030420

Khouri C, Petit C, Tod M, Lepelley M, Revol B, Roustit M, Cracowski JL (2021) Adverse drug reaction risks obtained from meta-analyses and pharmacovigilance disproportionality analyses are correlated in most cases. J Clin Epidemiol 134:14–21. https://doi.org/10.1016/j.jclinepi.2021.01.015

Kumar A (2023) Meta-analysis in clinical research: principles and procedures, 1st edn. Springer, Singapore; ISBN: 978-981-99-2369-4

Lucas S, Ailani J, Smith TR, Abdrabboh A, Xue F, Navetta MS (2022) Pharmacovigilance: reporting requirements throughout a product's lifecycle. Ther Adv Drug Saf 13:20420986221125006. https://doi.org/10.1177/20420986221125006

Malikova MA (2020) Practical applications of regulatory requirements for signal detection and communications in pharmacovigilance. Ther Adv Drug Saf 11:2042098620909614. https://doi.org/10.1177/2042098620909614

Menachemi N, Collum TH (2011) Benefits and drawbacks of electronic health record systems. Risk Manag Healthc Policy 4:47–55. https://doi.org/10.2147/RMHP.S12985

Osborne CA (2010) Adverse drug reactions: investigating to reporting. J Can Acad Child Adolesc Psychiatry 19(1):46–47

Salvador MR, Monteiro C, Pereira L, Duarte AP (2022) Quality of spontaneous reports of adverse drug reactions sent to a regional pharmacovigilance unit. Int J Environ Res Public Health 19(7):3754. https://doi.org/10.3390/ijerph19073754

Samara C, Garcia A, Henry C, Vallotton L, Cariolato L, Desmeules J, Pinçon A (2023) Safety surveillance during drug development: comparative evaluation of existing regulations. Adv Ther 40(5):2147–2185. https://doi.org/10.1007/s12325-023-02492-3

Sartori D, Aronson JK, Onakpoya IJ (2020) Signals of adverse drug reactions communicated by pharmacovigilance stakeholders: protocol for a scoping review of the global literature. Syst Rev 9(1):180. https://doi.org/10.1186/s13643-020-01429-z

Sharma R, Kumar A, Majeed J, Thakur AK, Aggarwal G (2022) Drugs acting on the renin-angiotensin-aldosterone system (RAAS) and deaths of COVID-19 patients: a systematic review and meta-analysis of observational studies. Egypt Heart J 74(1):64. https://doi.org/10.1186/s43044-022-00303-8

Suke SG, Kosta P, Negi H (2015) Role of pharmacovigilance in India: an overview. Online J Public Health Inform 7(2):e223. https://doi.org/10.5210/ojphi.v7i2.5595

Ventola CL (2018) Big data and pharmacovigilance: data mining for adverse drug events and interactions. P T 43(6):340–351

Vogler M, Ricci Conesa H, de Araújo Ferreira K, Moreira Cruz F, Simioni Gasparotto F, Fleck K, Maciel Rebelo F, Kollross B, Silveira Gonçalves Y (2020) Electronic reporting systems in pharmacovigilance: the implementation of Vigi flow in Brazil. Pharmaceut Med 34(5):327–334. https://doi.org/10.1007/s40290-020-00349-6

Wisniewski AF, Bate A, Bousquet C, Brueckner A, Candore G, Juhlin K, Macia-Martinez MA, Manlik K, Quarcoo N, Seabroke S, Slattery J, Southworth H, Thakrar B, Tregunno P, Van Holle L, Kayser M, Norén GN (2016) Good signal detection practices: evidence from IMI PROTECT. Drug Saf 39(6):469–490. https://doi.org/10.1007/s40264-016-0405-1

Yao B, Zhu L, Jiang Q, Xia HA (2013) Safety monitoring in clinical trials. Pharmaceutics 5(1):94–106. https://doi.org/10.3390/pharmaceutics5010094

Role of Artificial Intelligence in Pharmacovigilance

17

Jyoti Upadhyay, Mukesh Nandave, and Anoop Kumar

Abstract

Pharmacovigilance ensures the safety and efficacy of any pharmaceutical drug products or medical devices throughout their lifecycle. Traditional methods available for monitoring of adverse drug reactions (ADRs) are resource limited and prone to cause underreporting of ADRs. Recent technological advancement in pharmacovigilance reporting is the integration of artificial intelligence (AI) and ADR reporting. In this chapter we investigated the role of AI technologies in pharmacovigilance, emphasizing its potential benefits. AI technologies cover machine learning, deep learning, and natural learning processing (NLP) that have shown remarkable ability in automation of pharmacovigilance data like signal detection, risk assessment, and regulatory compliance. AI algorithms help in analyzing the extensive amounts of unstructured data from different sources like electronic health records (EHRs), medical literature and identification of real-time ADR data. In addition, AI models help in facilitating early detection of ADRs and give valuable insights in identifying risk–benefit profile of drug. Although AI technologies have several advantages, there are also some challenges related to the quality of data, transparency, bias, and regulatory compliance. All these challenges need to be addressed to entirely use the potential of AI technology in pharmacovigilance. Combined efforts are required between AI

J. Upadhyay (✉)
Department of Pharmaceutical Sciences, School of Health Sciences and Technology, UPES University, Dehradun, Uttarakhand, India
e-mail: jupadhyay@ddn.upes.ac.in

M. Nandave · A. Kumar
Department of Pharmacology, Delhi Pharmaceutical Sciences and Research University, New Delhi, India
e-mail: mukeshnandave@gmail.com; anoopdpsru@dpsru.edu.in

M. Nandave, A. Kumar (eds.), *Pharmacovigilance Essentials*,
https://doi.org/10.1007/978-981-99-8949-2_17

technologies, regulatory agencies, and pharmaceutical companies to establish the standard guidelines and safeguard the ethical and responsible use of AI technology in pharmacovigilance. There is a need to refine the AI-driven pharmacovigilance strategies by developing healthcare and drug safety decision-making, ultimately benefiting the patients.

Keywords

Pharmacovigilance · Patient safety · Adverse drug reactions · Electronic health record system

17.1 Introduction

Pharmacovigilance (PV) is the science and activities of the healthcare system that ensure patient safety through collection, detection, assessment, researching, monitoring, evaluation, and prevention of adverse drug reactions (ADRs) caused using medicine, vaccines, or medical devices that are observed during clinical trial phases or in the post-marketing surveillance studies (Liang et al. 2022). PV plays a significant role in safety management and encompasses a set of critical components designed to detect, understand, evaluate, and prevent adverse effects or any medication related issues. The primary function of PV is ensuring safety of healthcare products consumers and patients. By examining the medication safety profile, healthcare providers and regulators can detect the potential risks caused by the medication, thereby minimizing the harm caused to the consumers or patients (Stevenson and Green 2016). Underestimation of adverse drug reaction reporting is the major global setback that may be attributed to the shortage of time and documentation. The World Health Organization has initiated ADRs reporting program that has played an important role in enriching the significance of the science and practice of pharmacovigilance, fostering awareness, and advancing the knowledge of monitoring and managing the ADRs. PV has a significant role in clinical settings and communities in drug use and regulations and preventing potential harm caused by approved medicines (Jeetu and Anusha 2010). There are limited resources available for PV in middle- and low-income countries. Healthcare professionals are overwhelmed with huge job responsibilities. A study in China reported that healthcare professionals involved in OPD (outpatient department) of big hospitals serves around hundred patients per day (Li and Xie 2013). It is difficult for healthcare professionals to spend extra time on filling out the ICSR manually. In addition, the pharmacovigilance system or electronic health record (EHR) system might lack the information required to support healthcare professionals. A study reported that a well-trained healthcare professional took an average of 53 s to document an adverse event in the EHR system (Linder et al. 2010). Because of inadequate investment and training opportunities in PV education, many significant adverse drug reactions remain undocumented. A report investigated the percentage of unreported adverse event in clinical practice might reach as high as 90% (Tatonetti et al. 2012). Inadequate EHRs, real-world data, and databases related to insurance claims make it difficult to determine the real risks of drug use (Kiguba et al. 2021). Insufficient fund issues reflect another problem. Though ICSR reporting in middle- and low-income countries is currently rising with limited resource availability, still the progress in reporting is going on. Many middle- and low-income countries have started their national ADR reporting systems and linked with WHO's global pharmacovigilance systems. ADR event monitoring is constantly increased at cohort level and continues with post-marketing surveillance event monitoring (Agyapong et al. 2021). With the advancement of technologies like artificial intelligence (AI), there is a widespread integration of automatic processes that have been developed in different domains of medicines (He et al. 2019). Furthermore, it is commendable that PV community generally adopt AI-based technology. There are several databases, tutorials, and the latest software accessible from open resources. This provides a unique opportunity for middle- and low-income countries to enhance all facets of healthcare by using AI. For instance, in Africa, AI technologies have been used to predict birth asphyxia in resource-constrained settings and in the diagnosis of communicable as well as non-communicable diseases like tuberculosis and diabetic retinopathy (Owoyemi et al. 2020). Another study during COVID-19 pandemic shows that in South America, the web-platforms and mobile applications employed AI algorithms like decision tree to assess the symptoms and offer counseling related to the pandemic (Chatterjee et al. 2020). AI-based technologies like deep learning, machine learning, natural language processing have been implemented to advance ADR reporting systems (Murali et al. 2019; Hauben and Hartford 2021). Natural language processing helps in detecting and extracting ADR from an unstructured text (Henry et al. 2020; Bian et al. 2012; Li et al. 2016) and identifying PV signals in extensive databases through unsupervised Bayesian techniques (Bihan et al. 2020).

17.2 AI in Healthcare Settings

Recent advancements in AI technology have revealed the possibilities for addressing several healthcare tasks. However, AI systems have encountered many challenges in achieving their deliberate practical outcomes. These systems are constructed in a way so that their primary focus is on the technical aspects with the integration of real-world data. United Nations (UN) in 2017 conducted a meeting to deliberate the deployment of AI technology to deliver a wide range of critical public services (AI for Good Global Summit, Geneva 2017). Another recent UN meeting convened diverse stakeholders to assess the potential contribution of AI toward achieving sustainable development goals (SDGs) (Anon n.d.). Data serves as an important tool for AI technology and therefore in healthcare systems this technology helps in establishing a comprehensive PV database system. Many countries worldwide face a unique circumstance while forming their PV database. In general, this database is initiated by healthcare professionals beginning with the spontaneous reporting of ADR. Multiple large scale PV databases have been developed in middle- and low-income countries. Vaccine Adverse Event Reporting System (VAERS) and Food and Administration Adverse Event Reporting System (FAERS) are the database used in USA (FDA 2023; VAERS 2023). Another database used globally is VigiBase maintained by Uppsala Monitoring Centre and contains the aggregate data from over 150 countries. But the main problem while working with PV databases in middle- and low-income countries is the underreporting. This happens because of limited availability of resources like lack of infrastructure, funds, human resources, and policies. An examination of study data reveals that Western countries like European Union and USA have furnished approximately 70% of the ADR data in VigiBase, while other countries like Africa contributed only 0.9% of ADR in 2019. The number of ADR received from National Medicine Regulatory Authorities in Ethiopia, Kenya, and Tanzania were 6.7, 35, and 4.1 per million of population (Bihan et al. 2020).

AI in the medical field holds the promise of improving both effectiveness and accuracy of patient diagnosis and evaluation ultimately leading to improved health outcomes. In a healthcare setting, patients receive diagnosis by describing their symptoms and concerns and the vital signs were monitored by advanced super-computerized nurses that may appear to be something out of science fiction. Moreover, such medical care has attained the possibility by the integration of AI into the field of medicine. Nonetheless, AI in diagnostic medical field holds the probability of enhancing quality and efficiency of medical care, diagnosis and ultimately, they are subjected to be patented when put into practice and closely observed by experienced healthcare experts and professionals (Nagam 2023).

17.3 Types of AI

AI can be categorized into three main parts, i.e., artificial narrow intelligence (ANI), artificial general intelligence (AGI), artificial super intelligence (ASI). ANI is also known as weak AI characterized by its target-oriented nature, designed to excel in well-defined tasks. It lacks the capability of performing tasks outside its narrow domain. Highly specialized ANI machines operate within limitations and constraints; therefore, it is defined as weak ANI (Page et al. 2018). Artificial general intelligence (AGI) is the competence of an intelligent system that possesses the quality to understand and adapt to virtually any task those humans or other animals can achieve. This system proficiently undertakes a widespread sequence of tasks, in parallel with the cognitive adaptability of humans (Goertzel 2014). Artificial super intelligence (ASI) is a hypothetical aspect in AI, representing the development of AI where machines surpass human intelligence and possess skills that are recently beyond human knowledge. With ASI, machines can think of probable interpretations that are difficult for humans to think, as the human brain has a limitation in thinking ability that is constrained to several neurons (Baum and Tonn 2015).

17.4 AI Technologies in Pharmacovigilance

There are many regulations governing the responsibilities that clinical trial sponsors must fulfill and Marketing Authorization Holders (MAH) for the approved pharmaceutical products. This requires the collection of large data related to clinical trials safety data with specific MAHs including ADR reporting, poor quality medicinal products, medication errors, and medicine exposure during pregnancy (European Medicines Agency (EMA) 2017). All this data comprises single patient records from different sources composed, arranged, and assessed as per the standard procedure. These challenges led to the adoption of advanced AI technology impacting several regulatory contexts and raise concern about individual data safety and usage (Lewis and McCallum 2020). These technologies include:

17.5 Natural Learning Processing (NLP)

NLP in healthcare enables professionals to extract valuable information from a large amount of recorded data. NLP is the ability of the machines that understand and explain human language both in written and spoken form and that enable to interpret human language efficiently (Cambria and White 2014). In modern healthcare system, the EHRs are experiencing rapid development on a large scale like in China in 2011, the government invested US $97 million to perform a study project on healthcare information systems OPD management, EHR and electronic medical record (EMR) (Deng et al. 2018; Li and Hu 2012). NLP has the potential to convert unstructured medical records to structured data containing important medical insights so that medical professionals can easily extract useful information (Jung et al. 2018), thereby reducing the operational cost and improving the data quality in the healthcare system. NLP has resolved a number of challenges occurring in the medical field like ADR detection, EHR data classification and extraction (Guo et al. 2017). NLP provides easy accessibility to extract repositories of encoded data and this coded information gives valuable information for advancing patient safety (Bates et al. 2003). Rather than converting all the text content into coded formats, NLP focusses on identifying data that most likely contain relevant types. For example, if one wants to seek out occurrences of "aspiration pneumonia" and its several verbal expressions to determine the number of patients who might suffer from complications linked with sedation in a conscious state. However, some studies showed that NLP can attain a higher degree of precision as compared to these search techniques. In many studies inconsistency in accuracy was observed because of decreased specificity as the search tool includes studies where a condition was explicitly denied, "e.g., no data to suggest aspiration pneumonia" (Hripcsak et al. 2003). Two independent research studies show that NLP can attain the same level of accuracy as skilled human coders when it codes for radiographic information. In addition, this technique is also found to be more accurate than basic text methods like searching specific phrases within the reports (Fiszman et al. 2000). A study on patient safety investigated the use of NLP system on medical terminology lexicon that determines adverse events in outpatient department (OPD) (Honigman et al. 2001). This study shows promising results, but some limitations have also been observed in this approach. It depends solely on the lexical analysis method without in-depth understanding of NLP causing a significant number of false positives. The issue observed in the system is difficulty in identifying negative terms, differentiating crucial medical differentiators. Another study involves applied informatics health information network (AIHIN) where they estimated patient's risk associated with active form of tuberculosis by generating Arden Syntax modules and triggered a notification to the hospital epidemiologist when a patient at high risk placed in a shared hospital (Hripcsak et al. 1999). NLP system modifications are important to handle text associated with patient safety and the method of these modifications completely dependent upon the processor's underlying techniques. Like, for instance, Medical Language Extraction and Encoding System (MEDLEE) employs lexicon for categorizing words and phrases into semantic types and utilizes semantic grammar to analyze sentences and generate a structured output (Friedman et al. 1995).

17.6 Machine Learning (ML) Algorithm for Adverse Event Detection

ML techniques is a promising approach for clinical findings support especially while dealing with unstructured complicated data. ML plays an important role in data interpretation to predict adverse drug reactions. This technique uses different types of data inputs like gene expression, chemical structure of drugs, and text mining. Data categories are then processed subsequently through algorithmic methods utilizing random forest approach in ML or by employing deep learning methods for generating predictive models (Vamathevan et al. 2019). Deep learning approach in ML combines and examines the different biological data and creates a new hypothesis. This technique is efficiently used in the field of drug repurposing and drug discovery. Though its use in gene expression associated ADR prediction is limited (Wang et al. 2020). Mohsen et al. (2021) designed framework that combines two different databases, i.e., ADR event information FAERS and toxicogenomic (TG)-genomics assisted toxicity evaluation systems databases (GATEs). They have incorporated features like data feature selection, cleaning, filtering, and fine tuning of hyperparameters. In their study they have designed fourteen predictive models by using deep neural networks (DNN) with average validation precision of 89.4% representing that their technology has significantly and consistently predicts ADR from a broad range of drugs (Mohsen et al. 2021). Database like Open TG-GATEs is extensive toxicogenomic database that compiles data related to gene expression profiles of both in vivo and in vitro samples subjected to diverse drug treatments. This is the part of Japanese TG project that aimed to develop drug toxicities database for drug development. This database also collects other parameters like biochemical, physiological, and pathological data of animal studies (Mohsen et al. 2021; Uehara et al. 2009). The Library of Integrated Network-Based Cellular

Signatures (LINCS) database has been employed to forecast numerous ADRs within a single research study (Wang et al. 2016).

17.7 Predictive Analytics (PA) for Risk Assessment

PA for risk assessment in ADR reporting refers to the technique of integrating statistical and analytical techniques to predict or forecast the adverse events associated with the use of pharmaceutical drug product or medical devices. Ensuring the patient safety, the handling of ADRs reporting holds a great significance for public health. For instance, where the ADRs go unnoticed or underreported leads to preventable human suffering and financial loss and wears away public trust in adherence to pharmaceutical therapy. The basic requirement for ADR monitoring and immediately issuing alerts is primarily related to the principle of data mining that involves data exploration and extraction employing statistical and mathematical techniques. For assessing drug safety an ideal system must be robust and straightforward in maintaining precision. In context of this, the system would receive comprehensive information related to the structure of drug molecules and deliver notifications for any potential harm or specific ADR that may occur (Hammann et al. 2010). Currently several preclinical studies are employed to predict the safety and pharmacology of the drug compounds in pharmaceutical industries. Thorough identification of possible issues with limited set of compounds is required in safety pharmacological studies. Predictive safety pharmacology (PSP) encompasses the regular screening of a significant number of compounds using cost-effective reliable assays (Food and Drug Administration, FDA 2023). The term "predictive" means accurate documentation of active compounds against any target within a comprehensive assay focusing on safety profile. It includes 80–120 receptors (enzymes, nuclear, ion channels. and transporters). The active compounds could trigger ADR in clinical settings and the situation becomes complicated because of the interaction of compounds with multiple targets. Therefore, it shows captivating scientific challenge to design predictive models capable of capturing risk assessment, identifying ADR using a limited number of compounds with decreased number of target proteins to be screened (Curran et al. 1995). Hammann et al. (2010) investigated the relationship between chemical structures and occurrence of ADR in brain, liver, kidney, and skin. They have examined different sets of medicinal compounds (507), sourced from Swiss drug registry. By using decision tree model and machine learning approach they have identified physical, chemical, and structural features of drug compounds that are prone to have ADRs. Remarkably their model shows a high level of predictive accuracy in projecting ADR associated with nervous, hepatic renal tissues, and allergies. Their model demonstrates the practicality of using straightforward techniques that entail no computationally intensive processes. This can be applied at early drug development stage, drug interaction with specific target organ and generating alerts for drug compounds during post-marketing surveillance and pharmacovigilance (Hammann et al. 2010). Bender et al. (2007) focuses on the advancement of ADR detection through computer assisted determination of compounds with unwanted effects. They developed and validated in silico models for a set of preclinical studies and ADR, which serves as an important tool for prioritizing and streamlining compounds in routine processes. They developed independent models that establish connections between molecular structure, target proteins, and also link molecular structures to adverse drug reactions. Target models were developed by using information from databases like WOMBAT and their in-house repository. The side effects annotations are sourced from World Drug Index (Bender et al. 2007).

17.8 AI-Driven Data Sources

EHR is the digital record of patient information like patient ID, contact information, medication history, disease, medication, diagnostic results, and treatment. EHR offers several advantages like improving operational efficiency, contributing to better patient outcomes, impacting public health in a positive way by efficiently managing and analyzing large patient data (WebCite® 2017). EHR offers access to this data that can be leveraged to survey overall health of the population, identifying opportunities for public health improvements and serves as a safety measure against potential risk associated with drug use. A novel initiative named "DiSTRIBuTE" utilizes EHR for monitoring public health data. Implementation of this initiative has demonstrated that EHRs excel in continuously tracking influenza trends twice in a week as compared to traditional manual reporting of the patient information. This program was launched by the International Society for Disease Surveillance (ISDS), categorized data by age group and helps in decision-making on public health safety, cost-effectiveness, health outcomes, and quality of life. The categorized data is analyzed and interpreted in real-time. Information privacy is accurately maintained by adhering to the Fair Information Practice Principles (FIPPs) and the de-personalized information is shared electronically to address accurate queries related to public health. In 2009, CDC executed EHRs to strengthened efforts in tracing H1N1 pandemic among other noticeable instances. It offers valuable health record screening extending beyond surveillance and possibly paving the way for future research (Diamond et al. 2009). Health surveillance programs using EHRs will monitor overall health of the population highlighting associated health risk, threats and provide an accurate report to healthcare officials (WHO 2023). Nowadays, EHRs are generated, employed, modified, and assessed by several independent entities like hospitals, insurance companies, patients, and physicians themselves. They are gaining importance within primary care where patient records are documented and retrieved in conjunction with online medical resources and supporting tools facilitating the medication prescriptions. These EHRs can be significantly transformed into changing aspects of patient–clinician interactions like email communication, consultation, and telemedicine (Asan et al. 2015). AI-driven data sources have been integrated into four independent "workspaces" within the system, (a) ICSR reports are sourced from Open FDA, (b) RWD utilizes OMOP-CDM data model, (c) social media data collected through Twitter, and (d) scientific literature data retrieved from PubMed. An independent workspace is equipped with data analytics adapted to its content. openFDA is analysis metrics, whereas OMOP-CDM and Twitter data is descriptive statistical analysis among other methods. In each of these workspaces, end users configure "investigations scenarios" identified by Drug Event Combinations (DEC). The platforms provide specialized characteristics like comprehensive reporting suitable for regulatory purposes. In the context of real-world data, many organizations committed to drug safety are actively investigating the potential of emerging data resources. Like in 2014, IMI WEB-RADR 1 and 2 were initiated that utilizes the capabilities of new technologies and social media for ADR reporting. It developed mobile apps that enable healthcare professionals and patients to report ADRs and get news alerts and up to date information (Dimitriadis et al. 2023). Country specific mobile applications were initiated in Croatia, Netherlands, and UK. A joint collaborative effort involving WHO, UMC, and MHRA, has developed generic Med Safety app, which is now available in several countries involving Armenia, Zambia, Burkina Faso, Ghana, Ethiopia, Uganda, Botswana, and Cote d'Ivoire (WEB-RADR 2023).

17.9 Automated Adverse Event Detection

For enhancing patient safety, the healthcare team requires a reliable, effective, and valuable tools for detecting and evaluating adverse events. Many tools are available that help in identifying ADR but are constrained and none has gained acceptance (Ausserhofer et al. 2014). Global Trigger Tool (GTT) is one of the promising tools designed by Institute of Healthcare Improvement (Stockwell et al. 2013). This tool is retrospective data that provides structured process for determining ADR from patient data. GTT focusses on triggering agents from patient data to alert reviewers about the presence of potential ADR. This tool has been established to determine up to ten folds as many as ADR than other methods of detection. Several studies have used GTT platform where they also revised the methods like by altering review process or triggers. The modified version of GTT is renamed as Trigger Tool Methodology (Adler et al. 2008). Traditional method of manually recording ADR was developed by healthcare professionals to review patient data, the trigger tool has increased interest in adopting semi- or fully automated ADR detection methods utilizing EHRs. These detection methods are found to be advantageous in terms of resources efficiency and time for identification of ADR (Menendez et al. 2016). Execution of automated surveillance system that utilizes HER has significantly streamlined the process for determining ADRs (Murff et al. 2003). Such prospective ADR detecting technology can offer real-time feedback and enable healthcare providers to promptly use the interventions when necessary.

17.10 Current Challenges Faced by AI-Driven Pharmacovigilance in Resource-Constrained Environments

ADR underreporting is observed mainly in remote and rural areas where self-medication plays an important role in the usage of medicines in middle- and low-income countries where reporting of such cases remains unnoticed and undocumented. Lack of training and education opportunities in PV leads to a shortage of health care providers in middle- and low-income countries. Also, traditional PV uses healthcare professionals in four domains, i.e., PV operations, systems, surveillance, and qualified person for PV (QPPV). We need experts in different fields of AI in PV like drug safety physician, supervisors, system administrators, engineers for NLP development and ML algorithms. Another huge challenge for ADR reporting in middle- and low-income countries is to provide training for AI dependent PV as it possesses cross languages, cross-specialty and is given in only few numbers of countries with few middle- and low-income countries on the list. Limited funding opportunities for healthcare providers to attend and understand AI-based PV system at global scale is another challenge in putting AI technologies into use for PV (Luo et al. 2017). In education, AI-based PV would be implemented in the teaching institutions for undergraduate student as it helps in cultivating interdisciplinary professionals and progresses awareness of PV. A study in China reported that despite of having established online system of spontaneous reporting of ADR, the ADR reporting rate was very low because of poor understanding of seriousness of ADR and indistinct feedback pathways (Chen et al. 2021a). Higher education and interdisciplinary approach are the challenges observed in AI dependent PV system as it requires experts in computer science engineers with the knowledge of medical science. Technological challenges involve data annotation and data integration as every healthcare institution supports its own data model that may differ from others as they are unique with different value representation and terminologies. The data collection, data integration, and conversion of data into a common data model must be done into a compatible form from different institutions. All the data compilation requires health care team and engineers to give time and efforts for transforming this data. It was observed that in middle- and low-income countries, language is one of the major barriers for data transformation as it must be monitored in different local language formats (Chen et al. 2021b).

For AI dependent PV, data annotation is very crucial as the training models and algorithms completely rely on annotated data to make predictions. For training models, poor high-quality data and high cost limit the research on AI dependent PV. Even in structured database, the data annotation of PV signals is not present, despite of this a large ICSR database exists. In addition, it was observed that the unstructured data like medical records, literature, clinical data, and social media posts augment PV information more than the structured database. In some research studies, 28.6% of ADR related to the use of statins were reported in a structured format database whereas rest of the data was presented in unstructured format (Skentzos et al. 2011). "Variation" is one of the major technological problems associated with AI dependent PV. The terminologies used like "drug name," "disease" are highly variable and less formal, as well as the description of ADR is unclear, grammatical and spelling errors may be common. Diverse language may cause difficulty in data collection, integration, and normalization (Li et al. 2021). Government funding and regulation for PV is another major challenge for AI dependent PV program as it plays an important role in decision-making. Several middle- and low-income countries are young and are not supported by regulatory authorities and require strong regulations for engaging health care professionals and local industries (Olsson et al. 2015).

17.11 Proposed Strategies to Address AI-Driven Pharmacovigilance Challenges in Resource-Constrained Environments

Improving EHRs and creating a database for AI-driven PV system helps to manage and restore the clinical data. The improvement should focus on implementing regulations that ensure EHR employment in healthcare department and workforce training and education for AI dependent PV system. Critical information like patient laboratory data, medical history, and medication orders can be integrated in EHRs and used for AI dependent PV system. The effectiveness of AI dependent PV detection can be enhanced by integration of databases, incorporating AI algorithm with EHR system enabling proactive management of PV signals, automates form completion, and send reminders (Wang et al. 2018). Apart from EHRs, biomedical literature and social sites provide alternative solutions for collecting PV information. These additional data sources have represented their importance in public health (Sloane et al. 2015), enriching the PV database and providing significant solutions in implementing AI dependent PV database by reducing gaps in information. National PV projects at an early stage rely completely on a limited pool of skilled healthcare professionals and their ability to educate and motivate others. It is important to include PV education program in the curricula of the healthcare training institutions like India which has mandated the inclusion of PV training program for UG students in medical programs (Olsson et al. 2015).

For introducing AI dependent PV system in middle- and low-income countries there is a requirement of increased investment and infrastructure development, presenting a significant opportunity to align data driven era with cutting edge technology. Incorporation of global medical vocabularies like RxNorm, MeDRA, SNOMED, CT, and LOINC (Liang et al. 2022) help in standardization of concepts and uniformity in data processing in the field of PV. This in turn enhances the effectiveness of ADR reporting and detection systems. In resource limited settings the process of representing local and non-standard terminology to these standardized medical vocabularies holds great potential for improving data quality and advancing research in PV. Highlighting the significance and cost-effectiveness of an AI-dependent pharmacovigilance (PV) system is important to raise government awareness. AI's ability to streamline data processing and enable extensive analysis

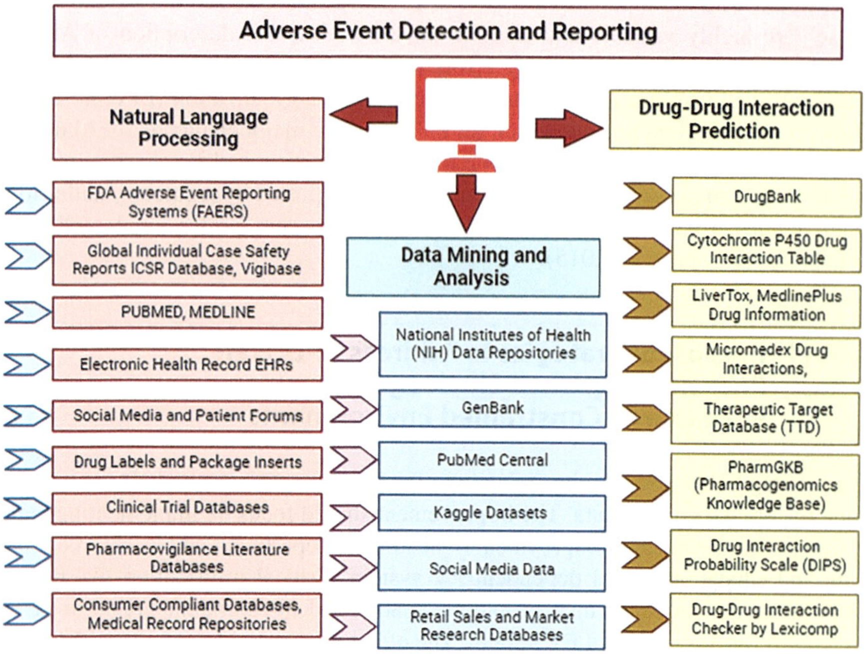

Fig. 17.1 Adverse event detection and reporting databases

can cause significant reduction in human workload, that ultimately enhances the potential for preventive and predictive healthcare measures. With a comprehensive knowledge of the potential benefits of implementing these systems it is important to establish regulatory frameworks that should encompass: (a) increased support for developing AI dependent PV system, (b) ensuring the efficient operations and maintenance of AI dependent PV systems, (c) effective supervision and compliance oversight, (d) data and personal information security.

Figure 17.1 represents databases used in ADR detection and reporting. PubMed (NIH 2023a) and Medline (NLM 2023) contain scientific information in the form of research articles, case studies, and clinical studies. Drug labels and package inserts are used to identify reported ADRs, warnings, and safety precautions. Clinical Trial Databases (Classic 2023) are used to extract adverse event narratives from clinical report data providing deeper insights into safety profiles. Consumer complaint databases (Onlinelegalindia n.d.) regulated by regulatory authorities contain text data related to ADRs reported by consumers. Big hospitals maintain repositories of medical records describing patient experiences with medications. NIH (NIH 2023b) provides data related to biomedical and genomic information. GenBank (NCBI 2023) provides genetic sequence information maintained by NCBI. Kaggle dataset (KAGGLE 2023) is a platform for data science competitions and collaborations, hosting a wide range of datasets. Retail Sales and Market Research Datasets (DATARADE 2023) provide sales and market research data that businesses use for market analysis, consumer behavior studies, and product development. Drug Bank (DRUGBANK 2023) is a comprehensive dataset providing information on drug–drug interactions, pharmacokinetics, and dynamics. Cytochrome P450 Drug Interaction Dataset (DRUG 2023) provides information on drug interactions with cytochrome P450 (CYP) enzymes that are important in drug metabolism. LiverTOx (Livertox 2023) database provides information on drug induced liber diseases. MedlinePlus Drug Information (Medlineplus 2023) provides information on drug interactions and side effects. Micromedex (Micromedexsolutions 2023) is a drug interaction database that helps in identifying potential drug interactions, drug–food, and drug–disease interactions. Therapeutic Target Database (Idrblab 2023) is useful in predicting drug–drug interactions. Pharmacogenomics Knowledge Base PharmaGkB (Pharmgkb 2023) provides information on genetic variations and its effect on drug response and interactions. Drug Interaction Probability Scale (Horn et al. 2007) is used to assess the likelihood of drug interactions. Lexicomp (Wolterskluwer 2023) provides a tool that permits healthcare professionals to check potential drug interactions including severity and management of interactions.

17.12 Conclusion and Outlook

AI impact on ADR reporting is transformative process and these technologies have revolutionizing impact in the way ADRs are identified, monitored, and assessed. AI technologies enable early detection of ADR by analyzing extensive data sources showing immediate response to patient safety concerns. AI algorithms and automation help in saving time and reducing workload on health care professionals and improve operational efficiency. AI technologies facilitate real-time monitoring of patient safety by employing rapid actions when ADR related issues arise. Integration of data sources like EHRs, literature, social media provides a comprehensive analysis of drug safety. Predictive analysis of ADRs and drug interactions supports proactive risk management of ADRs. AI technologies offer significant benefits but challenges like data quality, data privacy, ethical considerations, and interpretability must be addressed. There is a need for collaborative efforts between healthcare providers, regulatory agencies, and pharmaceutical industries to maximize potential benefits of AI in pharmacovigilance. Overall, AI technologies are poised to play an important role in safeguarding public health and patient safety.

References

Adler L, Denham CR, McKeever M, Purinton R, Guilloteau F, Moorhead JD et al (2008) Global trigger tool: implementation basics. J Patient Saf 4(4):245–249

Agyapong PD, Akite EJ, Ansah NA, Ansah PO, Asante KP, Awuni DA et al (2021) Baseline incidence of meningitis, malaria, mortality and other health outcomes in infants and young sub-Saharan African children prior to the introduction of the RTS, S/AS01E malaria vaccine. Malar J 20(1):197

AI for Good Global Summit, Geneva (2017). http://www.itu.int/en/ITU-T/AI/Pages/201706-default.aspx
Anon (n.d.) Looking to the future UN to consider how artificial intelligence could help achieve economic growth and reduce inequalities. http://www.un.org/sustainabledevelopment/blog/2017/10/looking-to-future-un-to-consider-how-artificial-intelligence-could-help-achieve-economic-growth-and-reduce-inequalities/2017
Asan O, Young HN, Chewning B, Montague E (2015) How physician electronic health record screen sharing affects patient and doctor non-verbal communication in primary care. Patient Educ Couns 98(3):310–316
Ausserhofer D, Zander B, Busse R, Schubert M, De Geest S, Rafferty AM, RN4CAST Consortium (2014) Prevalence, patterns and predictors of nursing care left undone in European hospitals: results from the multicountry cross-sectional RN4CAST study. BMJ Qual Saf 23(2):126–135
Bates DW, Evans RS, Murff H, Stetson PD, Pizziferri L, Hripcsak G (2003) Detecting adverse events using information technology. J Am Med Inform Assoc 10:11528
Baum SD, Tonn BE (2015) Confronting future catastrophic threats to humanity. Futures 72:1–3
Bender A, Scheiber J, Glick M, Davies JW, Azzaoui K, Hamon J, Urban L, Whitebread S, Jenkins JL (2007) Analysis of pharmacology data and the prediction of adverse drug reactions and off-target effects from chemical structure. ChemMedChem 2(6):861–873
Bian J, Topaloglu U, Yu F (2012) Towards large-scale twitter mining for drug-related adverse events. SHB12 (2012) 2012:25–32
Bihan K, Lebrun-Vignes B, Funck-Brentano C, Salem JE (2020) Uses of pharmacovigilance databases: an overview. Therapie 75(6):591–598
Cambria E, White B (2014) Jumping NLP curves: a review of natural language processing research [review article]. IEEE Comput Intell Mag 9(2):48–57
Chatterjee P, Tesis A, Cymberknop LJ, Armentano RL (2020) Internet of things and artificial intelligence in healthcare during COVID-19 pandemic-A South American perspective. Front Public Health 8:600213
Chen Y, Wang Y, Wang N, Xiang Y, Zhang R, Xiao J et al (2021a) Knowledge, attitude, and practice regarding pharmacovigilance among the general public in Western China: a cross-sectional study. Curr Med Res Opin 37(1):101–108
Chen R, Zhang Y, Dou Z, Chen F, Xie K, Wang S (2021b) Data sharing and privacy in pharmaceutical studies. Curr Pharm Des 27(7):911–918
Classic (2023). https://classic.clinicaltrials.gov/ct2/. Accessed 25 Sept 2023
Curran ME, Splawski I, Timothy KW, Vincen GM, Green ED, Keating MT (1995) A molecular basis for cardiac arrhythmia: HERG mutations cause long QT syndrome. Cell 80(5):795–803
DATARADE (2023). https://datarade.ai/search/products/retail-datasets. Accessed 25 Sept 2023
Deng H, Wang J, Liu X, Liu B, Lei J (2018) Evaluating the outcomes of medical informatics development as a discipline in China: a publication perspective. Comput Methods Prog Biomed 164:75–85. https://doi.org/10.1016/j.cmpb.2018.07.001
Diamond CC, Mostashari F, Shirky C (2009) Collecting and sharing data for population health: a new paradigm. Health Aff (Millwood) 28(2):454–466
Dimitriadis VK, Dimitsaki S, Chytas A, Gavriilidis GI, Kakalou C, Bonotis P, Natsiavas P (2023) An open-source platform integrating emerging data sources to support multi-modal active pharmacovigilance. Front Drug Saf Regul 2:1016042
DRUG (2023). https://drug-interactions.medicine.iu.edu/MainTable.aspx. Accessed 25 Sept 2023
DRUGBANK (2023). https://go.drugbank.com/. Accessed 25 Sept 2023
European Medicines Agency (EMA) (2017) EMA/873138/2011 rev 2—guideline on good pharmacovigilance practices (GVP). Module VI—collection, management and submission of reports of suspected adverse reactions to medicinal products. http://www.ema.europa.eu/docs/en_GB/document_library/Regulatory_and_procedural_guideline/2017/08/WC500232767.pdf. Accessed 16 Sept 2023
FDA (2023). https://open.fda.gov/data/faers/. Accessed 12 Sept 2023
Fiszman M, Chapman WW, Aronsky D, Evans RS, Haug PJ (2000) Automatic detection of acute bacterial pneumonia from chest X-ray reports. J Am Med Inform Assoc 7:593–604

Food and Drug Administration (2023) S7A safety pharmacology studies for human pharmaceuticals. U. S. Department of Health and Human Services. Food and Drug Administration, United States of America. http://www.fda.gov/Cder/guidance/4461fnl.htm
Friedman C, Hripcsak G, DuMouchel W, Johnson SB, P.D. (1995) Clayton natural language processing in an operational clinical information system. Nat Lang Eng 1:83–108
Goertzel B (2014) Artificial general intelligence: concept, state of the art, and future prospects. J Artif Gen Intell 5(1):1
Guo H, Na X, Hou L, Li J (2017) Classifying Chinese questions related to health care posted by consumers via the internet. J Med Internet Res 19(6):e220. https://doi.org/10.2196/jmir.7156
Hammann F, Gutmann H, Vogt N, Helma C, Drewe J (2010) Prediction of adverse drug reactions using decision tree modeling. Clin Pharmacol Ther 88(1):52–59
Hauben M, Hartford CG (2021) Artificial intelligence in pharmacovigilance: scoping points to consider. Clin Ther 43(2):372–379
He J, Baxter SL, Xu J, Xu J, Zhou X, Zhang K (2019) The practical implementation of artificial intelligence technologies in medicine. Nat Med 25(1):30–36
Henry S, Buchan K, Filannino M, Stubbs A, Uzuner O (2020) 2018 n2c2 shared task on adverse drug events and medication extraction in electronic health records. J Am Med Inform Assoc 27(1):3–12
Honigman B, Light P, Pulling RM, Bates DW (2001) A computerized method for identifying incidents associated with adverse drug events in outpatients. Int J Med Inform 61:21–32
Horn JR, Hansten PD, Chan LN (2007) Proposal for a new tool to evaluate drug interaction cases. Ann Pharmacother 41(4):674–680
Hripcsak G, Knirsch C, Jain NL, Stazesky RC, Pablos-Mendez A, Fulmer T (1999) A health information network for managing inner-city tuberculosis: bridging clinical care, public health, and home care. Comput Biomed Res 32:67–76
Hripcsak G, Bakken S, Stetson PD, Patel VL (2003) Mining complex clinical data for patient safety research: a framework for event discovery. J Biomed Inform 36(1–2):120–130
Idrblab (2023). https://db.idrblab.net/ttd/. Accessed 25 Sept 2023
Jeetu G, Anusha G (2010) Pharmacovigilance: a worldwide master key for drug safety monitoring. J Young Pharm 2(3):315–320
Jung KY, Kim T, Jung J, Lee J, Choi JS, Mira K, Chang DK, Cha WC (2018) The effectiveness of near-field communication integrated with a mobile electronic medical record system: emergency department simulation study. JMIR Mhealth Uhealth 6(9):e11187. https://doi.org/10.2196/11187
KAGGLE (2023). https://www.kaggle.com/datasets. Accessed 25 Sept 2023
Kiguba R, Olsson S, Waitt C (2021) Pharmacovigilance in low- and middle-income countries: a review with particular focus on Africa. Br J Clin Pharmacol 89:491. https://doi.org/10.1111/bcp.15193
Lewis DJ, McCallum JF (2020) Utilizing advanced technologies to augment pharmacovigilance systems: challenges and opportunities. Ther Innov Regul Sci 54:888–899
Li Y, Hu J (2012) Health informationization of China: status and development. Chin J Health Inform Manag 1:001
Li Q, Xie P (2013) Outpatient workload in China. Lancet 381(9882):1983–1984
Li J, Sun Y, Johnson RJ, Sciaky D, Wei CH, Leaman R et al (2016) BioCreative V CDR task corpus: a resource for chemical disease relation extraction. Database (Oxford) 2016:baw068
Li Z, Yang Z, Wang L, Zhang Y, Lin H, Wang J (2021) Lexicon knowledge boosted interaction graph network for adverse drug reaction recognition from social media. IEEE J Biomed Health Inform 25(7):2777–2786
Liang L, Hu J, Sun G, Hong N, Wu G, He Y, Li Y, Hao T, Liu L, Gong M (2022) Artificial intelligence-based pharmacovigilance in the setting of limited resources. Drug Saf 45(5):511–519
Linder JA, Haas JS, Iyer A, Labuzetta MA, Ibara M, Celeste M et al (2010) Secondary use of electronic health record data: spontaneous triggered adverse drug event reporting. Pharmacoepidemiol Drug Saf 19(12):1211–1215
Livertox (2023). https://ncbi.nlm.nih.gov/books/n/livertox. Accessed 25 Sept 2023

Luo Y, Thompson WK, Herr TM, Zeng Z, Berendsen MA, Jonnalagadda SR et al (2017) Natural language processing for HER based pharmacovigilance: a structured review. Drug Saf 40(11):1075–1089

Medlineplus (2023). https://medlineplus.gov/druginformation.html. Accessed 25 Sept 2023

Menendez ME, Janssen SJ, Ring D (2016) Electronic health record-based triggers to detect adverse events after outpatient orthopaedic surgery. BMJ Qual Saf 25(1):25–30

Micromedexsolutions (2023). https://www.micromedexsolutions.com/micromedex2/librarian/deeplinkaccess. Accessed 25 Sept 2023

Mohsen A, Tripathi LP, Mizuguchi K (2021) Deep learning prediction of adverse drug reactions in drug discovery using open TG–GATEs and FAERS databases. Front Drug Discov 1:768792

Murali K, Kaur S, Prakash A, Medhi B (2019) Artificial intelligence in pharmacovigilance: practical utility. Indian J Pharmacol 51(6):373

Murff HJ, Forster AJ, Peterson JF, Fiskio JM, Heiman HL, Bates DW (2003) Electronically screening discharge summaries for adverse medical events. J Am Med Inform Assoc 10(4):339–350

Nagam VM (2023) Diagnostic medical artificial intelligence: futuristic prospects for implementation in healthcare settings. Front Artif Intell 6:1169244

NCBI (2023). https://www.ncbi.nlm.nih.gov/genbank/. Accessed 25 Sept 2023

NIH (2023a). PubMed (nih.gov). Accessed 25 Sept 2023

NIH (2023b). https://www.nih.gov/. Accessed 25 Sept 2023

NLM (2023). https://www.nlm.nih.gov/medline/index.html. Accessed 25 Sept 2023

Olsson S, Pal SN, Dodoo A (2015) Pharmacovigilance in resource-limited countries. Expert Rev Clin Pharmacol 8(4):449–460

Onlinelegalindia (n.d.). https://www.onlinelegalindia.com/services/consumer-complaint-campaign/?utm_source=bing&utm_content=OLI_ConsumerComplaint&msclkid=7ab56a4f71411d11cf8b0f5ff2e2a600&utm_medium=cpc&utm_campaign=OLI_Consumer%20Complaint%20%232&utm_term=consumer%20complaint%20database#2&Campaignid=428330907&Adgroupid=1330410526219504&device=c&Adposition=&physical=149209&match_type=e&network=consumer%20complaint%20database&target_name=kwd-83151744118938:loc-90&placement=&keyword_id=consumer%20complaint%20database. Accessed 25 Sept 2023

Owoyemi A, Owoyemi J, Osiyemi A, Boyd A (2020) Artificial intelligence for healthcare in Africa. Front Digit Health 2:6

Page J, Bain M, Mukhlish F (2018) The risks of low level narrow artificial intelligence. In: 2018 IEEE International conference on intelligence and safety for robotics (ISR). IEEE, pp 1–6

Pharmgkb (2023). https://www.pharmgkb.org/. Accessed 25 Sept 2023

Skentzos S, Shubina M, Plutzky J, Turchin A (2011) Structured vs unstructured: factors affecting adverse drug reaction documentation in an EMR repository. AMIA Annu Symp Proc 2011:1270–1279

Sloane R, Osanlou O, Lewis D, Bollegala D, Maskell S, Pirmohamed M (2015) Social media and pharmacovigilance: a review of the opportunities and challenges. Br J Clin Pharmacol 80(4):910–920

Stevenson JG, Green L (2016) Biologics, pharmacovigilance, and patient safety: it's all in the name. J Manag Care Spec Pharm 22(8):927–930

Stockwell DC, Kirkendall E, Muething SE, Kloppenborg E, Vinodrao H, Jacobs BR (2013) Automated adverse event detection collaborative: electronic adverse event identification, classification, and corrective actions across academic pediatric institutions. J Patient Saf 9(4):203–210

Tatonetti NP, Ye PP, Daneshjou R, Altman RB (2012) Data-driven prediction of drug effects and interactions. Sci Transl Med 4(125):125ra31

Uehara T, Ono A, Maruyama T, Kato I, Yamada H, Ohno Y et al (2009) The Japanese toxicogenomics project: application of toxicogenomics. Mol Nutr Food Res 54:218–227. https://doi.org/10.1002/mnfr.200900169

VAERS (2023). https://vaers.hhs.gov/. Accessed 12 Sept 2023

Vamathevan J, Clark D, Czodrowski P, Dunham I, Ferran E, Lee G et al (2019) Applications of machine learning in drug discovery and development. Nat Rev Drug Discov 18:463–477. https://doi.org/10.1038/s41573-019-0024-5

Wang Z, Clark NR, Ma'ayan A (2016) Drug-induced adverse events prediction with the LINCS L1000 data. Bioinformatics 32:2338–2345. https://doi.org/10.1093/bioinformatics/btw168

Wang L, Rastegar-Mojarad M, Ji Z, Liu S, Liu K, Moon S et al (2018) Detecting pharmacovigilance signals combining electronic medical records with spontaneous reports: a case study of conventional disease-modifying antirheumatic drugs for rheumatoid arthritis. Front Pharmacol 9:875

Wang X, Zhao Y, Pourpanah F (2020) Recent advances in deep learning. Int J Mach Learn Cyber 11:747–750. https://doi.org/10.1007/s13042-020-01096-5

WebCite® (2017) U.S Department of Health and Human Services URL: https://www.healthit.gov/providers-professionals/faqs/what-electronic-healthrecord-ehr. Accessed 3 Oct 2017. Archived by WebCite® at http://www.webcitation.org/6twtffZwS

WEB-RADR (2023). WEB-RADR. Accessed 17 Sept 2023

WHO (2023) Public health surveillance. World Health Organization. http://www.who.int/topics/public_health_surveillance/en/. Accessed 17 Sept 2023. Archived by WebCite® at http://www.webcitation.org/6wCf3xH19

Wolterskluwer (2023). https://www.wolterskluwer.com/en/solutions/lexicomp. Accessed 25 Sept 2023

Current Challenges and Future Perspectives: Pharmacovigilance

18

Alishan Zia, Mukesh Nandave, and Anoop Kumar

Abstract

With the identification and prevention of adverse drug events, pharmacovigilance increases patient safety. Although there are obstacles that limit the detection of adverse drug events, many adverse drug events go unreported or are reported incorrectly. Large data sets from diverse sources, such as wearable medical devices and electronic health records, are one difficulty. Artificial intelligence, which includes machine learning techniques like deep learning and natural language processing, can identify and gather data on adverse medication reactions, automating the pharmacovigilance process and enhancing the monitoring of well-known and well-documented adverse drug reactions. In addition, artificial intelligence techniques can help in identifying and preventing adverse medication events due to the rising demand for telehealth services for treating both acute and chronic disorders. In this review, we discuss the current and future perspectives of pharmacovigilance that may be useful to improve the quality of pharmacovigilance and the role of artificial intelligence in telehealth practices.

Keywords

Pharmacovigilance · Adverse drug event · Artificial intelligence · Telemedicine

A. Zia (✉) · M. Nandave · A. Kumar
Department of Pharmacology, Delhi Pharmaceutical Sciences and Research University, New Delhi, India
e-mail: mukeshnandave@gmail.com; anoopdpsru@dpsru.edu.in

M. Nandave, A. Kumar (eds.), *Pharmacovigilance Essentials*,
https://doi.org/10.1007/978-981-99-8949-2_18

18.1 Introduction

Pharmacovigilance was first introduced in December of 1961 with a case report/letter published by W. McBride, an Australian doctor in The Lancet. He was the first person to suspect a link between phocomelia, a limb deformity, and thalidomide which was a drug that was prescribed during pregnancy as an anti-emetic as well as sedative drug (McBride 1961).

World Health Organization (WHO) in the year, 1968 promoted the "Program for International Drug Monitoring" which was a pilot study project aimed toward centralizing global data related to adverse drug reactions toward identifying early steps of pharmacovigilance. The terminology "pharmacovigilance" was introduced in the mid-1970s by a group of French pharmacologists and toxicologists for the promotion of a project titled "Assessment of Risks of Side-Effects That Had the Potential to be Associated with Use of Drugs During Treatment" (Bégaud et al. 1994).

Pharmacovigilance is a science dealing with the collection, monitoring, research, assessment, and evaluation of information concerning adverse effects of drugs, various biologically derived products, blood-derived products, herbal products, different vaccines, medical devices, any traditional and/or complementary drugs by healthcare professionals and patients in order to identify novel information involving any hazards that may be associated with above-mentioned products which may prevent harm to patients. Pharmacovigilance determines challenges in maximization of drug safety and maintenance regarding public confidence.

Hence, pharmaceutical as well as biotechnology firms must monitor as well as estimate and manage risk related with drugs (WHO 2002a). Pharmacovigilance is primarily associated with adverse drug reactions that include responses toward drug which are noxious in nature and mostly accidental in nature. These drug reactions occur at dosages that are normally prescribed as prophylactic, diagnostic, or therapeutic (Shuka et al. 2012).

Continuously monitoring the effectiveness of drugs and their side-effects can reduce associated morbidity as well as mortality along with maximization of benefits and minimization of associated risks. It should be acknowledged that even after taking utmost precautions at pre-clinical as well as clinical tests, no pharmaceutical company can provide absolute drug safety.

Since most clinical trials incorporate few patients, less commonly associated side-effects as well as ADRs are known when a new drug is introduced in the market. Hence, post-marketing pharmacovigilance makes use of tools like data mining and studying case reports to identify adverse drug effects. Governmental drug regulation agencies have pharmacovigilance systems for monitoring adverse drug reactions.

18.2 Current Scenario of Pharmacovigilance

Safety profile and quality of medicines are of greatest concern for each stakeholder in the healthcare system which includes physicians, pharmacists, and nurses, among others. Adverse drug reaction can be defined as "an appreciable harmful and unpleasant response that may result from any intervention by making use of a medicinal agent that can help in predicting any potential hazard arising following its future prescription and by warranting the prevention as well as a specific type of treatment or any alteration in dosages or product withdrawal" (Edwards and Aronson 2000).

Adverse drug reactions are mostly associated with an increase in mortality as well as hospitalization and often may have economic implications (Butt et al. 2011; Lazarou et al. 1998; Ahmad 2003; Xu and Wang 2014).

Pharmacovigilance constitutes activities that are associated with recognizing, assessing, understanding as well as preventing adverse drug effects (WHO 2002b). Thus, post-marketed surveillance of drugs is increasingly becoming important for pharmaceutical companies.

Thus, in many countries' organizations have been set up that are completely functioning as pharmacovigilance units. Clinical drug trials are important for the evaluation and safety of new medical products and devices. There are rare occurrences of adverse events that are mostly discovered before reaching market or most of them are mostly reported when the drug is under pharmacovigilance, i.e., during phase IV clinical study trial. Each pharmacovigilance drug study is an essential part of Phase 4 trial and is an important part of the process of drug development (Suvarna 2010).

Studies of Phase IV are further different in the design than the earlier clinical preliminaries which is the principal thing to note about studies of Phase IV (Carreiro et al. 2015). All Phase IV has common set of objectives and is proof that health-associated intervention may be effectively coordinated within public general health as well as clinical practice (Smith et al. 2015).

Post-marketed adverse drug effect report systems are mainly under-utilized both by caregivers and patients in developing nations. As a result, most of the adverse effects are not reported to drug regulating agencies (Pierce et al. 2017).

Hence, currently though there are drug regulatory agencies that keep a watch over adverse drug reactions by means of pharmacovigilance, there does exist a lack of knowledge in many clinicians and health caregivers that produces a significant drawback in studying complete safety profile of any drug that is marketed.

18.3 Recent Advancements by PvPI (Pharmacovigilance Programme of India)

The Central Drugs Standard Control Organization and Directorate General of Health Services under aegis of the Ministry of Health and Family Welfare, Government of India with Indian Pharmacopeia Commission, Ghaziabad (U.P.)

National Coordinating Centre has initiated the Pharmacovigilance Program pan India for the protection of patient health by ensuring safety of drugs (Yang et al. 2014; Carreiro et al. 2015; Pivovarov et al. 2015).

The Pharmacovigilance Programme of India or PvPI was initiated by the Government of India on 14th of July 2010, in association with the All India Institute of Medical Sciences (AIIMS), New Delhi as a National Coordination Centre for monitoring of adverse drug reactions (ADRs) in India (Huang et al. 2015; Zhang et al. 2015; Alvaro et al. 2015). In 2010, twenty-two centers for monitoring ADRs were set up which included AIIMS, New Delhi. In order to implement it in a better and coordinated manner, National Coordination Centre was then shifted from All India Institute of Medical Sciences (AIIMS), New Delhi, to Indian Pharmacopoeia Commission located in Ghaziabad, Uttar Pradesh, on 15th of April, 2011 (Ben Abacha and Zweigenbaum 2011; Fong et al. 2015; Ben Abacha et al. 2015).

The primary purpose of PvPI is a collation of available gathered data, its processing and analysis and using these inferences for recommending various regulatory guidelines alongside communicating risks associated with drugs to healthcare professionals as well as the general public (Kim et al. 2015; Lopez Pineda et al. 2015).

The mission statement of Pharmacovigilance Programme of India is to safeguard the health of Indian general population by making sure that the beneficial uses of various medicinal agents outweigh risks that may be associated with their use.

Vision of this program is improvement of safety of patients and their welfare in India by means of monitoring of safety of drugs and also reducing risks associated with medicines.

Objectives of this program are as follows: (a) Creating national system for reporting of patient's safety; (b) identification and analysis of newly reported adverse drug reactions; (c) for analyzing ratio between drug benefit and risk of medications which are in market; (d) for generating evidence- based information concerning safety of drugs; (e) for supporting regulatory drug agencies in decisions involving using medications; (f) for communicating information involving drug safety to stakeholders for minimizing any risk; (g) to evolve as center of excellence for pharmacovigilance at national level; (h) for collaborating with another national center for exchanging information and management of data; and (e) to act as training as well as consultancy center for other pharmacovigilance centers located around the world (WHO 2004).

In a big country like India which has a population of approximately 1.2 billion and has variability in ethnicities, differences in prevalence of diseases, existing different systems of practice, difference in socioeconomic status, it is important that a standardized as well as strong system of pharmacovigilance as well as drug safety program monitoring exists.

Short term goals of the Pharmacovigilance Programme of India

(a) Development of MCI-approved medical hospitals and colleges.
(b) Encouraging healthcare professionals to report adverse reactions to drugs or vaccines or medical devices as well as biological medicinal products.
(c) Collecting case-reports along with data.

Long term goals of the Pharmacovigilance Programme of India

(a) Expansion of this program to all government as well as private hospitals and public health program centers across India.
(b) Development and implementation of electronic reporting or e-reporting system.
(c) Development of habit of reporting of adverse effects among health professionals.
(d) To eventually make adverse drug effects reporting a mandatory requisite for health professionals.

Pharmacovigilance system is not successful in India due to the following multiple reasons:

(a) Lack of funding as well as systematization in India.
(b) Data collected from various peripherally located zonal medical centers is of poor quality and is not analyzed properly.
(c) There is no research on adverse drug effects in India, hence, it is difficult to ascertain the actual incidence of ADRs.
(d) There is negligible involvement of health professionals from both rural and urban areas.
(e) There is very limited knowledge with motivation regarding pharmacovigilance among doctors as well as in common public.

Recently, systematic tools for recognizing safety concerning signals from different case reports have been introduced. Most of these methods are at present static in nature and their utility in the identification of drug safety is currently being assessed. These methods calculate the proportional reporting ratio, using Bayesian techniques (Waller and Arlett 2002; DuMouchel 1999; Bate et al. 1998).

Data mining tools are currently being used to facilitate the evaluation of reported drug effects by use of statistical techniques for the detection of potential adverse effects of any drug post-marketing.

18.4 Current Challenges and Future Strategies

The safety of data associated with drugs, its analysis and the willingness of the industry to accept these changes is the main challenges at present. Big-sized data as well as cloud-based solutions are currently utilized by different companies to some extent, while only few companies have completely accepted these. Among deep concerns are security of data and safeguarding its integrity.

Data fed in safety-acquired databases must have good quality and should be structured for appropriate analysis. Only a few stakeholders readily accept the latest form of developments as well as regulation guidelines in maintaining standard data and hence, there is a pressing need for remaining stakeholders to begin using these advancements.

There is an increasing awareness regarding use of artificial intelligence-based methods for analyzing pharmacovigilance-related data. Most companies have already started to utilize this technology already, while others are in the process of accepting the change. Hence, one can expect pharmacovigilance to become fully automated in future.

Hence, in the near future, there will be a greater need to accept automated artificial intelligence-based analysis in the field of pharmacovigilance. Hence, the field of pharmacovigilance in the near future shall evidence massive changes in processing methods and shall be a welcome shift from tedious and repetitive types of manual processing of available medical knowledge as a value-added task.

Therefore, it is critical that everyone involved, including the pharmaceutical industry, healthcare providers, and drug regulatory agencies, establish an appropriate setting for these changes to be accepted in which such a transformation can take place with no compromises over public health/safety and ideally providing alongside providing benefits to patients.

Therefore, developing new automated technologies that will enable the early integration of these tools into the pharmacovigilance industry for better adaptation from the outset is one of the challenges facing pharmacovigilance in the future (Thole and Enejo n.d.).

18.5 Healthcare Profession

Following the launch of first model of iPhone in the year, 2007, an eco-system started to form which enabled monitoring of clinical situations in a real world along with collection of clinical and research-based data that was associated with health. This was made possible with the most commonly used mobile systems.

In today's integration system that is constituted by computational, social, mobile as well as cloud computing, a social fabric comprised of customers who are adept in technology got created. The digital technological revolution gave birth to significant numbers of developments in medicine.

A significant medical revolution that has a significant effect over the healthcare system involves the newest technologies like artificial intelligence or AI, the use of biosensors, advanced robotic systems, and medical internet of things or MIoT (Manogaran et al. 2017; Pace et al. 2018; Hathaliya et al. 2019).

These modern innovations have helped in digitalizing major services in medical health sector for enhancing healthcare (Yan et al. 2015; Reinhardt et al. 2020; Aceto et al. 2020).

Hence, main aim of this digital and automated revolution is planning and building of artificially intelligent healthcare system for an effective and efficient function and for creating better platform of technology for visualizing and making decisions in real-time (Mavrogiorgou et al. 2019; Suman et al. 2020).

Novel technologies like internet of services are capable of creating newer possibilities in field of medicine by reduction of operating time and involved risks. By making use of these technologies, doctors anticipate outcomes of administering any drug to patients.

These modern technologies are intelligent enough to solve a variety of issues in healthcare, particularly involved with detection, simulation of process, data analysis, and selection of appropriate therapy. Virtual healthcare consultation is an important innovation in healthcare as doctors are capable of using internet-based technological advancements for digital monitoring of patients who are staying at distant and remote locations and will have the capacity to address any adverse drug reactions, especially ones with emergencies (Kernebeck et al. 2020).

18.5.1 Self-Medication

Self-medication is practiced all around the world and is considered the major culprit in the development of resistance toward antibiotics. This rampant usage of antibiotics has led to development of major health issues due to various factors like the inability to diagnose the cause behind any disease which eventually leads to a delayed diagnosis. This further delays the treatment which might eventually result in increased morbidity and mortality.

Self-medication may be defined as "consuming drugs, herbal formulations or home-based remedies as self-initiative or after following advice of different individual without any consultation from doctor" (Hernandez-Juyol and Job-Quesada 2002).

Self-medication is a commonly followed practice in economically backward populations due to costly healthcare facilities. This may be partly attributed to free access to "over-the-counter" drugs in India. There might be other reasons for any person to engage in self-medication such as- self-care, sympathetic attitude toward ailing family members, less time, toward family members in sickness, lack of time, no health facilities, financial constraints, lack of knowledge, misbelief, influenced by advertisements, etc. (Geissler et al. 2000).

OTC Committee of "Organisation of Pharmaceutical Producers of India" has been striving toward promoting responsible behavior in self-medication. Its aim is to provide regulation for issues like accessibility of household remedies and to increase awareness regarding self-medication in public as well as government (Verma et al. 2010).

As per the World Health Organization's positional statement on self-medication, "It is now of wide acceptance that self-medication is important in health system." People's confidence in self-medication has grown as a result of awareness of their own responsibility for their health. Self-medication has increased due to higher public understanding, education, and socioeconomic status (WHO 1995).

Risks involved with self-medication are (Bennadi 2014):

1. Not consulting with a doctor may result in wrong diagnosis.
2. Stubborn behavior in seeking medical advice.
3. Wrong therapy choice.

4. Inability to recognize pharmacological interactions and risks associated.
5. Severe forms of adverse drug effects.
6. Failure to recognize if the same drug is repeatedly being taken under different names.
7. Not reporting self-medication drugs to the attending physician.
8. Less or overdosage.
9. Long use.
10. Risk of developing drug dependence.
11. Interactions between diet and drug taken.

18.6 Clinical Trial Monitoring

Clinical trial monitoring is an important part of conducting a clinical trial that improves safety of study participants while at the same time upgrading quality of clinical data and integrity of clinical trial. Monitoring of these trials is performed by team monitors, teams that assess quality assurance and trial associated managers (Love et al. 2020).

International Council for Harmonisation of Technical Requirements for Pharmaceuticals for Human Use or ICH Good Clinical Practice (GCP) has clearly outlined purpose of monitoring clinical trials.

The purpose of clinical monitoring of trials is verifying (Love et al. 2022):

1. Rights as well as well-being of humans to be protected;
2. Reported data must be accurate, verifiable as well as complete.
3. Trial conduct must be in compliance with current protocols or amendment(s) in accordance with good clinical practice.

Guidelines on monitoring of clinical trial are distributed mostly in technical language and do not deal with practical framework for achieving aims in clinical trial monitoring. Since there are different specialities that are involved in monitoring, there are bound to be disparities that can lead to misunderstanding as well as errors in communication (National Research Council 2012).

All of this can result in poor monitoring that can massively impact patient rights as well as their safety. Additionally, there may be an impact over data integrity. This can result in repeated monitoring that might not add to the value of trial and can result in extra burdening of clinical research-associated teams while at the same time, increasing the overall cost involved.

In such conditions, it becomes difficult to discuss research methodology and deliver clinical tools in a congenial atmosphere wherein all specialities can work together.

Thus, in the absence of common consensus, the research grant committees do not provide monetary benefits to clinical trials. When each of the clinical trial group creates its own strategy for trial monitoring along with different language, difficulty in communication exists between trial groups (Dietrich et al. 2020).

18.7 Implementing AI in Adverse Event Case Processing

Artificial intelligence simulates human intelligence by making use of informatics as well as mathematical methodologies. This system analyzes data for improvement of processing of data. Ultimate aim of artificial intelligence is handling of tasks in timed as well as efficient way. Applying artificial intelligence to pharmacovigilance requires newer methods for improving management of reported cases and monitoring of risk and benefit balance.

Artificial intelligence can be used for automated repetition of processing of data. This technique also helps in identifying clinical situations that have similarity with any particular case being studied.

Artificial intelligence works by automation of data-based entry by converting telephonic calls and electronic mails to data related points. For example, screening of social networking sites for newly reported cases or for importing telephonic calls in previously existing database related to pharmacovigilance. Artificial intelligence processes all screened data to valid data entries.

Artificial intelligence can be utilized in variety of pharmacovigilance fields such as:

(a) Identification of patient clusters for identification of best possible medication which is achievable by analysis of the patient's profile and adverse drug-related events in a particular case.
(b) Detecting missing data-based information in any adverse drug effect report in real-time whenever any report gets registered by means of artificial intelligence-based algorithms.
(c) Automatically reviewing social network for detecting any adverse drug events reported publicly. This may compensate for missing reports at pharmacovigilance website in official manner.

18.8 Telehealth in Pharmacovigilance

Telemedicine can be defined as usage of electronic technologies pertaining to information as well as communication for providing and supporting health care system. Telehealth is remote system of health care that may include video conferencing, case monitoring, maintaining electronic health-based records, observing as well as reporting adverse drug responses, continued health education as well as training programs for health care professionals (Patil et al. 2002).

World Health Organization or WHO has defined telemedicine as "delivering health services, wherein distance is a critical underlying reason for all health system professionals who use information as well as communication technology for exchanging important information related to diagnostics, treatment as well as prevention of occurrence of disease or injuries, research, evaluation and continuing education of health professionals for advancement in health" (WHO 1997).

18.8.1 Milestones in Telemedicine

Health care in home settings is a long story and has existed for many decades in clinics. For example, in 1879, an article in "the *Lancet*" mentioned use of the telephone for reducing unnecessary clinical visits. In the 1920s, radio services were utilized for giving medical advices on ships. In 1925, a magazine *known as "Science and Invention"* illustrated doctor using the radio to provide a diagnosis to a patient.

In the year 1960, the National Aeronautics and Space Administration or NASA implemented telemedicine system for the purpose of monitoring the physiological health parameters of astronauts. This led to the beginning of an era of modernized telemedicine. This led to the launch of a pioneer telemedicine project undertaken by NASA for providing health care services in rural areas. The project was termed as "Space Technology applied in Rural Papago Advanced Health Care" (Bashshur and Lovett 1977; Brown 1995).

The 1980s were revolutionary times for developing telecommunication as well as internet-based services that supported the fast growth of this field. The main focus was on diagnostic health services such as tele-pathology, tele-radiology, and tele-dermatology (Latifi and Ganapathy 2004).

In India, the first telemedicine unit began its work in Aragonda, AP. It was inaugurated in 2001 by former United States President, Mr. Bill Clinton. At present, there are approximately 400 centers of telemedicine existing across India (Mathew 2005).

18.8.2 Objectives of Telemedicine

These are as under

(a) **Making high-quality healthcare facilities available for underprivileged population:** In India, a large section of the population based in rural areas is separated from cities by large distance, hence accessibility to the standard quality of health care. Telemedicine increases the availability of medical health care services along with clinical care in spite of economic as well as geographical barriers.
(b) **Saving time:** Use of telemedicine saves time that either a patient or doctor can spend in traveling from one location to another for availing health services.
(c) **Monitoring of cases, providing home-based care along with remote critical health care:** Telemedicine may help in monitoring any patient from any distance by a specialist and it allows remotely regulating critical and home-based care.
(d) **Reducing cost of medical health care:** Increasing healthcare cost has become a critical concern in today's world. Incidental expense that is related with health care includes cost which is linked with factors like traveling, accommodation, food expenses, etc. These contribute significantly to complete treatment cost.

(e) **Surveying and tracking of diseases:** Telemedicine is an important application that can help in surveying as well as collecting data related to epidemic and endemic conditions. This will help in efficiently managing diseases within any given community by helping disaster management program (Mathew 2005).
(f) **Continuing medical education as well as training programs:** Health science is undergoing evolution at a rapid rate on a day-to-day basis. Hence, it is important for practitioners to remain updated with latest data so as to provide safe as well as effective medical care to all stakeholders. Hence, CMEs are important for health professionals, training for health professionals along with educational programs for general public. These educational programs can be efficiently delivered with telemedicine.

Most importantly, telehealth or telemedicine may act as a major link between the nodal and referral centers for providing health care to patients staying at remote locations with less time expenditure and by spending less money.

18.8.3 Telemedicine or Telehealth Services Types

Telehealth or telemedicine services have different types such as

(a) **Storage and forwarding type:** This telehealth service is practiced in areas where direct contact with remote centers is not possible or immediate message transmission. In such cases, patient interviews can be recorded, clinical examinations as well as investigations are conducted and all data forwarded to remotely situated specialized centers for evaluation and if required, expert opinions, for non-emerging cases.
(b) **Interaction-based services:** With the availability of high-speed telecommunication services, direct interaction with any specialized referral center is possible in real-time situation. Patients visiting remotely situated health care centers may directly interact in face-to-face sessions with doctors with specific specializations present in a remote referral center. Video conferencing sessions among professionals help in providing health care from multiple speciality experts.
(c) **Remotely possibility of patient monitoring:** This process uses audio-visual aids and various types of telecommunication and technologies for electronic processing of information for monitoring health of a patient from distant location.
(d) **Mobile-based telemedicine/health:** Mobile-based telehealth monitoring is important in natural disaster settings like earthquakes and floods since under these conditions medical health facilities may not be available fast enough. Telehealth medicine equipment may be specifically installed in ambulances that have satellite connections. This is especially important in providing health care in remotely situated sites (Mishra et al. 2004). At present, there are 10 mobile-based telemedicine functional units in India which is equipped with an ultra-

sound, X-ray facility, echocardiography, electrocardiography, biochemistry, and ophthalmic facilities. Each unit has a para-medical/technical staff who conducts required investigations. The test results are examined by a medical specialist present in a tertiary health care center by making use of direct link from satellites with internet connectivity.

18.8.4 Tele-Pharmacy and Telehealth

Tele-pharmacy can be defined as "long distanced supervision by senior pharmacists of technicians appointed in pharmacies located at any distant site." Tele-pharmacy is done by the computerized entry of physician's prescription, then the appointed technician will view and dispense the drugs (Casey et al. 2006).

However, there may be errors in medications when reviewed from a remote site resulting in ADRs. Most hospitals have an internal system for tracking medication errors at internal level and much inconvenience can be avoided with this system.

18.8.5 Social Networking Sites and Their Role in Pharmacovigilance

In recent years, it has been observed that an increasing number of individuals are reporting adverse drug responses on various social media platforms. This phenomenon is termed as "experience cloud." Most of the time clinicians do not go through these reflective reports on these platforms which can lead to patient non-compliance and poor behavior. Use of artificial intelligence-based software for extracting medical information concerning adverse drug effects is an important step toward pharmacovigilance reporting (Boon 2007).

18.8.6 Specialized Healthcare Social Networks and Forums

Using social media for the purpose of pharmacovigilance is slowly gaining importance. As a result, different resources are being studied for identifying adverse drug reactions. Specialized healthcare social networking sites and forums for reporting of ADRs are DailyStrength, PatientsLikeMe®, and MedHelp® (Liu and Chen 2015).

Social networking media is enriched with real-time sources of data which might help in identifying newer issues associated with drug safety along with uses of medicines in conditions like pregnancy, proper reading of drug labels, drug misuse, errors of medication, and efficacy of medicinal products. Doctors are increasingly recognizing the requirement of incorporation of needs as well as concerns related to patients; thus, there is more patient-centric health care.

Specialized healthcare-associated social media platforms or forums aid in the collection of important posts over social media regarding treatment-based outcomes and give regulators and the pharmaceutical business early access to reported adverse events related to drugs.

Popular social networking sites such as Twitter and Facebook are user-friendly interfaces which are used by patients to report their clinical conditions as well as adverse drug reactions (Shukla et al. 2022).

18.8.7 Recommendation: The Way Forward

Extracting adverse drug effect-related information from different types of databases has various challenges involved, which include proper management, storage, querying, and analysis of entire extracted data. The resolution of a particular drug-related adverse event may be related to the interpretation of medical dictionary problems and the miscoding of data.

Various methods for analysis should be capable of systematically screening various databases for identification of serious types of adverse drug events that may be of potential concern in the background of large amounts of data which may balance concerns regarding excess signaling.

Also, after identifying these signals, the pharmacovigilance system must be capable of triggering an alert that might signal a potential safety risk involved with a particular drug. Data mining analytical can calculate the inter-relationship between any particular drug and adverse events caused by it.

Thus, in recent times, it has been a requirement for pharmacovigilance agencies to incorporate automated artificial intelligence-based tools that can perform data mining processes from various sites such as official websites, social networking sites such as Facebook, Twitter, or Instagram, channelize it into high-quality input data, and then be able to provide an alert in form of a signal so as to alert a physician or pharmacist to possible adverse response to any drug.

However, these modern techniques can be used as adjunct tools to traditional systems of pharmacovigilance. Hence, pharmacovigilance may be utilized to study the potency of different drugs including vaccines, administering right doses, and monitoring of any adverse drug reactions. Thus, an excessive of warnings might undermine real risk factors hidden for a long period of time, however, a low information output may severely dent the trust of the general public in medicinal drugs and the system of pharmaco-surveillance. Properly implementing technology associated with pharmacovigilance requires specific expertise in communicating a variety of information concerning risks that may be beneficial to clinicians as well as patients.

18.8.8 Conclusion: The Way Forward

Pharmacovigilance is a primary responsibility of physicians as well as the general public who must report any adverse reaction following intake of drugs. Doctors must keep themselves abreast with recent developments in the pharmaceutical world and must be able to recognize any drug effects easily so as to provide correct management at the right time, hence this is the need of the current situation to ensure the proper management and reporting of unwanted drug reactions.

References

Aceto G, Persico V, Pescapé A (2020) Industry 4.0 and health: internet of things, big data, and cloud computing for healthcare 4.0. J Ind Inf Integr 18:100129–100132

Ahmad SR (2003) Adverse drug event monitoring at the Food and Drug Administration: your report can make a difference. J Gen Intern Med 18(1):57–60

Alvaro N, Conway M, Doan S, Lofi C, Overington J, Collier N (2015) Crowdsourcing twitter annotations to identify first- hand experiences of prescription drug use. J Biomed Inform 58:280–287

Bashshur R, Lovett J (1977) Assessment of telemedicine: results of the initial experience. Aviat Space Environ Med 48:65–70

Bate A, Lindquist M, Edwards IR (1998) A Bayesian neural network method for adverse drug reaction signal generation. Eur J Clin Pharmacol 54:315–321

Bégaud B, Chaslerie A, Haramburu F (1994) Organization and results of drug vigilance in France. Rev Epidemiol Sante Publique 42:416–423

Ben Abacha A, Zweigenbaum P (2011) A hybrid approach for the extraction of semantic relations from MEDLINE abstracts. In: 12th International conference on computational linguistics and intelligent text processing. CICLing, Tokyo. https://doi.org/10.1007/978-3-642-19437-5_11

Ben Abacha A, Mahbub Chowdhury F, Karanasiou A, Mrabet Y, Lavelli A, Zweigenbaum P (2015) Text mining for pharmacovigilance: using machine learning for drug name recognition and drug- drug interaction extraction and classification. J Biomed Inform 58:122–132

Bennadi D (2014) Self medication. J Basic Clin Pharm 5(1):19–23

Boon A (2007) Telepharmacy at a critical access hospital. Am J Health Syst Pharm 64:242–244

Brown N (1995) A brief history of telemedicine. Telemed Inform Exchange 105:833–835

Butt TF, Cox AR, Lewis H, Ferner RE (2011) Patient experiences of serious adverse drug reactions and their attitudes to medicines. Drug Saf 34(4):319–328

Carreiro AV, Amaral PMT, Pinto S, Tomas P, de Carvalho M, Madeira SC (2015) Prognostic models based on patient snapshots and time windows: predicting disease progression to assisted ventilation in amyotrophic lateral sclerosis. J Biomed Inform 58:133–144

Casey M, Moscovice I, Davidson G (2006) Pharmacist staffing, technology use and implementation of medication safety practices in rural hospitals. J Rural Health 22:321–330

Dietrich J, Gattepaille LM, Grum BA, Jiri L, Lerch M, Sartori D, Wisniewski A (2020) Adverse events in twitter-development of a benchmark reference dataset: results from IMI WEB-RADR. Drug Safe 43:467–478

DuMouchel W (1999) Bayesian data mining in large frequency tables, with an application to the FDA spontaneous reporting system. Am Stat 53:177–190

Edwards IR, Aronson JK (2000) Adverse drug reactions: definitions, diagnosis, and management. Lancet 356(9237):1255–1259

Fong A, Hettinger AZ, Ratwani RM (2015) Exploring methods for identifying related patient safety events using structured and unstructured data. J Biomed Inform 58:89–95

Geissler PW, Nokes K, Prince RJ, Odhiambo RA, Aagaard-Hansen J, Ouma JH (2000) Children and medicines: self-treatment of common illnesses among Luo schoolchildren in Western Kenya. Soc Sci Med 50:1771–1783

Hathaliya J, Sharma P, Tanwar S, Gupta R (2019) Blockchain-based remote patient monitoring in healthcare 4.0. In: Proceedings of the 2019 IEEE 9th International conference on advanced computing. IACC, Tiruchirappalli, pp 87–91

Hernandez-Juyol M, Job-Quesada JR (2002) Dentistry and self-medication: a current challenge. Med Oral 7:344–347

Huang Z, Dong W, Duan H (2015) A probabilistic topic model for clinical risk stratification from electronic health records. J Biomed Inform 58:28–36

Kernebeck S, Busse TS, Böttcher MD, Weitz J, Ehlers J, Bork U (2020) Impact of mobile health and medical applications on clinical practice in gastroenterology. World J Gastroenterol 26:4182–4197

Kim S, Liu H, Yeganova L, Wilbur JW (2015) Extracting drug- drug interactions from literature using a rich feature- based linear kernel approach. J Biomed Inform 58:23–30

Latifi R, Ganapathy K (2004) Telemedicine in the Indian context: an overview. In: Establishing telemedicine in developing countries: from inception to implementation. Studies in health technology and informatics, India IOS Press, pp 178–181

Lazarou J, Pomeranz BH, Corey PN (1998) Incidence of adverse drug reactions in hospitalized patients: a meta-analysis of prospective studies. JAMA 279(15):1200–1205

Liu X, Chen H (2015) A research framework for pharmacovigilance in health social media: identification and evaluation of patient adverse drug event reports. J Biomed Inform 58:268–279

Lopez Pineda A, Ye Y, Visweswaran S, Cooper GF, Wagner MM (2015) Comparison of machine learning classifiers for influenza detection from emergency department free- text reports. J Biomed Inform 58:60–69

Love SB, Yorke-Edwards V, Lensen S et al (2020) Monitoring in practice—how are UK academic clinical trials monitored? A survey. Trials 21:59–64

Love SB, Yorke-Edwards V, Ward E, Haydock R, Keen K, Biggs K et al (2022) What is the purpose of clinical trial monitoring? Trials 23:836–845

Manogaran G, Thota C, Lopez D, Sundarasekar R (2017) Big data security intelligence for healthcare industry 4.0. In: Thames L, Schaefer D (eds) Cybersecurity for industry 4.0. Springer series in advanced manufacturing; Springer International Publishing, Cham; ISBN 9783319506593

Mathew D (2005) Information technology and public health management of disasters- a model for South Asian countries. Prehosp Disaster Med 20:54–60

Mavrogiorgou A, Kiourtis A, Perakis K, Miltiadou D, Pitsios S, Kyriazis D (2019) Analyzing data and data sources towards aunified approach for ensuring end-to-end data and data sources quality in healthcare 4.0. Comput Methods Prog Biomed 181:104967

McBride WG (1961) Thalidomide and congenital abnormalities. Lancet 278:1358–1360. https://doi.org/10.1016/S0140-6736(61)90927-8

Mishra SK, Ayyagari A, Bhandari M, Bedi BS, Shah R (2004) Telemedicine application in Maha Kumbhmela (Indian festival) with large congregation. Telemed J E Health 10:S107–S108

National Research Council (2012) The role of telehealth in an evolving health care environment: workshop summary. The National Academies Press, Washington, DC

Pace P, Aloi G, Gravina R, Caliciuri G, Fortino G, Liotta A (2018) An edge-based architecture to support efficient applications for healthcare industry 4.0. IEEE Trans Ind Inform 15:481–489

Patil AV, Somasundaram KV, Goyal RC (2002) Current health scenario in rural India. Aust J Rural Health 10:129–135

Pierce CE, Bouri K, Pamer C, Proestel S, Rodriguez HW, Van Le H et al (2017) Evaluation [17] of facebook and twitter monitoring to detect safety signals for medical products: an analysis of recent FDA safety alerts. Drug Saf 40(4):317–331

Pivovarov R, Perott AJ, Brave E, Angiolillo J, Wiggins CH, Elhadad N (2015) Learning probabilistic phenotypes from heterogeneous EHR data. J Biomed Inform 58:156–165

Reinhardt IC, Oliveira JC, Ring DT (2020) Current perspectives on the development of industry 4.0 in the pharmaceutical sector. J Ind Inf Integr 18:100131–100133

Shuka SS, Gidwani B, Pandey R, Rao SP, Singh V et al (2012) Importance of pharmacovigilance in Indian pharmaceutical industry. Asian J Res Pharm Sci 2:4–8

Shukla A, Dwivedi S, Sharma UK (2022) Prospective role of social media in pharmacovigilance: a review of stance from limited resources. Int J Pharm Res Appl 7(3):989–999

Smith PG, Morrow RH, Ross DA (2015) Field trials of health interventions: a [16] toolbox, 3rd edn. OUP Oxford, Oxford; Chapter 22, Phase IV studies. https://www.ncbi.nlm.nih.gov/books/NBK305508/

Suman R, Javaid M, Haleem A, Vaishya R, Bahl S, Nandan D (2020) Sustainability of coronavirus on different surfaces. J Clin Exp Hepatol 10:386–390
Suvarna V (2010) Phase IV of drug development. Perspect Clin Res 1(2):57
Thole JS, Enejo B (n.d.) The future of pharmacovigilance; www.adlittle.com
Verma RK, Mohan L, Pandey M (2010) Evaluation of self-medication among professional students in North India: proper statutory drug control must be implemented. Asian J Pharm Clin Res 3:60–64
Waller PC, Arlett PA (2002) Responding to signals. In: Mann RD, Andrews E (eds) Pharmacovigilance. John Wiley and Sons Ltd, Chichester, pp 105–128
WHO (1995) World Health Organization: report of the WHO expert committee on National drug policies; http://www.who.int/medicines/library/dap/who-dap-95-9/who-dap-95.9.shtml
WHO (1997) A health telematics policy in support of WHO's health-for-all strategy for global health development: report of the WHO group consultation on health telematics. World Health Organization, Geneva, p 1998
WHO (2002a) The importance of pharmacovigilance, safety monitoring of medicinal products. World Health Organization
WHO (2002b) The importance of pharmacovigilance-safety monitoring of medicinal [12] products; [cited 2018 August 29]; http://apps.who.int/medicinedocs/en/d/Js4893e/1.html
WHO (2004) Pharmacovigilance: ensuring the safe use of medicines. WHO, Geneva
Xu R, Wang Q (2014) Large-scale combining signals from both biomedical literature and the FDA adverse event reporting system (FAERS) to improve post-marketing drug safety signal detection. BMC Bioinform 15(1):17–20
Yan H, Da Xu L, Bi Z, Pang Z, Zhang J, Chen Y (2015) An emerging technology wearable wireless sensor networks with applications in human health condition monitoring. J Manag Anal 2:121–137
Yang CC, Yang H, Jiang L (2014) Postmarketing drug safety surveillance using publicly available health consumer contributed content in social media. ACM Trans Manag Inf Syst 5:2–21
Zhang Y, Padma R, Patel N (2015) Paving the COWpath: learning and visualizing clinical pathways from electronic health records. J Biomed Inform 58:186–197

Annexure 1: ADR Forms for India

M. Nandave, A. Kumar (eds.), *Pharmacovigilance Essentials*,
https://doi.org/10.1007/978-981-99-8949-2

Version-1.3

SUSPECTED ADVERSE DRUG REACTION REPORTING FORM

For VOLUNTARY reporting of Adverse Drug Reaction by Healthcare Professionals

INDIAN PHARMACOPOEIA COMMISSION(National Coordination Centre-Pharmacovigilance Programme of India)
Ministry of Health & Family Welfare, Government of India Sector-23, Raj Nagar, Ghaziabad-201002

A. PATIENT INFORMATION

1. Patient Initials ________	2. Age at the time of Event or Date of Birth ____________	3. M ☐ F ☐ Other ☐ 4. Weight________Kgs

Reg. No. /IPD No. /OPD No. /CR No. :

AMC Report No. :

Worldwide Unique No. :

B. SUSPECTED ADVERSE REACTION

5. Event/Reaction start date (dd/mm/yyyy)

6. Event/Reaction stop date (dd/mm/yyyy)

6 (A). Onset Lag Time

7. Describe Event/Reaction with treatment details, if any

12. Relevant tests/ laboratory data with dates

13. Relevant medical/medication history (e.g. allergies, race, pregnancy, smoking, alcohol use, hepatic/renal dysfunction, past surgery etc.)

14. Seriousness of the reaction: No ☐ if Yes ☐(please tick anyone)

☐ Death (dd/mm/yyyy) ☐ Congenital-anomaly
☐ Life threatening ☐ Disability
☐Hospitalization/Prolonged ☐ Other Medically important

15. Outcomes

☐ Recovered ☐ Recovering ☐ Not recovered
☐ Fatal ☐ Recovered with sequelae ☐ Unknown

C. SUSPECTED MEDICATION(S)

S.No	8. Name (Brand/Generic)	Manufacturer (if known)	Batch No. / Lot No.	Exp. Date (if known)	Dose used	Route used	Frequency (OD, BD etc.)	Therapy dates		Indication	Causality Assessment
								Date started	Date stopped		
i											
ii											
iii											
iv*											

S.No as per C	9. Action Taken (please tick)						10. Reaction reappeared after reintroduction (please tick)			
	Drug withdrawn	Dose increased	Dose reduced	Dose not changed	Not applicable	Unknown	Yes	No	Effect unknown	Dose (if reintroduced)
i										
ii										
iii										
iv										

11. Concomitant medical product including self-medication and herbal remedies with therapy dates (Exclude those used to treat reaction)

S.No	Name (Brand/Generic)	Dose used	Route used	Frequency (OD, BD, etc.)	Therapy dates		Indication
					Date started	Date stopped	
i							
ii							
iii*							

Additional Information:

D. REPORTER DETAILS

16. Name and Professional Address:_______________________
____
Pin:___________E-mail_______________________________
Tel. No. (with STD code)____________________________
Occupation:__________________ Signature:________________

17. Date of this report (dd/mm/yyyy):

Sig. and Name of Receiver-

Confidentiality: The patient's identity is held in strict confidence and protected to the fullest extent. Submission of a report does not constitute an admission that medical personnel or manufacturer or the product caused or contributed to the reaction. Submission of an ADR report does not have any legal implication on the reporter.

*use separate page for more information

National Coordination Centre for Pharmacovigilance Programme of India

Ministry of Health & Family Welfare, Government of India
Sector-23, Raj Nagar, Ghaziabad-201002
Tel.: 0120-2783400, 2783401, 2783392, Fax: 0120-2783311
www.ipc.nic.in

ADVICE ABOUT REPORTING

A. What to report?

- Report serious adverse drug reactions. A reaction is serious when the patient outcome is:
  - Death
  - Life-threatening
  - Hospitalization (initial or prolonged)
  - Disability (significant, persistent or permanent)
  - Congenital anomaly
  - Required intervention to prevent permanent impairment or damage
- Report non-serious, known or unknown, frequent or rare adverse drug reactions due to Medicines, Vaccines and Herbal products etc.

  Note- Adverse Event Following Immunization can also be reported in Serious AEFI case Notification Form available on http://www.ipc.gov.in)

B. Who can report?

- All healthcare professionals (Clinicians, Dentists, Pharmacists and Nurses etc) can report adverse drug reactions

C. Where to report?

- Duly filled inSuspected Adverse Drug Reaction Reporting Form can be sent to the nearest Adverse Drug Reaction Monitoring Centre (AMC) or directly to the National Coordination Centre (NCC) for PvPI.
- Call on Helpline (Toll Free) 1800 180 3024 to report ADRs or directly mail this filled form to pvpi.ipc@gov.in
- A list of nationwide AMCs is available at:
  http://www.ipc.gov.in, http://www.ipc.gov.in/PvPI/pv_home.html

D. What happens to the submitted information?

- Information provided in this form is handled in strict confidence. The causality assessment is carried out at AMCs by using WHO-UMC scale. The analyzed forms are forwarded to the NCC through ADR database. Finally the data is analyzed and forwarded to the Global Pharmacovigilance Database managed by WHO Uppsala Monitoring Centre in Sweden.
- The reports are periodically reviewed by the NCC-PvPI. The information generated on the basis of these reports helps in continuous assessment of the benefit-risk ratio of medicines.
- The Signal Review Panel of PvPI to review the data and suggest any interventions that may be required.

E. Mandatory fields for suspected ADR reporting form

- Patient initials, age at onset of reaction, reaction term(s), date of onset of reaction, suspected medication(s) and reporter information.

For ADRs Reporting

- **E-mail:pvpi.ipc@gov.in**
- ***PvPI Helpline (Toll Free):1800 180 3024****(9:00 AM to 5:30 PM, Monday-Friday)*
- ***ADR Mobile App: "ADR PvPI"***

Annexure 2: ADR Forms for EU

M. Nandave, A. Kumar (eds.), *Pharmacovigilance Essentials*,
https://doi.org/10.1007/978-981-99-8949-2

EUROPEAN MEDICINES AGENCY
SCIENCE MEDICINES HEALTH

Insert lead inspector's competent authority logo / emblem

PHARMACOVIGILANCE INSPECTION REPORT

Pharmacovigilance system name: Company Name:

PSMF :

Inspection number: PV 12345**/0206**INS/PHV/XXXX/XXX

[Enter EMA inspection reference number and/or NCA inspection reference as applicable]

[Delete guidance notes and other non-applicable parts of this document before finalising]

Version number:

Date of issuance:

Table of contents

Abbreviations

ADR	Adverse Drug Reaction
AE	Adverse Event
CA	Competent Authority
CAPA	Corrective Action Preventive Action
CHMP	Committee for Medicinal Products for Human Use
CRO	Contract Research Organisation
CSR	Clinical Study Report
CSU	Central Safety Unit
EMA	European Medicines Agency
GVP	Good Vigilance Practice
ICH	International Conference on Harmonisation
ICSR	Individual Case Safety Report
IR	Inspection Report
MAH	Marketing Authorization Holder
PhV/PV	Pharmacovigilance
PSMF	Pharmacovigilance System Master File
PSUR	Periodic Safety Updates Reports
QA	Quality Assurance
QPPV	Qualified Person for Pharmacovigilance
RA	Regulatory Authority
SAE	Serious Adverse Event
SAR	Serious Adverse Reaction
SOP	Standard Operating Procedure
SUSAR	Suspected Unexpected Serious Adverse Reaction
TBA	To Be Announced

SECTION A: Administrative information

Inspection type:	*National routine, etc*
Name and address(es) of site(s) inspected:	
Contact person:	*If different from QPPV*
Date(s) of inspection:	
Lead inspector if any:	
Reporting inspector if any:	
Accompanying inspector(s) and experts:	
Previous PhV inspections : **Date and competent authority (inspectorates)**	
Purpose of inspection:	
Products selected to provide system examples:	*As part of the general systems review, there are products chosen for close evaluation of ADR reports, PSURs, etc.* *Note also: CAPs, MRPs, NAs as appropriate*
Name and location of EU/EEA qualified person for pharmacovigilance:	*Name:* *Contact details:*
Date of first issue of report to MAH:	*Date of submission*
Deadline for submission of responses by MAH:	
Date(s) of receipt of responses from MAH:	
Date of final version of report:	
Report author:	*Name* *Job title*

SECTION B: General information

B.1. Scope and reason for the inspection

System inspection or product inspection, or combined – supervisory authority inspection, local inspection, particular focus, etc reasons for the inspection for the particular inspectee or any other particular reason.

B.2. Reference texts and documents for the inspection

- Directive 2010/84/EU amending Directive 2001/83/EC
- EU Regulation 1235/10 amending Regulation (EU) No 726/2004
- Commission implementing Regulation 520/2012 on the performance of PhV activities
- Directive 2001/20/EC
- Directive 2005/28/EC
- CPMP/ICH/287/95: E2B (M) "Note for Guidance on Clinical Safety Data Management: Data Elements for Transmission of Individual Case Safety Reports" and ICH E2B/M2 "Note for Guidance on Electronic Transmission of Individual Case Safety Reports Message Specification"
- CPMP/ICH/288/95: E2C (R1) "Note for Guidance on Clinical Safety Data Management: Periodic Safety Update Reports for Marketed Drugs"
- CPMP/ICH/3945/03: E2D "Post-Approval Safety Data Management: Definitions and standards for Expedited Reporting"
- CHMP/313666/05: "Guideline on the exposure to medicinal products during pregnancy: need for post-authorization data"
- CHMP/235910/05: "Guideline on conduct of pharmacovigilance for medicines used by the pediatric population"

B.3. Conduct of the inspection with summary of the organisation and any significant changes and action taken since the last inspection

The inspection was performed in accordance with the inspection plan (attached as Appendix II). If necessary include the adjustments or changes.

A closing meeting was held to review the inspection findings, at place and date and attendance record (Appendix III).

Brief summary of the pharmacovigilance system with presentation of changes, if any.

SECTION C: Inspected items

Refer to Appendix 1- Summary of items inspected.

SECTION D: Findings

D.1. Definitions of inspection finding grading

Critical (CR): a deficiency in pharmacovigilance systems, practices or processes that adversely affects the rights, safety or well-being of patients or that poses a potential risk to public health or that represents a serious violation of applicable legislation and guidelines.

Major (MA): a deficiency in pharmacovigilance systems, practices or processes that could potentially adversely affect the rights, safety or well-being of patients or that could potentially pose a risk to public health or that represents a violation of applicable legislation and guidelines.

Minor (MI): a deficiency in pharmacovigilance systems, practices or processes that would not be expected to adversely affect the rights, safety or well-being of patients or pose a risk to public health.

Comment: the observations might lead to suggestions on how to improve quality or reduce the potential for a deviation to occur in the future.

The factual matter contained in the inspection report relates only to those things that the inspection team saw and heard during the inspection process. The inspection report is not to be taken as implying a satisfactory state of affairs in documentation, premises, equipment, personnel or procedures not examined during the inspection.

D.2. Guidance for responding to inspection findings

Responses to inspection findings should be clear, concise and include proposed actions to address both the identified deficiency and the root cause of the deficiency. Consideration should also be given to identifying and preventing other potential similar deficiencies within the pharmacovigilance system.

Responses should be entered directly into the table(s) in section D.3.1., without changes to the inspectors' text that describes the findings. The following text is intended as guidance when considering the information that should be entered into each of the fields within the table(s). 'Not applicable' should be entered into the relevant field if the requested information is not appropriate for the finding in question.

Root cause analysis Identify the root cause(s) which, if adequately addressed, will prevent recurrence of the deficiency. There may be more than one root cause for any given deficiency.
Further assessment Assess the extent to which the deficiency exists within the pharmacovigilance system and what impact it may have for all products. Where applicable, describe what further assessment has been performed or may be required to fully evaluate the impact of the deficiency e.g. retrospective analysis of data may be required to fully assess the impact.
Corrective action(s) Detail the action(s) taken / proposed to correct the identified deficiency.
Preventative action(s) Detail the action(s) taken / proposed to eliminate the root cause of the deficiency, in order to prevent recurrence. Action(s) to identify and prevent other potential similar deficiencies should also be considered.
Deliverable(s) Detail the specific outputs from the proposed / completed corrective and preventative action(s). For example, updated procedure/work instruction, record of re-training, IT solution.
Due date(s) Specify the actual / proposed date(s) for completion of each action. Indicate when an action is completed.

D.3. Inspection findings

D.3.1. Critical findings

Present the critical findings as corresponding to the definition.

Finding CR1	**Use the categories (and subcategories) listed in Appendix I followed by a short title for the finding**
<<Inspector to add text>> **References:** Directive 2001/83/EC as amended, Article 104(3). Commission Implementing Regulation (EU) No. 520/2012, Article 10. GVP Module xxx (as appropriate) Add any local requirement (if appropriate)	
Root cause analysis	
<<MAH to add text>>	
Further assessment	
<<MAH to add text>>	
Corrective action(s)	
<<MAH to add text>>	
Deliverable(s) <<MAH to add text>>	**Due date(s)** <<MAH to add text>>
Preventative Action(s)	
<<MAH to add text>>	
Deliverable(s) <<MAH to add text>>	**Due date(s)** <<MAH to add text>>

Recommendation / Observation (amend as necessary)

D.3.2. Major findings

Present the major findings as corresponding to the definition

Finding MA1	**Use the categories (and subcategories) listed in Appendix I followed by a short title for the finding**
<<Inspector to add text>> **References:** Directive 2001/83/EC as amended, Article 104(3). Commission Implementing Regulation (EU) No. 520/2012, Article 10.	

GVP Module xxx (as appropriate)
Add any local requirement (if appropriate)

Root cause analysis

<<MAH to add text>>

Further assessment

<<MAH to add text>>

Corrective action(s)

<<MAH to add text>>

Deliverable(s)	**Due date(s)**
<<MAH to add text>>	<<MAH to add text>>

Preventative action(s)

<<MAH to add text>>

Deliverable(s)	**Due date(s)**
<<MAH to add text>>	<<MAH to add text>>

Recommendation / Observation (amend as necessary)

D.3.3. Minor findings

Present the minor findings as corresponding to the definition

Finding MI1	**Use the categories (and subcategories) listed in Appendix I followed by a short title for the finding**

<<Inspector to add text>>

References:

Directive 2001/83/EC as amended, Article 104(3).

Commission Implementing Regulation (EU) No. 520/2012, Article 10.

GVP Module xxx (as appropriate)
Add any local requirement (if appropriate)

Root cause analysis

<<MAH to add text>>

Further assessment

<<MAH to add text>>

Corrective action(s)

<<MAH to add text>>

Deliverable(s)	Due date(s)
<<MAH to add text>>	<<MAH to add text>>
Preventative action(s)	
<<MAH to add text>>	
Deliverable(s) <<MAH to add text>>	**Due date(s)** <<MAH to add text>>

Recommendation / Observation (amend as necessary)

D.3.4. Comments

Issues the inspectors would like to communicate to the inspectee– but that do not necessarily represent any finding.

SECTION E:

E.1 Conclusions

E.2 Recommendations

E.3 Evaluation by the inspectors of the response from the inspectee

E.4 Final conclusions and recommendations

SECTION F: Date and signatures of lead and other inspectors, experts if applicable

APPENDIX I - Summary of items inspected -*optional*

If the list of items covered during the inspection has been provided in section (B.1), Appendix I is optional and may be deleted.

(Please enter, which areas were inspected during the inspection, if necessary enter comments or specify).

	Extent* Yes	Extent* No	Findings (Y/N) CR	MA	Comments
1. QPPV					
Qualifications					
Job description					
System oversight					
Back-up process and delegation					
Others					
2. PSMF					
Format					
Content					
Maintenance and submission					
Others					
3. Written instructions (SOPs, manuals, etc)					
Procedures					
Manuals					
Process for SOP training					
Others					
4. Contracts, agreements					
Contracts					
Agreements					
Others					
5. Periodic safety update reports					
PSUR scheduling					
Format and content					
Quality control of PSURs					

	Extent* Yes	Extent* No	Findings (Y/N) CR	MA	Comments
Timeliness of submission					
Assessment report comments					
Others					
6. Risk-management system					
Risk-management plan format and content					
Compliance with risk-minimisation measures which are beyond routine pharmacovigilance					
Others					
7. Management and reporting of adverse reactions					
Receipt of ICSRs from all sources and collection and collation at one point within the EU					
Assessments of seriousness, causality and expectedness					
Medical review and MedDRA coding					
QC process					
Submissions and follow up processes					
Reporting procedures for PSP, PASS, PAES, other non-interventional trials					
Literature screening					
Others					
8. Computerised systems used for					

	Extent* Yes	Extent* No	Findings (Y/N) CR	MA	Comments
pharmacovigilance activities					
Process for ensuring computerised systems					
Documentation of fitness for purpose					
Backup and disaster recovery process					
Process for migration of database					
Others					
9. Clinical trials					
SUSAR reporting					
Consistency between the IB and SPC when marketed products are used in CT					
Reconciliation of SAEs between clinical trial and pharmacovigilance databases.					
Others					
10. Signal management					
Dataset used for conducting signal detection (inclusion of information from all relevant sources)					
Periodicity of data review					
Cumulative review					
Process for further validation and investigation					
Timely update of SmPCs and PILs following signal confirmation					
Others					
11. Product quality					

	Extent* Yes	Extent* No	Findings (Y/N) CR	MA	Comments
Review of quality complaints and trend analyses					
Reconciliation between the complaints and safety databases					
Others					
12. Archiving					
Record management					
Archiving facilities					
Others					
13. Quality management system					
Quality system and compliance management					
Facilities and equipment for pharmacovigilance					
Audit (internal- and external) and CAPA process					
Others					
14. Training					
Initial and on-going training					
Evaluation of training					
Maintenance of training records					
15. Regulatory affairs					
Creation and updates of product information					
Answer to questions from competent authorities					
16. Medical information					

	Extent* Yes	Extent* No	Findings (Y/N) CR	MA	Comments
Reconciliation between medical information request and safety database					
17. Additional issues if any					

** Yes – this means an assessment of this area was undertaken that was considered sufficient by the inspector to make an assessment of compliance and identify any issues.*

No – this area was not looked at. This could be because it wasn't necessary to address the scope of the inspection or answer any concerns/questions in the inspection request.

A comment should be provided. This could be because it was not applicable.

Please note that the above items are not an exhaustive list, and other areas should be examined, as appropriate to ensure the scope and objectives of the inspection are met.

APPENDIX II - Pharmacovigilance inspection plan

{Add inspection plan}

APPENDIX III - Closing meeting attendance record

Annexure 3(a): Side Effect Reporting Form Canada

M. Nandave, A. Kumar (eds.), *Pharmacovigilance Essentials*,
https://doi.org/10.1007/978-981-99-8949-2

SIDE EFFECT REPORTING FORM

FAX completed form to 1-866-678-6789
For more information call 1-866-234-2345

PROTECTED "B" WHEN COMPLETED"

Reporting suspected side effects (also known as adverse reactions) to marketed health products in Canada may contribute to the identification of previously unrecognized rare or serious side effects, which may lead to changes in the product's safety information.

Instructions on how to complete and submit this form and information about confidentiality can be found on Page 2.
Complete all mandatory fields, marked by a *, and provide as much detail as possible for the remaining fields.

A) About the person who had the side effect

Reference # (if applicable)

1. Age*	2. Sex*	3. Height	4. Weight
______ Years ______ Months	☐ Male ☐ Female	______ cm ______ ft ______ in	______ kg ______ lbs ______ oz

5. Medical history and other related information (allergies, pregnancy, smoking/alcohol use, liver disease, etc.)

B) Reporter information

1. Name*	2. Telephone*	3. Province/Territory

4. Address	5. E-mail

6. Preferred language	7. Organization (if applicable)
☐ English ☐ French	

8. Select one that best describes you

☐ Consumer or other non-health professional ☐ Physician ☐ Pharmacist

☐ Other health professional (specify) ____________

9. Has this also been reported to the manufacturer?

☐ Yes ☐ No

C) Side Effect

1. Seriousness of the side effect

☐ Death (yyyy-mm-dd) ____________
☐ Life-threatening ☐ Disability
☐ Admitted to hospital ☐ Birth defect
☐ Lengthened hospital stay ☐ Needed medical attention

2. Recovered after the side effect*

☐ Yes ☐ No ☐ Unknown

☐ Recovering (explain) ____________

3. Side effect start date* (yyyy-mm-dd)	4. Side effect end date (yyyy-mm-dd)

5. Describe the side effect (timeliness, treatment, etc.)*

D) Suspected health product

1. Product name*	2. Strength	3. Manufacturer

4. Lot #	5. DIN #/NPN #

6. Country of purchase	7. Where it was purchased/obtained
☐ Canada ☐ United States ☐ Other (specify): ____________	☐ Pharmacy ☐ Grocery store ☐ Internet ☐ Other (specify): ____________

8. Product start date (yyyy-mm-dd)*	9. Product end date (yyyy-mm-dd)

At the time of the side effect, specify:

10. Dosage* (strength and quantity)	11. Frequency (e.g. twice daily)	12. How the product was taken* (e.g. by mouth)

13. What was the product prescribed/taken for?*

14. Did use of the product stop after the side effect appeared?	15. If the product was stopped did the side effect stop?
☐ Yes ☐ No	☐ Yes ☐ No ☐ Does not apply

16. Was the product restarted after the side effect stopped?	17. If the product was restarted, did the side effect return?
☐ Yes ☐ No ☐ Does not apply	☐ Yes ☐ No ☐ Does not apply

18. Likelihood that the product caused the side effect

☐ Certain ☐ Not available/Unable to assess
☐ Probably/Likely ☐ Unlikely
☐ Possible ☐ Unrelated

19. Other health products taken at the time of the side effect, excluding treatment (length of use, timelines, etc.)

20. Related test/laboratory results

" As per the Treasury Board of Canada Secretariat Government Security Policy.

Pub.: 150142 | Date: April 2020

Health Canada Santé Canada

Canada

How to complete the Side Effect Reporting Form

- All sections of the form should be filled in as completely as possible. Use a separate form for each patient. Attach an additional form if there is more than one suspected health product. Additional pages may be attached if more space is required. Please provide the product label where possible.
- Follow-up information for a side effect that has already been reported can be submitted using a new form, indicating that it consists of follow-up information, including, if known, the date of the original report and the report number provided in the acknowledgement.

What is a side effect?

A side effect (also known as adverse reaction) is a harmful and unintended response to a health product. Health products include prescription and non-prescription medications; natural health products; biologics (includes biotechnology products, vaccines, fractionated blood products, human blood and blood components, as well as human cells, tissues and organs) radiopharmaceuticals; and disinfectants and sanitizers with disinfectant claims. This includes any undesirable patient effect suspected to be associated with health product use. An unintended effect, health product abuse, overdose, interaction (including drug-drug and drug-food interactions) and unusual lack of therapeutic efficacy are all considered to be reportable side effects.

What is considered a serious side effect?

A serious side effect is one that requires in-patient hospitalization or prolongation of existing hospitalization, causes congenital malformation, results in persistent or significant disability or incapacity, is life-threatening or results in death. Side effects that result in significant medical intervention to prevent one of these listed outcomes are also considered to be serious.

What types of side effects should be reported?

All suspected side effects should be reported, especially those that are:

- *unexpected*, regardless of their severity (i.e. not consistent with product information or labelling;
- *serious*, whether expected or not;
- reactions to *recently marketed* health products (on the market less than five years), regardless of their nature or severity.

How to submit your completed form	Other ways to report a side effect
Fax: 1-866-678-6789 **Mail:** Canada Vigilance Program Marketed Health Products Directorate Health Canada Address locator 1908C Ottawa ON K1A 0K9	**Online:** canada.ca/medeffect **Telephone:** 1-866-234-2345 ***Do not send reports by e-mail.** Health Canada is not able to ensure secure transfer of information by e-mail.*

Other information

- Reporting a side effect does not constitute an admission that medical personnel or the product caused or contributed to it.
- Side effect reports are, for the most part, only suspected associations. A temporal or possible association is sufficient for a report to be made. Reporting of a side effect does not imply a definitive causal link.
- Health professionals and consumers may also report side effects to the market authorization holder. Indicate on your form sent to Health Canada if a case was also reported to the product's market authorization holder.

For more information about side effect reporting, call Health Canada at 1-866-234-2345 or contact a regional office directly:	
British Columbia CanadaVigilance_BC@hc-sc.gc.ca **Alberta, Northwest Territories and Yukon** CanadaVigilance_AB@hc-sc.gc.ca **Saskatchewan and Nunavut** CanadaVigilance_SK@hc-sc.gc.ca **Manitoba** CanadaVigilance_MB@hc-sc.gc.ca	**Ontario** CanadaVigilance_ON@hc-sc.gc.ca **Québec** CanadaVigilance_QC@hc-sc.gc.ca **New Brunswick, Nova Scotia, Prince Edward Island, and Newfoundland and Labrador** CanadaVigilance_ATL@hc-sc.gc.ca

Confidentiality

In the context of Health Canada's side effect reporting program (the Canada Vigilance Program), personal information is collected pursuant to section 4 of the *Department of Health Act*, for the purpose of monitoring licensed products, detecting potential emerging safety issues and trends, mitigating the risks and improving the safe use and efficacy of the health products. Information related to the identity of the patient and/or reporter will be protected as personal information under the *Privacy Act*, and in the case of an access to information request, under the *Access to Information Act*. Suspected health product side effect-related information that is voluntarily submitted to Health Canada is maintainedin a secure computerized database. The program endeavours to use and disclose only de-identified information but may use and disclose personal information that is not de-identified as permitted under the *Privacy Act*. For further details regarding the personal information collected under this program, visit the Personal Information Bank; Health Canada; Health Products and Food Branch; Branch Incident Reporting System; PIB#PPU 417 at: **https://www.canada.ca/en/health-canada/corporate/about-health-canada/activities-responsibilities/access-information-privacy/info-source-federal-government-employee-information.html#a25** Every Canadian individual has the right to access their own personal information and is entitled to request correction to ensure accuracy of their information. If you wish to exercise this right, contact the Treasury Board of Canada Secretariat (**www.tbs-sct.gc.ca/tbsf-fsct/350-58-eng.ASP**).

Annexure 3(b): ADR Reporting Forms for Non-EU

M. Nandave, A. Kumar (eds.), *Pharmacovigilance Essentials*,
https://doi.org/10.1007/978-981-99-8949-2

SIDE EFFECT REPORTING FORM

Reporting suspected side effects (also known as adverse reactions) to marketed health products in Canada may contribute to the identification of previously unrecognized rare or serious side effects, which may lead to changes in the product's safety information.

FAX completed form to 1-866-678-6789
For more information call 1-866-234-2345

PROTECTED "B" WHEN COMPLETED"

Instructions on how to complete and submit this form and information about confidentiality can be found on Page 2. Complete all mandatory fields, marked by a *, and provide as much detail as possible for the remaining fields.

A) About the person who had the side effect

Reference # (if applicable)

1. Age* ______ Years ______ Months
2. Sex* ☐ Male ☐ Female
3. Height ______ cm ______ ft ______ in
4. Weight ______ kg ______ lbs ______ oz
5. Medical history and other related information (allergies, pregnancy, smoking/alcohol use, liver disease, etc.)

B) Reporter information

1. Name*
2. Telephone*
3. Province/Territory
4. Address
5. E-mail
6. Preferred language ☐ English ☐ French
7. Organization (if applicable)
8. Select one that best describes you
   ☐ Consumer or other non-health professional ☐ Physician ☐ Pharmacist
   ☐ Other health professional (specify) ______
9. Has this also been reported to the manufacturer?
   ☐ Yes ☐ No

C) Side Effect

1. Seriousness of the side effect
   ☐ Death (yyyy-mm-dd) ______
   ☐ Life-threatening ☐ Disability
   ☐ Admitted to hospital ☐ Birth defect
   ☐ Lengthened hospital stay ☐ Needed medical attention
2. Recovered after the side effect*
   ☐ Yes ☐ No ☐ Unknown
   ☐ Recovering (explain) ______
3. Side effect start date* (yyyy-mm-dd)
4. Side effect end date (yyyy-mm-dd)
5. Describe the side effect (timeliness, treatment, etc.)*

D) Suspected health product

1. Product name*
2. Strength
3. Manufacturer
4. Lot #
5. DIN #/NPN #
6. Country of purchase
   ☐ Canada
   ☐ United States
   ☐ Other (specify): ______
7. Where it was purchased/obtained
   ☐ Pharmacy
   ☐ Grocery store
   ☐ Internet
   ☐ Other (specify): ______
8. Product start date (yyyy-mm-dd)*
9. Product end date (yyyy-mm-dd)

At the time of the side effect, specify:

10. Dosage* (strength and quantity)
11. Frequency (e.g. twice daily)
12. How the product was taken* (e.g. by mouth)
13. What was the product prescribed/taken for?*
14. Did use of the product stop after the side effect appeared?
    ☐ Yes
    ☐ No
15. If the product was stopped did the side effect stop?
    ☐ Yes
    ☐ No
    ☐ Does not apply
16. Was the product restarted after the side effect stopped?
    ☐ Yes
    ☐ No
    ☐ Does not apply
17. If the product was restarted, did the side effect return?
    ☐ Yes
    ☐ No
    ☐ Does not apply
18. Likelihood that the product caused the side effect
    ☐ Certain ☐ Not available/Unable to assess
    ☐ Probably/Likely ☐ Unlikely
    ☐ Possible ☐ Unrelated
19. Other health products taken at the time of the side effect, excluding treatment (length of use, timelines, etc.)
20. Related test/laboratory results

"As per the Treasury Board of Canada Secretariat Government Security Policy.

Pub.: 150142 | Date: April 2020

Health Canada Santé Canada

Canada

How to complete the Side Effect Reporting Form

- All sections of the form should be filled in as completely as possible. Use a separate form for each patient. Attach an additional form if there is more than one suspected health product. Additional pages may be attached if more space is required. Please provide the product label where possible.
- Follow-up information for a side effect that has already been reported can be submitted using a new form, indicating that it consists of follow-up information, including, if known, the date of the original report and the report number provided in the acknowledgement.

What is a side effect?

A side effect (also known as adverse reaction) is a harmful and unintended response to a health product. Health products include prescription and non-prescription medications; natural health products; biologics (includes biotechnology products, vaccines, fractionated blood products, human blood and blood components, as well as human cells, tissues and organs) radiopharmaceuticals; and disinfectants and sanitizers with disinfectant claims. This includes any undesirable patient effect suspected to be associated with health product use. An unintended effect, health product abuse, overdose, interaction (including drug-drug and drug-food interactions) and unusual lack of therapeutic efficacy are all considered to be reportable side effects.

What is considered a serious side effect?

A serious side effect is one that requires in-patient hospitalization or prolongation of existing hospitalization, causes congenital malformation, results in persistent or significant disability or incapacity, is life-threatening or results in death. Side effects that result in significant medical intervention to prevent one of these listed outcomes are also considered to be serious.

What types of side effects should be reported?

All suspected side effects should be reported, especially those that are:

- *unexpected*, regardless of their severity (i.e. not consistent with product information or labelling;
- *serious*, whether expected or not;
- reactions to *recently marketed* health products (on the market less than five years), regardless of their nature or severity.

How to submit your completed form	Other ways to report a side effect
Fax: 1-866-678-6789 **Mail:** Canada Vigilance Program Marketed Health Products Directorate Health Canada Address locator 1908C Ottawa ON K1A 0K9	**Online: canada.ca/medeffect** **Telephone:** 1-866-234-2345 ***Do not send reports by e-mail.*** *Health Canada is not able to ensure secure transfer of information by e-mail.*

Other information

- Reporting a side effect does not constitute an admission that medical personnel or the product caused or contributed to it.
- Side effect reports are, for the most part, only suspected associations. A temporal or possible association is sufficient for a report to be made. Reporting of a side effect does not imply a definitive causal link.
- Health professionals and consumers may also report side effects to the market authorization holder. Indicate on your form sent to Health Canada if a case was also reported to the product's market authorization holder.

For more information about side effect reporting, call Health Canada at 1-866-234-2345 or contact a regional office directly:	
British Columbia CanadaVigilance_BC@hc-sc.gc.ca **Alberta, Northwest Territories and Yukon** CanadaVigilance_AB@hc-sc.gc.ca **Saskatchewan and Nunavut** CanadaVigilance_SK@hc-sc.gc.ca **Manitoba** CanadaVigilance_MB@hc-sc.gc.ca	**Ontario** CanadaVigilance_ON@hc-sc.gc.ca **Québec** CanadaVigilance_QC@hc-sc.gc.ca **New Brunswick, Nova Scotia, Prince Edward Island, and Newfoundland and Labrador** CanadaVigilance_ATL@hc-sc.gc.ca

Confidentiality

In the context of Health Canada's side effect reporting program (the Canada Vigilance Program), personal information is collected pursuant to section 4 of the *Department of Health Act*, for the purpose of monitoring licensed products, detecting potential emerging safety issues and trends, mitigating the risks and improving the safe use and efficacy of the health products. Information related to the identity of the patient and/or reporter will be protected as personal information under the *Privacy Act*, and in the case of an access to information request, under the *Access to Information Act*. Suspected health product side effect related information that is voluntarily submitted to Health Canada is maintainedin a secure computerized database. The program endeavours to use and disclose only de-identified information but may use and disclose personal information that is not de-identified as permitted under the *Privacy Act*. For further details regarding the personal information collected under this program, visit the Personal Information Bank; Health Canada; Health Products and Food Branch; Branch Incident Reporting System; PIB#PPU 417 at: **https://www.canada.ca/en/health-canada/corporate/about-health-canada/activities-responsibilities/access-information-privacy/info-source-federal-government-employee-information.html#a25** Every Canadian individual has the right to access their own personal information and is entitled to request correction to ensure accuracy of their information. If you wish to exercise this right, contact the Treasury Board of Canada Secretariat (**www.tbs-sct.gc.ca/tbsf-fsct/350-58-eng.ASP**).

Annexure 4(a): MedWatch Form 3500

M. Nandave, A. Kumar (eds.), *Pharmacovigilance Essentials*, https://doi.org/10.1007/978-981-99-8949-2

Reset Form

FDA

DEPARTMENT OF HEALTH AND HUMAN SERVICES
Food and Drug Administration

MEDWATCH

The FDA Safety Information and Adverse Event Reporting Program

Form FDA 3500

Form Approved: OMB No. 0910-0291, Expires: 06-30-2025
See PRA statement on page 6.

FDA USE ONLY
Triage unit sequence #
FDA Rec. Date

For VOLUNTARY reporting of adverse events, product problems and product use/medication errors

Note: For date prompts of "dd-mmm-yyyy" please use 2-digit day, 3-letter month abbreviation, and 4-digit year; for example, 01-Jan-1900.

A. PATIENT INFORMATION

1. **Patient Identifier** *(In confidence)*

2. Age ☐ Year(s) ☐ Week(s) ☐ Month(s) ☐ Day(s)

or Date of Birth *(e.g., 01-Jan-1900)*

3a. **Sex:** Enter the patient's sex at birth *(the sex that a person has or was assigned to at birth).*
☐ Male ☐ Undifferentiated
☐ Female ☐ Decline to answer

3b. **Gender:** Enter the patient's current gender *(how the patient thinks of themself).*
☐ Cisgender man/boy (gender corresponds with birth sex)
☐ Cisgender woman/girl (gender corresponds with birth sex)
☐ Transgender man/trans man/ female-to-male (FTM)
☐ Transgender woman/trans woman/ male-to-female (MTF)
☐ Other gender category; please specify:
☐ Decline to answer

4. **Weight** ☐ lb ☐ kg

5. **Ethnicity** *(Check one)*
☐ Hispanic/Latino
☐ Not Hispanic/Latino

6. **Race** *(check all that apply)*
☐ American Indian/Alaska Native
☐ Asian
☐ Black or African American
☐ Native Hawaiian/ Other Pacific Islander
☐ White

B. ADVERSE EVENT, PRODUCT PROBLEM

1. **Type of Report** *(check all that apply)*
☐ Adverse Event
☐ Product Use/Medication Error
☐ Product Problem *(e.g., defects/malfunctions)*
☐ Problem with Different Manufacturer of Same Medicine

2. **Outcome Attributed to Adverse Event** *(check all that apply)*
☐ Death – Date of death *(e.g., 01-Jan-1900)*:
☐ Life-threatening
☐ Hospitalization (initial or prolonged)
☐ Other Serious or Important Medical Events
☐ Required Intervention to Prevent Permanent Impairment/Damage
☐ Disability or Permanent Damage
☐ Congenital Anomaly/Birth Defects

3. **Date of Event** *(e.g., 01-Jan-1900)*

4. **Date of this Report** *(e.g., 01-Jan-1900)*

5. **Describe Event, Problem or Product Use/Medication Error**

Characters Remaining (max. 4,000):

(field continues on next page)

Submission of a report does not constitute an admission that medical personnel or the product caused or contributed to the event.
* Please see instructions

6. **Relevant Test/Laboratory Data**	**Date** *(e.g., 01-Jan-1900)*	**Relevant Test/Laboratory Data**	**Date** *(e.g., 01-Jan-1900)*

Additional comments Characters Remaining (max. 2,000):

7. **Other Relevant History, Including Preexisting Medical Conditions** *(e.g., allergies, pregnancy, tobacco product use, liver/kidney problems, etc.)* Characters Remaining (max. 2,000):

 (continued on next page)

C. PRODUCT AVAILABILITY

1. **Product Available for Evaluation?** *(Do not send product to FDA)*
☐ Yes ☐ No ☐ Returned to Manufacturer on *(e.g., 01-Jan-1900)* ☐

2. **Do you have a picture of the product?** *(Check if you are including a picture)* ☐ Yes

D. SUSPECT PRODUCTS

SUSPECT PRODUCT #1

This report involves: ☐ Cosmetic ☐ Dietary supplement ☐ Food/medical food ☐ Other

1. **Name, Strength, Manufacturer/Compounder** *(from product label).*

Product Name | Strength | Unit

NDC # or Unique ID | Manufacturer/ Compounder Name | Lot #

2. **Dose or Amount** | **Frequency** | **Route**

Unit | **Other Frequency** | **Other Route**

3. **Treament Dates/Therapy Dates** *(give best estimate of length of treatment (start/stop) or date of dose reduction.)*

Therapy started on *(e.g., 01-Jan-1900)* | Therapy stopped on *(e.g., 01-Jan-1900)* | Dose reduced on *(e.g., 01-Jan-1900)* **OR** | Duration | Unit

Is therapy still on-going? ☐ Yes ☐ No

4. **Diagnosis for use** *(indication)*

5. **Product Type** *(check all that apply)*
☐ OTC ☐ Generic
☐ Compounded ☐ Biosimilar

6. **Expiration Date** *(e.g., 01-Jan-1900)*

7. **Event Abated after use Stopped or Dose Reduced?**
☐ Yes ☐ No ☐ Doesn't apply

8. **Event Reappeared after Reintroduction?**
☐ Yes ☐ No ☐ Doesn't apply

SUSPECT PRODUCT #2

This report involves: ☐ Cosmetic ☐ Dietary supplement ☐ Food/medical food ☐ Other

1. **Name, Strength, Manufacturer/Compounder** *(from product label).*

Product Name | Strength | Unit

NDC # or Unique ID | Manufacturer/ Compounder Name | Lot #

2. **Dose or Amount** | **Frequency** | **Route**

Unit | **Other Frequency** | **Other Route**

3. **Treament Dates/Therapy Dates** *(give best estimate of length of treatment (start/stop) or date of dose reduction.)*

Therapy started on *(e.g., 01-Jan-1900)* | Therapy stopped on *(e.g., 01-Jan-1900)* | Dose reduced on *(e.g., 01-Jan-1900)* **OR** | Duration | Unit

Is therapy still on-going? ☐ Yes ☐ No

4. **Diagnosis for use** *(indication)*

5. **Product Type** *(check all that apply)*
☐ OTC ☐ Generic
☐ Compounded ☐ Biosimilar

6. **Expiration Date** *(e.g., 01-Jan-1900)*

7. **Event Abated after use Stopped or Dose Reduced?**
☐ Yes ☐ No ☐ Doesn't apply

8. **Event Reappeared after Reintroduction?**
☐ Yes ☐ No ☐ Doesn't apply

 (continued on next page)

E. SUSPECT MEDICAL DEVICE

1. **Brand Name**

2a. **Common Device Name**

2b. **Procode**

3. **Manufacurer Name, City and State**

4. **Model #**

Lot #

Catalog #

Expiration Date *(e.g., 01-Jan-1900)*

Serial #

Unique Device Identifier *(UDI)* **#**

5. **Operator of device**

☐ Health Professional ☐ Patient/Consumer ☐ Other

6a. **If Implanted, Give Date** *(e.g., 01-Jan-1900)*

6b. **If Explanted, Give Date** *(e.g., 01-Jan-1900)*

7a. **Is this a single-use device that was reprocessed and reused on a patient?**

☐ Yes ☐ No

7b. **If Yes to Item 7a, Enter Name, Address of Reprocessor**

8. **Was this device ever serviced by a third-party servicer?**

☐ Yes ☐ No ☐ Unknown

F. OTHER (CONCOMITANT) MEDICAL PRODUCTS

1. **Product names and therapy dates** *(Exclude treatment of event)*

	Product Name	Therapy Start Date *(e.g., 01-Jan-1900)*	Therapy End Date *(e.g., 01-Jan-1900)*
1.			
2.			
3.			
4.			
5.			
6.			
7.			
8.			
9.			
10.			

 (continued on next page)

G. REPORTER *(See confidentiality section on next page)*

1. **Name and Address**

Last Name	First Name

Address

City	State/Province/Region	ZIP/Postal Code

Country

Phone #	Email

2. **Health Professional?**	3. **Occupation**	4. **Also Reported to:**
☐ Yes ☐ No		☐ Manufacturer/Compounder ☐ User Facility ☐ Distributor/Importer

5. **If you do NOT want your identity disclosed to the manufacturer, please mark this box:** ☐

ADVICE ABOUT VOLUNTARY REPORTING

Detailed instructions available at:

https://www.fda.gov/safety/medwatch-forms-fda-safety-reporting/instructions-completing-form-fda-3500

Report adverse events, product problems or product use errors with:

- Medications(drugs or biologics)
- Medical devices (including diabetes glucose-test kit, hearing aids, breast pumps, and many more)
- Combination products(medication & medical devices)
- Blood transfusions, gene therapies, and human cells and tissue transplants (for example, tendons, bone, and corneas)
- Special nutritional products(dietary supplements, medical foods, infant formulas)
- Cosmetics (such as moisturizers, makeup, shampoos and conditioners, face and body washes, deodorants, nail care products, hair dyes and relaxers, and tattoos)
- Food (including beverages and ingredients added to foods)

Report product problems – quality, performance or safety concerns such as:

- Suspected counterfeit product
- Suspected contamination
- Questionable stability
- Defective components
- Poor packaging or labeling
- Therapeutic failures (product didn't work)

Report SERIOUS adverse events. An event is serious when the patient outcome is:

- Death
- Life-threatening
- Hospitalization (initial or prolonged)
- Disability or permanent damage
- Congenital anomaly/birth defect
- Required intervention to prevent permanent impairment or damage
- Other serious (important medical events)

Report even if:

- You're not certain the product caused the event
- You don't have all the details
- Just fill in the sections that apply to your report

How to report:

- Use section D for all products except medical devices
- Attach additional pages if needed
- Use a separate form for each patient
- Report either to FDA or the manufacturer (or both)

How to submit report:

- To report by phone, call toll-free: 1-800-FDA (332)-1088
- To fax report: 1-800-FDA (332)-0178
- To report online: www.fda.gov/medwatch/report.htm

If your report involves a serious adverse event with a device and it occurred in a facility outside a doctor's office, that facility may be legally required to report to FDA and/or the manufacturer. Please notify the person in that facility who would handle such reporting.

Where to submit adverse events related to the following products:

- If your report involves an animal drug, device, pet food and livestock feed problems, go to http://www.fda.gov/vetproductreporting
- If your report involves a health problem or a product problem with a tobacco product, go to https://www.safetyreporting.hhs.gov or call 1-877-287-1373 to report.
- If your report involves an adverse event with a vaccine, go to http://vaers.hhs.gov to report or call 1-800-822-7967.

Confidentiality:

The patient's identity is held in strict confidence by FDA and protected to the fullest extent of the law. The reporter's identity, including the identity of a self-reporter, may be shared with the manufacturer unless requested otherwise.

The information in this box applies only to requirements of the Paperwork Reduction Act of 1995

The burden time for this collection of information has been estimated to average 40 minutes per response, including the time to review instructions, search existing data sources, gather and maintain the data needed, and complete and review the collection of information. Send comments regarding this burden estimate or any other aspect of this collection of information, including suggestions for reducing this burden to:

Department of Health and Human Services
Food and Drug Administration
Office of Chief Information Officer
Office of Chief Information Officer
Paperwork Reduction Act (PRA) Staff
PRAStaff@fda.hhs.gov

Please DO NOT RETURN this form to the PRA Staff e-mail above.

OMB statement:

"An agency may not conduct or sponsor, and a person is not required to respond to, a collection of information unless it displays a currently valid OMB control number."

U.S. DEPARTMENT OF HEALTH
AND HUMAN SERVICES

Annexure 4(b): MedWatch Form FDA-3500A

M. Nandave, A. Kumar (eds.), *Pharmacovigilance Essentials*,
https://doi.org/10.1007/978-981-99-8949-2

Reset Form

FDA	**DEPARTMENT OF HEALTH AND HUMAN SERVICES** Food and Drug Administration **MEDWATCH** **FORM 3500A** For use by user-facilities, importers, distributors and manufacturers for MANDATORY reporting	Form Approved: OMB No. 0910-0291 Expires: 6-30-2025 See PRA statement on page 6. **FDA USE ONLY** Mfr report # UF/Importer Report # Exemption/Variance #

Note: For date prompts of "dd-mmm-yyyy" please use 2-digit day, 3-letter month abbreviation, and 4-digit year; for example, 01-JAN-1900.

A. PATIENT INFORMATION

1. **Patient Identifier** *(In confidence)*

2. Age
- ☐ Year(s) ☐ Week(s)
- ☐ Month(s) ☐ Day(s)

or Date of Birth *(e.g., 01-Jan-1900)*

3a. **Sex:** Enter the patient's sex at birth *(the sex that a person has or was assigned to at birth)*.
- ☐ Male ☐ Undifferentiated
- ☐ Female ☐ Decline to answer

3b. **Gender:** Enter the patient's current gender *(how the patient thinks of themself)*.
- ☐ Cisgender man/boy (gender corresponds with birth sex)
- ☐ Cisgender woman/girl (gender corresponds with birth sex)
- ☐ Transgender man/trans man/ female-to-male (FTM)
- ☐ Transgender woman/trans woman/ male-to-female (MTF)
- ☐ Other gender category; please specify:
- ☐ Decline to answer

4. **Weight**
- ☐ lb
- ☐ kg

5. **Ethnicity** *(Check one)*
- ☐ Hispanic/Latino
- ☐ Not Hispanic/Latino

6. **Race** *(check all that apply)*
- ☐ American Indian/Alaska Native
- ☐ Asian
- ☐ Black or African American
- ☐ Native Hawaiian/ Other Pacific Islander
- ☐ White

B. ADVERSE EVENT OR PRODUCT PROBLEM

1. **Type of Report** *(check all that apply)*
- ☐ Adverse Event
- ☐ Product Problem *(e.g., defects/malfunctions)*

2. **Outcome Attributed to Adverse Event** *(check all that apply)*
- ☐ Death – Date of death *(01-JAN-1900)*:
- ☐ Life-threatening
- ☐ Hospitalization (initial or prolonged)
- ☐ Other Serious or Important Medical Events
- ☐ Required Intervention to Prevent Permanent Impairment/Damage
- ☐ Disability or Permanent Damage
- ☐ Congenital Anomaly/Birth Defects

3. **Date of Event** *(01-JAN-1900)*

4. **Date of this Report** *(01-JAN-1900)*

Submission of a report does not constitute an admission that medical personnel or the product caused or contributed to the event.

* Please see instructions

(continued on next page)

5. **Describe Event or Problem**

6. **Relevant Test/Laboratory Data**	**Date** *(01-JAN-1900)*	**Relevant Test/Laboratory Data**	**Date** *(01-JAN-1900)*

Additional comments

 (continued on next page)

7. **Other Relevant History, Including Preexisting Medical Conditions** *(e.g., allergies, pregnancy, tobacco product use, alcohol use, and liver/kidney problems, etc.)*

C. SUSPECT PRODUCTS

SUSPECT PRODUCT #1

1. **Name, Strength, Manufacturer/Compounder**

Product Name	Strength	Unit
		--

NDC # or Unique ID	Manufacturer/Compounder Name	Lot #

2. **List Medical Product and Treatment Given at the Same Time of the Event and Date** *(Do not include treatment for initial event)*

3. **Dose or Amount**	**Frequency**	**Route**
	--	--
Unit	**Other Frequency**	**Other Route**
--		

4. **Treament Dates/Therapy Dates** *(give best estimate of length of treatment (start/stop) or date of dose reduction.)*

Therapy started on *(e.g., 01-Jan-1900)*	Therapy stopped on *(e.g., 01-Jan-1900)*	Dose Reduced *(e.g., 01-Jan-1900)* **OR**	Duration	Unit
				--

5. **Diagnosis for use** *(indication)*	6. **Product Type** *(check all that apply)*	7. **Expiration Date** *(e.g., 01-Jan-1900)*
	☐ OTC ☐ Generic ☐ Compounded ☐ Biosimilar	

8. **Event Abated after use Stopped or Dose Reduced?**	9. **Event Reappeared after Reintroduction?**
☐ Yes ☐ No ☐ Doesn't apply	☐ Yes ☐ No ☐ Doesn't apply

(continued on next page)

SUSPECT PRODUCT #2

1. **Name, Strength, Manufacturer/Compounder**

Product Name	Strength	Unit
		--

NDC # or Unique ID	Manufacturer/Compounder Name	Lot #

2. **List Medical Product and Treatment Given at the Same Time of the Event and Date** *(Do not include treatment for initial event)*

3. **Dose or Amount**	**Frequency**	**Route**
Unit --	-- **Other Frequency**	-- **Other Route**

4. **Treament Dates/Therapy Dates** *(give best estimate of length of treatment (start/stop) or date of dose reduction.)*

Therapy started on *(e.g., 01-Jan-1900)*	Therapy stopped on *(e.g., 01-Jan-1900)*	Dose Reduced *(e.g., 01-Jan-1900)* **OR**	Duration	Unit --

5. **Diagnosis for use** *(indication)*

6. **Product Type** *(check all that apply)*

☐ OTC ☐ Generic
☐ Compounded ☐ Biosimilar

7. **Expiration Date** *(e.g., 01-Jan-1900)*

8. **Event Abated after use Stopped or Dose Reduced?**

☐ Yes ☐ No ☐ Doesn't apply

9. **Event Reappeared after Reintroduction?**

☐ Yes ☐ No ☐ Doesn't apply

D. SUSPECT MEDICAL DEVICE

1. **Brand Name**	2a. **Common Device Name**	2b. **Procode**

3. **Manufacurer Name, City and State**

4. **Model #**	**Lot #**	**Catalog #**
Expiration Date *(01-JAN-1900)*	**Serial #**	

(continued on next page)

Unique Device Identifier *(UDI)* **#**

5. **Operator of Device**
☐ Health Professional ☐ Patient/Consumer
☐ Other

6a. **If Implanted, Give Date** *(01-JAN-1900)*

6b. **If Explanted, Give Date** *(01-JAN-1900)*

7a. **Is this a single-use device that was reprocessed and reused on a patient?**
☐ Yes ☐ No

7b. **If yes, enter the name and address of the reprocessor**

8. **Was this device ever serviced by a third-party servicer?**
☐ Yes ☐ No ☐ Unknown

9. **Is this Device Available for Evaluation?** *(Do not send to FDA)*
☐ Yes ☐ No
☐ Returned to manufacturer on *(01-JAN-1900)*

10. **Concomitant Medical Products and Therapy Dates** *(Exclude treatment of event)*

Product Name	Therapy Start Date *(01-JAN-1900)*	Therapy End Date *(01-JAN-1900)*
1.		
2.		
3.		
4.		
5.		
6.		
7.		
8.		
9.		
10.		

E. INITIAL REPORTER

1. **Name and Address**

Last Name | First Name

Address

City | State/Province/Region | ZIP/Postal Code | Country
--

Phone # | Email

2. **Health Professional?**
☐ Yes ☐ No

3. **Occupation** *(Select from list)*
--

4. *Initial reporter also sent report to FDA*
☐ Yes ☐ No ☐ Unknown

(continued on next page)

F. FOR USE BY USER FACILITY/IMPORTER *(Devices Only)*

1. **Check One**
☐ User Facility ☐ Importer

2. **User Facility/Importer Report Number**

3. **User Facility or Importer Name/Address**

4. **Contact Person**

5. **Phone Number**

6. **Date User Facility or Importer Became Aware of Event** *(01-JAN-1900)*

7. **Type of Report**

8. **Date of This Report** *(01-JAN-1900)*

9. **Approximate Age of Device**

10. **Adverse Event Problem** *(Refer to coding manual)*

Health Effect – Clinical Code	Health Effect – Impact Code	Medical Device Problem Code	Component Code

11. **Report Sent to FDA?**
(If Yes, enter date (01-JAN-1900))
☐ Yes ☐ No

12. **Location Where Event Occurred**
☐ Ambulatory Surgical Facility ☐ Outpatient Treatment Facility ☐ Other *(Specify)*
☐ Home ☐ Outpatient Diagnostic Facility
☐ Hospital ☐ Nursing Home

13. **Report Sent to Manufacturer?**
(If Yes, enter date (01-JAN-1900))
☐ Yes
☐ No

14. **Manufacturer Name/Address**

G. ALL MANUFACTURERS

1. **Contact Office** *(and Manufacturing Site for Devices)* **or Compounding Outsourcing Facility**

Name	Email Address	Phone Number

Address

Compounding Outsourcing Facility 503B?
☐ Check box if applicable

Outsourcing Facility

2. **Report Source** *(check all that apply)*
☐ Foreign ☐ Literature ☐ Health Professional ☐ Company Representative
☐ Study ☐ Consumer ☐ Use Faciltiy ☐ Distributor/Importer ☐ Other *(Please list)*

3. **Date Received by Manufacturer** *(01-JAN-1900)*

4. **NDA #**	**ANDA #**	**IND #**	**BLA #**	**PMA/510***(k)* **#**

Check all that apply:
☐ Combination product ☐ Pre-ANDA ☐ Pre-1938 ☐ OTC ☐ Compounded Product

5. **If IND/Pre-ANDA, Give Protocol #**

6. **Type of Report** *(Check all that apply)*
☐ 5-day ☐ 15-day ☐ Periodic ☐ Follow-up #
☐ 7-day ☐ 30-day ☐ Initial

7. **Adverse Event Term***(s)*

8. **Manufacturer Report Number**

Form FDA-3500A MEDWATCH (11/22)
(PREVIOUS EDITION OBSOLETE)

Page 6 of 7

(continued on next page)

H. DEVICE MANUFACTURERS ONLY

1. **Type of Reportable Event** *(check all that apply.)*
☐ Death ☐ Malfunction
☐ Serious Injury ☐ Summary Report
No. of events summarized

2. **If Follow-up, What Type?**
☐ Correction
☐ Additional Information
☐ Response to FDA Request
☐ Device Evaluation

3. **Device Evaluated by Manufacturer?**
☐ Yes ☐ No

4. **Device Manufacture Date** *(01-JAN-1900)*

5. **Labeled for Single Use?**
☐ Yes ☐ No

6. **Adverse Event Problem** *(Refer to coding manual)*

Health Effect – Clinical Code	Health Effect – Impact Code	Medical Device Problem Code	Component Code

Type of Investigation	Investigation Findings	Investigation Conclusions

7. **If Remedial Action Initiated, Check Type**
☐ Recall ☐ Relabeling ☐ Patient Monitoring
☐ Repair ☐ Notification ☐ Modification/Adjustment
☐ Replace ☐ Inspection ☐ Other:

8. **Usage of Device**
☐ Initial Use of Device
☐ Reuse
☐ Unknown

9. **If action reported to FDA under 21 USC 360i(g), list correction/ removal reporting number:**

10. **Related Report Number**

11. **Additional Manufacturer Narrative**

PRIVACY ACT STATEMENT

Authority: The information collected in this form is provided to comply with the Privacy Act of 1974 (P.L. 93-579) for individuals seeking non-employee student, post-graduate or senior scientist training opportunities from the Food and Drug Administration. Purpose and Uses: All information collected in this form is required to begin the Traineeship. Completed forms are used by the Staff to meet program selection and on-boarding requirements. Information is also shared with the FDA personnel authorized to administer the program. Effects of nondisclosure: Disclosure of the information is voluntary; however, collection of this information is necessary to continue with the FDA.

PRA Info

This section applies only to requirements of the Paperwork Reduction Act of 1995.

DO NOT SEND YOUR COMPLETED FORM TO THE PRA STAFF EMAIL ADDRESS BELOW.

The burden time for this collection of information is estimated to average 15 minutes per response, including the time to review instructions, search existing data sources, gather and maintain the data needed and complete and review the collection of information. Send comments regarding this burden estimate or any other aspect of this information collection, including suggestions for reducing this burden, to:

Department of Health and Human Services
Food and Drug Administration
Office of Operations
Paperwork Reduction Act (PRA) Staff
PRAStaff@fda.hhs.gov

"An agency may not conduct or sponsor, and a person is not required to respond to, a collection of information unless it displays a currently valid OMB control number."

Form FDA-3500A **MedWatch** (11/22) **Page 7 of 7**
(PREVIOUS EDITION OBSOLETE)

Annexure 4(c): MedWatch Form FDA-3500B

M. Nandave, A. Kumar (eds.), *Pharmacovigilance Essentials*,
https://doi.org/10.1007/978-981-99-8949-2

FDA

DEPARTMENT OF HEALTH AND HUMAN SERVICES
Food and Drug Administration

MEDWATCH

Consumer Voluntary Reporting
(FORM FDA 3500B)

Form Approved: OMB No. 0910-0291
Expiration Date: 06/30/2025
(See PRA Statement below)

When do I use this form?

- You were hurt or had a bad side effect (including new or worsening symptoms) after taking a drug or using a medical device or product.
- You used a drug, product, or medical device incorrectly which could have or led to unsafe use.
- You noticed a problem with the quality of the drug, product or medical device.
- You had problems with how a drug worked after switching from one maker to another maker.

Don't use this form to report:

- Vaccines – report problems to the Vaccine Adverse Event Reporting System (VAERS).
- Investigational drugs or medical devices (those being studied) – report problems to your doctor or to the contact person listed in the clinical trial.
- Animal Drug, Device, Pet Food and Livestock Feed Problems – report problems to FDA's Center for Veterinary Medicine.
- Tobacco products – report health or product problems to the Safety Reporting Portal (SRP) https://www.safetyreporting.hhs.gov or call 1-877-287-1363.
- Food, cosmetic or dietary supplement products – report problems to the SRP https://www.safetyreporting.hhs.gov/SRP2.

Will the information I report be kept private?

The FDA recognizes that privacy is an important concern, so you should know:

- We ask only for the name and contact information of the person filling out the form in case we need more information.
- Your name and contact information may be shared with the company that makes the product to help them better understand the problem you are reporting, unless you request otherwise (see Section F).

What types of products should I use this form for?

- Prescription and over-the-counter drugs, therapeutic biologics and biosimilars including monoclonal antibodies, and biologics, such as human cells and tissues used for transplantation (for example, tendons, ligaments, and bone) allergenics and gene therapies.
- Medical devices, including any health-related kit, test, tool, or piece of equipment (such as breast implants, pacemakers, diabetes glucose-test kits, hearing aids, breast pumps, and many others)
- Cosmetics such as moisturizers, makeup, shampoos and conditioners, face and body washes, deodorants, nail care products, hair dyes and relaxers, and tattoos
- Foods (including beverages and ingredients added to foods)

Are there specific instructions for filling out the form?

- Fill in as much information as possible and send in the report even if you do not have all the information.
- You can fill out this form yourself or have someone fill it out for you. If you need help, you may want to talk with your health professional.
- Feel free to include or attach an image of the product. Please do not send the products to the FDA.

How will I know the FDA has received my form?

- You will receive a reply from the FDA after we receive your report. We will personally contact you only if we need additional information.
- Your report will become part of a database so that it can be reviewed and compared to other reports by an FDA safety evaluator who will determine what steps to take.

How can I contact the FDA if I have questions?

Toll-free line: 1-800-332-1088
To report online: www.fda.gov/medwatch/report.htm

The information below applies only to requirements of the Paperwork Reduction Act of 1995.

The burden time for this collection of information is estimated to average 30 minutes per response, including the time to review instructions, search existing data sources, gather and maintain the data needed and complete and review the collection of information. Send comments regarding this burden estimate or any other aspect of this information collection, including suggestions for reducing this burden to the address to the right:

OMB Statement: "An agency may not conduct or sponsor, and a person is not required to respond to, a collection of information unless it displays a currently valid OMB number."

Department of Health and Human Services
Food and Drug Administration
Office of Chief Information Officer
Paperwork Reduction Act (PRA) Staff
PRAStaff@fda.hhs.gov

DO NOT SEND YOUR COMPLETED FORM TO THIS PRA STAFF ADDRESS.

FORM FDA 3500B (11/22) MedWatch **Consumer Voluntary Reporting** **General Information Page**

EF

FDA

DEPARTMENT OF HEALTH AND HUMAN SERVICES
Food and Drug Administration

MEDWATCH

Consumer Voluntary Reporting
(FORM FDA 3500B)

Form Approved: OMB No. 0910-0291
Expiration Date: 06/30/2025
(See PRA Statement on preceding general information page)

Note: *For date prompts of "dd-mmm-yyyy" please use 2-digit day, 3-letter month abbreviation, and 4-digit year; for example, 01-Jan-1900.*

Section A – About the Problem

1. What kind of problem was it? *(Check all that apply)*

- ☐ Were hurt or had a bad side effect *(including new or worsening symptoms)*
- ☐ Used a product incorrectly which could have or led to a problem
- ☐ Noticed a problem with the quality of the product
- ☐ Had problems after switching from one product maker to another maker

2. Did any of the following happen? *(Check all that apply)*

- ☐ Hospitalization – admitted or stayed longer
- ☐ Required help to prevent permanent harm
- ☐ Disability or health problem
- ☐ Birth defect
- ☐ Life-threatening
- ☐ Death *(include date) (e.g., 01-Jan-1900)*: ______
- ☐ Other serious/important medical incident

3. Date the problem occurred *(e.g., 01-Jan-1900)*

4. Tell us what happened, how it happened or why it happened. *(Include as many details as possible. FDA may reach out to you for any additional documents if necessary)*
Characters Remaining (max. 4,000):

For more information, visit http://www.fda.gov/MedWatch

Submission of a report does not constitute an admission that medical personnel or the product caused or contributed to the event.

5. Relevant Tests/Laboratory Results	Date (e.g., 01-Jan-1900)	Relevant Tests/Laboratory Results	Date (e.g., 01-Jan-1900)

Additional Comments Characters Remaining (max. 2,000):

Section B – Product Availability

1. Do you still have the product in case we need to evaluate it? *(Do not send the product to FDA. We will contact you directly if we need it.)* ☐ Yes ☐ No

2. Do you have a picture of the product? *(check yes if you are including a picture)* ☐ Yes

For a problem with a product, including

- prescription or over-the-counter medicine
- biologics, such as blood transfusions, gene therapies, and human cells and tissue transplants (for example, tendons, bone, and corneas)
- nutrition products, such as vitamins and minerals, herbal remedies, infant formulas, and medical foods
- cosmetics or make-up products
- foods (including beverages and ingredients added to foods)

➡ Go to Section C

For a problem with a medical device, including

- any health-related test, tool, or piece of equipment
- health-related kits, such as glucose monitoring kits or blood pressure cuffs
- implants, such as breast implants, pacemakers, or catheters
- other consumer health products, such as contact lenses, hearing aids, and breast pumps

➡ Go to Section D **(Skip Section C)**

For a health or product problem with a food, cosmetic, dietary supplement or tobacco product

➡ **Go to https://www.safetyreporting.hhs.gov/SRP2**

Section C – About the Products

1. This report is about ☐ Cosmetic ☐ Dietary Supplement ☐ Food/Medical Food ☐ Other

2. Name(s) of the product as it appears on the box, bottle, or package *(Include as many names as you see)*

3. Check if therapy is on-going ☐

4. Name(s) of the company that makes (or compounds) the product

For more information, visit http://www.fda.gov/MedWatch

Submission of a report does not constitute an admission that medical personnel or the product caused or contributed to the event.

5. Product Type *(check all that apply)*

☐ Over-the-Counter ☐ Compounded by a Pharmacy or an Outsourcing Facility ☐ Generic ☐ Biosimilar

6. Expiration date *(e.g., 01-Jan-1900)*	7. Lot number	8. NDC number

9. Strength *(for example, 800mg/160 mg or 20 mg)*

10. Quantity *(for example, 2 pills, 2 puffs, or 1 teaspoon, etc.)*	11. Frequency *(for example, twice daily or at bedtime)*	12. How was it taken or used *(for example, by mouth, injection, or on the skin)*?

13a. Date the person first started taking or using the product *(e.g., 01-Jan-1900)*:

13b. Date the person stopped taking or using the product *(e.g., 01-Jan-1900)*:

13c. Date the person reduced dose of the product *(e.g., 01-Jan-1900)*:

14. Give best estimate of duration Unit

15. Why was the person using the product? *(such as, what condition was it supposed to treat)*

16. Did the problem stop after the person reduced the dose or stopped taking or using the product? ☐ Yes ☐ No

17. Did the problem return if the person started taking or using the product again? ☐ Yes ☐ No ☐ Didn't restart

Go to Section E (Skip Section D)

Section D – About the Medical Device

1. Name of medical device

2. Name of the company that makes the medical device

3. Model number	4. Catalog number	5. Lot number	6. Serial number

7. Unique Device Identifier (UDI) number

8. Expiration date *(e.g., 01-Jan-1900)*

9. Was someone operating the medical device when the problem occurred? ☐ Yes ☐ No

If yes, who was operating it?

☐ The person who had the problem ☐ A health professional *(such as a doctor, nurse, or aide)*

☐ Someone else *(Please explain who)*

10. For implanted medical devices ONLY *(such as pacemakers, breast implants, etc.)*

Date the implant was put in *(e.g., 01-Jan-1900)* Date the implant was taken out *(If relevant) (e.g., 01-Jan-1900)*

Go to Section E

For more information, visit http://www.fda.gov/MedWatch

Submission of a report does not constitute an admission that medical personnel or the product caused or contributed to the event.

Section E – About the Person Who Had the Problem

1. Person's Initials	2a. Sex: Enter the patient's sex at birth (the sex that a person has or was assigned to at birth). ☐ Male ☐ Female ☐ Undifferentiated ☐ Decline to answer	2b. Gender: Enter the patient's current gender (how the patient thinks of themself). ☐ Cisgender man/boy (gender corresponds with birth sex) ☐ Cisgender woman/girl (gender corresponds with birth sex) ☐ Transgender man/trans man/ female-to-male (FTM) ☐ Transgender woman/trans woman/ male-to-female (MTF) ☐ Other gender category; please specify: ☐ Decline to answer

3. Age *(specify unit of time for age)* ☐ Year(s) ☐ Week(s) ☐ Month(s) ☐ Day(s)	4. Date of Birth *(e.g., 01-Jan-1900)*	5. Weight *(Specify lbs or kg)* ☐ lb ☐ kg

6. Ethnicity *(Choose only one)* ☐ Hispanic/Latino ☐ Not Hispanic/Latino	7. Race *(Choose all that apply)* ☐ American Indian or Alaska Native ☐ Black or African American ☐ White ☐ Asian ☐ Native Hawaiian or Other Pacific Islander

8. List known medical conditions. *(Such as diabetes, high blood pressure, cancer, heart disease, or others)*

Characters Remaining (max. 2,000):

9. Please list all allergies *(such as to drugs, foods, pollen or others)*

10. List any other important information about the person *(such as tobacco product use, pregnancy, alcohol use, etc.)*

11. List all current prescription medications and medical devices being used.

Characters Remaining (max. 2,000):

For more information, visit *http://www.fda.gov/MedWatch*	**Submission of a report does not constitute an admission that medical personnel or the product caused or contributed to the event.**

12. List all over-the-counter medications and any vitamins, minerals, supplements, and herbal remedies being used. Characters Remaining (max. 2,000):

Go to Section F

Section F – About the Person Filling Out This Form

We will contact you only if we need additional information.

1. Last name	2. First name
3. Number/Street	4. City and State/Province
5. ZIP or Postal code	6. Country

7. Telephone number	8. Email address	9. Today's date *(e.g., 01-Jan-1900)*

10. Did you report this problem to the company that makes the product (the manufacturer/compounder)? ☐ Yes ☐ No

11. If you do NOT want your identity disclosed to the manufacturer, place an "X" in this box: ☐

Send This Report by Mail or Fax

Keep the product in case the FDA wants to contact you for more information. Please do not send products to the FDA. Mail or fax the form to: MedWatch, Food and Drug Administration, 5600 Fishers Lane, Rockville, MD 20852; FAX: 800-332-0178 (toll-free).

Thank you for helping us protect the public health.

For more information, visit *http://www.fda.gov/MedWatch*	**Submission of a report does not constitute an admission that medical personnel or the product caused or contributed to the event.**

Annexure 5: Preliminary Investigation Report (PIR)

M. Nandave, A. Kumar (eds.), *Pharmacovigilance Essentials*,
https://doi.org/10.1007/978-981-99-8949-2

Adverse events following immunization- Reporting Forms

FIRST INFORMATION REPORT FORM

First Information Report

Adverse Events Following Immunization

(To be reported within 48 hrs to the GoI)

State	District
Block	Date of report
Name	
Age (DOB)	Sex: Male/ Female
Mother's / Father's Name	
Complete Address of the case	
Date & time of vaccination	Date & time of onset of symptoms
Complete address of place of vaccination	
Vaccines given	
Batch Number & Expiry date of each vaccine	
Type of reaction	
Date of Death	
Any other comment[1]	

Name of person filling the report

Signature and Designation

PRELIMINARY INVESTIGATION REPORT FORM
PRELIMINARY INVESTIGATION REPORT
Adverse Events Following Immunization

(To be reported within 7 DAYS to the GoI)

State	District
Block	Date of report
Name:	
Age (DOB):	Sex: Male/ Female
Mother's / Father's Name	
Complete Address of the case	
Date & time of vaccination	Date & time of onset of symptoms
Vaccines given	
Complete address of place of vaccination	
Batch Number & Expiry date of each vaccine	
Type of reaction	
Date of Death	
Probable cause of death:	
Probable cause of the AE: Programme error/ Vaccine reaction/ Coincidental/ Unknown	
Further action planned: Yes/ No (if Yes Details)	
Any other comment	

Name of person filling the report

Signature and Designation

DETAILED INVESTIGATION REPORT FORM

DETAILED INVESTIGATION REPORT

Adverse Events Following Immunization (AEFI)

(To be reported within three months)

Adverse event following Immunization or Death after Immunization

Date of Investigation: Case ID No.: IND (AEFI)/_ _ /_ _ _ /_ _ / _ _ _ Use same coding as done for AFP cases

1	Name of child affected (In Block Letters)	
2	Name of Parents	Father's name Mother's name
3	Age and Sex	— —/— —/— — Date of Birth Male/ Female yrsmo days (if know)
4	Full detailed address	
5	Place of immunization	Health facility/ Out reach session site/Field camp/ Hospital/ Maternity home/ Private clinic/ any other place
6	a. Date and time of immunization	
	b. Location of immunization session (Full address)	
7	No. of children immunized at the session	BCG___ DPT1___ DPT2___ DPT3___ DPT B___ OPV1___ OPV2___ OPV3___ OPV B___ HEPB 1___ HEPB 2___ HEPB 3___ MEASLES___ DT___ TT1___ TT2___ TT B___ VIT A___ OTHERS___
8	Date and time of onset of	
9	AEFI Date of Initial report	

9	Type of AEFI	
10	Was the patient admitted to hospital	Yes/ No/ Unknown
11	If Yes, date & Time of admission	
	Name of Hospital	
	Ward no	
	Centralized admission number	
	Outcome	Recovered/ still in hospital/ death/ unknown/ Residual problem
12	SYMPTOMS AND SIGNS	
	a. Time of onset	
	b. Sign of shock present/absent	
	c. Temperature	
	d. Pulse	
	e. Respiration	
	f. Convulsion	
	g. Vomiting	
	h. Diarrhoea	
	i. Altered sensorium	
	j. Rash	
	k. Any other symptoms & sign (pl specify)	
	l. Progress of symptoms and signs with brief history & chain of events (Please attach additional sheet if required or patient records if available)	

	m. Mention whether above sign and symptoms are seen by investigating officer or whether above sign and symptoms are noted from hospital record	
13	Treatment given (attach copy of case sheet, if available)	
14	GROWTH & DEVELOPMENT/PAST/ FAMILY HISTORY (please fill as relevant to case)	
	a. Type of Delivery	Normal delivery/ LSCS/ Assisted birth
	b. Gestation	Full term/Premature/Post dated
	c. Complications during birth	
	d. Birth weight (if possible)	
	e. Present Weight (if possible)	
	f. Present length/ height (if possible)	
	g. Present head circumference (if possible)	
	h. Developmental milestones	Gross motor
		Fine Motor
		Language
		Adaptive & Social
	i. Past illness like allergy, asthma, convulsion etc	
	j. Any previous history of similar event after immunization	Yes/ No/ Unknown
	k. Family history - history of epilepsy, allergy, asthma etc in the family	

	l. Any history of similar event in siblings	Yes/ No/ Unknown
	m. Was the child on any concurrent medication for any illness	Yes/ No/ Unknown If yes: Indication & Dosage
15	INFORMATION ON IMMUNIZATION (IN CASE PROGRAMME ERROR SUSPECTED)	
	a. Name of worker who administered vaccine	
	b. Designation	
	c. Length of service	
	d. Experience	
	e. When did worker receive the last training in immunization	
	f. Name of Health Assistant (Supervisor)	
	g. Designation	
	h. Length of service	
	i. Experience	
	j. When did Health Assistant (Supervisor) receive the last training in immunization	
16	k. Total number of mother and children immunized. Attached detailed list giving name/age/sex/vaccines given	
	l. Any history of similar event reported (among those vaccinated)	a. At same clinic: Yes/ No/ Unknown b. Using same vaccine type at previous clinic sessions: Yes/ No/ Unknown
	If Yes	Specify event Number Place

	m. Any history of similar event reported (among unimmunized)	a. At same clinic session: Yes/ No/ Unknown b. In the field: Yes/ No/ Unknown
	If Yes	Specify event Number Place
	n. At what stage was the index child immunized	a. Within the first few doses of the vial b. Within the last few doses of the vial c. Within the first vaccinations of the clinic session d. Within the last vaccinations of the clinic session e. Unknown
	o. Vaccination technique (observe the relevant vaccinator)	Reconstitution: Satisfactory/ Unsatisfactory/ Not observed
		Drawing of vaccine: Satisfactory/ Unsatisfactory/ Not observed
		Injection technique: Satisfactory/ Unsatisfactory/ Not observed
17	DETAILS OF VACCINE GIVEN PRIOR TO AEFI	
	a. Date of receipt of vaccine of implicated batch by	MoH/ State Regional Store District PHC/CHC/ Urban Health Center Sub center/ Out reach session site
	b. Status of maintenance of cold chain at	State
		Regional store
		District Head Quarter
		PHC/ Urban health post
		Subcenter
		Session Site
	c. Is there a suspicion of breach of cold chain as per records? (If so, when & where?)	

	m. Time of receipt of vaccine at field camp site (immunization session site)	
	n. Maintenance of cold chain during transit from Health Post/ PHC to field camp site	
	o. Name of person collecting vaccine from fixed centre to field camp site	
	p. Vaccines used	BCG/ DPT/ OPV/ Measles/ Hepatitis/ Vit A/ others (specify)
	q. If reconstituted, what diluent was used	
	r. Which type of syringe was used for reconstitution?	Reusable/ Disposable/ AD
	s. Practice of reconstitution	Same syringe used for multiple vials of same vaccine/ Same syringe used for reconstituting different vaccines/ Separate syringe for each vial/ Separate syringe for each vaccine
	t. Is the needle left in reconstituted vaccine vial	Yes/ No/ Not observed
	u. Whether label of vial intact i) Batch No ii) Expiry date iii) Manufactured by	
	v. Date and time when vial opened	
	w. Date of vaccine sent for testing	
	x. Result of sample of vaccine sent for testing	
	y. Is the vaccine collected by FDA or SRA	
	i) Name of the officer	
	ii) Date when vaccine sent for testing	

	iii) Place where vaccine sent for testing	
	iv) Result of vaccine sent for testing	
18	STERLISATION OF SYRINGE AND NEEDLE	
	a. Types of syringes used to vaccinate the child.	Reusable/ Disposable/ AD
	b. Method of sterilization if reusable syringes used	
	c. Name and Designation of person who was responsible for autoclaving/ boiling for 20 minutes	
	d. Date and time of autoclaving/ boiling started	
	e. Date and time of autoclaving/ boiling completed	
	f. Sterilization satisfaction as per records of Signolac strip register	
	g. No of syringes & needles autoclaved	
	h. No of syringes & needles used for the session.	
19	INVESTIGATIONS DONE	
	a. Whether any blood tests were done	
	b. If yes, results of blood tests	
	c. Whether CSF was examined	
	d. If yes, result of CSF tests	

Annexures 6: ADR Reporting Form for Geneva, Switzerland

M. Nandave, A. Kumar (eds.), *Pharmacovigilance Essentials*,
https://doi.org/10.1007/978-981-99-8949-2

CIOMS FORM

SUSPECT ADVERSE REACTION REPORT

I. REACTION INFORMATION

1. PATIENT INITIALS (first, last)	1a. COUNTRY	2. DATE OF BIRTH Day / Month / Year	2a. AGE Years	3. SEX	4-6 REACTION ONSET Day / Month / Year	8-12 CHECK ALL APPROPRIATE TO ADVERSE REACTION
				F		☐ PATIENT DIED ☐ INVOLVED OR PROLONGED INPATIENT HOSPITALISATION ☐ INVOLVED PERSISTENCE OR SIGNIFICANT DISABILITY OR INCAPACITY ☐ LIFE THREATENING

7 + 13 DESCRIBE REACTION(S) (including relevant tests/lab data)

II. SUSPECT DRUG(S) INFORMATION

14. SUSPECT DRUG(S) (include generic name)

20 DID REACTION ABATE AFTER STOPPING DRUG? ☐ YES ☐ NO ☐ NA

15. DAILY DOSE(S)

16. ROUTE(S) OF ADMINISTRATION

21. DID REACTION REAPPEAR AFTER REINTRODUCTION? ☐ YES ☐ NO ☐ NA

17. INDICATION(S) FOR USE

18. THERAPY DATES (from/to)

19. THERAPY DURATION

III. CONCOMITANT DRUG(S) AND HISTORY

22. CONCOMITANT DRUG(S) AND DATES OF ADMINISTRATION (exclude those used to treat reaction)

23. OTHER RELEVANT HISTORY (e.g. diagnostics, allergics, pregnancy with last month of period, etc.)

IV. MANUFACTURER INFORMATION

24a. NAME AND ADDRESS OF MANUFACTURER

24b. MFR CONTROL NO.

24c. DATE RECEIVED BY MANUFACTURER

24d. REPORT SOURCE ☐ STUDY ☐ LITERATURE ☐ HEALTH PROFESSIONAL

DATE OF THIS REPORT

25a. REPORT TYPE ☐ INITIAL ☐ FOLLOWUP

Annexure 7: ADR Reporting Forms for Vaccine or Medicine

M. Nandave, A. Kumar (eds.), *Pharmacovigilance Essentials*,
https://doi.org/10.1007/978-981-99-8949-2

Australian Government
Department of Health
Therapeutic Goods Administration

TGA use only

Report of suspected adverse reaction to medicines or vaccines

See statement about the collection and use of personal information overleaf, and please attach any additional data to this form

Patient initials or medical record number:	Sex: M ☐ F ☐ / Weight (kg):	Date of birth or age:

Suspected medicine(s)/vaccine(s)

Medicine/vaccine (please use trade names; include batch number and AUST R or AUST L number if known)	**Dosage** (Dose number for vaccines eg 1st DTP)	Date begun	Date stopped	Reason for use

Other medicine(s)/vaccine(s) taken at the time of the reaction

Medicine/vaccine	**Dosage**	Date begun	Date stopped	Reason for use

Reaction(s): Date of onset of reaction (for vaccines time after administration): / /

Describe: (please provide as much detail as possible and include any results of relevant laboratory data and other investigations)

Seriousness: Life threatening ☐ Hospitalised ☐ Required a visit to doctor ☐

Treatment of reaction:

Outcome: Recovered ☐ ▸ Date: / / | Not yet recovered ☐ | Fatal ☐ ▸ Date: / / | Unknown ☐

Sequelae? No ☐ Yes ☐ ▸ Describe:

Reporting: Doctor ☐ Pharmacist ☐ Other ☐

Contact details (email or phone)

Name:

Address:

Postcode:

Signature:

Date: / /

Thank you for taking the time to complete this form PTO

Report of suspected reaction to medicines or vaccines ("Blue card")

Privacy statement

For general privacy information, go to <www.tga.gov.au/privacy>.
Information in this report is collected to assist in the post market monitoring of the safety of therapeutic goods under the *Therapeutic Goods Act 1989* (the Act). All reports are entered into the Therapeutic Goods Administration's (TGA's) Adverse Event Management System (AEMS). Further information about how the TGA uses adverse event information that is reported to it is available at <www.tga.gov.au/reporting-adverse-events>.

The TGA collects personal information in this report to:
- monitor the safety of medicines and vaccines under the Act
- contact the reporter of the adverse event if further information is required
- contact representatives of entities that supply therapeutic goods, to discuss reported adverse events
- check that the same information has not been received multiple times for the same adverse event.

At times, this information is collected from someone other than the individual to whom the personal information relates. This can occur when an adverse event is reported to a person or an entity other than the TGA (such as a health professional, a hospital or a sponsor), and that person or entity passes the information on to the TGA. In those cases, ordinarily the TGA will not collect the name and contact details of patients. However, the TGA may collect other information relating to patients, including the date of birth or age, gender, weight, initials and information about the relevant adverse event.

Personal information collected in this report may be disclosed as permitted under the Privacy Act 1988, including by consent or where the disclosure is required by, or authorised under, a law (for example, under section 61 of the Act). Where a report relates to vaccine events, personal information about the reporter or the patient may be disclosed to State and Territory health agencies under subsection 61(3) of the Act.

Fold here first (Please do not use staples on this form)

www.tga.gov.au/reporting-problems Email: adr.reports@tga.gov.au Fax: 02 6232 8392

What to report
You do not need to be certain, just suspicious!
Any information related to the reporter and patient identifiers is kept strictly confidential.
Adverse drug reaction reports should be submitted for prescription medicines, vaccines, over-the-counter medicines (medicines purchased without a prescription), and complementary medicines (herbal medicines, naturopathic and/or homoeopathic medicines, and nutritional supplements such as vitamins and minerals). Please include timing of reactions relative to medicine administration where relevant.
The TGA particularly requests reports of:

- All suspected reactions to new medicines and vaccines
- All suspected drug interactions
- Unexpected reactions, that is not consistent with product information or labelling
- **Serious reactions which are suspected of significantly affecting a patient's management, including** reactions suspected of causing death, danger to life, admission to hospital, prolongation of hospitalisation, absence from productive activity, increased investigational or treatment costs, and birth defects.

Fold here second D1073 June 2018

Delivery Address:
PO Box 100
WODEN ACT 2606

No stamp required if posted in Australia

Medicines Safety Monitoring
Pharmacovigilance and Special Access Branch
Reply Paid 100
WODEN ACT 2606

Annexure 8: ADR Reporting Form in India for Herbal

M. Nandave, A. Kumar (eds.), *Pharmacovigilance Essentials*,
https://doi.org/10.1007/978-981-99-8949-2

Patient/consumer identification (please complete or tick boxes below as appropriate)

<table>
<tr><td>Last name</td><td>First name(s)</td><td rowspan="2">Patient/record number</td></tr>
<tr><td>Ethnicity</td><td></td></tr>
<tr><td colspan="2" rowspan="2">Address (place and region, or health facility may be used)</td><td>Date of birth</td></tr>
<tr><td>Sex ☐M ☐F</td></tr>
</table>

List of all medicines/vaccines/herbal medicines used by the patient. Please indicate suspected medicines with an asterisk (*) (please complete boxes below)

<table>
<tr><td>Medicine(s)Vaccine(s) + batch no.</td><td>Daily dose</td><td>Route of administration</td><td>Date started</td><td>Date stopped</td><td>Reason for use</td></tr>
<tr><td></td><td></td><td></td><td></td><td></td><td></td></tr>
<tr><td></td><td></td><td></td><td></td><td></td><td></td></tr>
<tr><td colspan="6">For herbal medicines please give detailed information on the product
Product name:

How was the product obtained?

List of product ingredients; attach product label if available:

Name and address of the manufacturer;

Name and address of the distributor:

Other relevant information:</td></tr>
</table>

Description of the suspected adverse reaction (please complete boxes below)

<table>
<tr><td>Date of onset of reaction (dd/mm/yy):</td></tr>
<tr><td>Description of reaction (please include results of laboratory tests if available):</td></tr>
</table>

Outcome of the suspected adverse reaction (please tick boxes as appropriate)

<table>
<tr><td>Recovered ☐</td><td>Not yet recovered ☐</td><td>Unknown ☐</td><td>Fatal ☐</td><td>Date of death</td></tr>
<tr><td colspan="2">Severe? Yes ☐ No ☐</td><td colspan="3">Rechallenge? Yes ☐ No ☐
Result:</td></tr>
<tr><td colspan="2">Was the patient admitted to hospital?
If yes, give name and address of hospital:</td><td colspan="3">Yes ☐ No ☐</td></tr>
</table>

Other factors (please tick box or describe as appropriate)

<table>
<tr><td>Kidney disease ☐</td><td>Liver disease ☐</td><td colspan="2">Allergy (please describe) ....
....</td></tr>
<tr><td colspan="3">Other illnesses (please describe):</td><td>Malnutrition ☐</td></tr>
</table>

Reporter identification

<table>
<tr><td>Type (please circle): nurse/doctor/pharmacist/other health worker /manufacturer/ distributor/supplier</td></tr>
<tr><td>Name:</td></tr>
<tr><td>Address:
Telephone:</td></tr>
<tr><td>E-mail address:</td></tr>
</table>

Signature of reporter: .... **Date:** ....

Please send completed form to: ....

Annexure 9(a): Medical Devices Adverse Event Form

M. Nandave, A. Kumar (eds.), *Pharmacovigilance Essentials*,
https://doi.org/10.1007/978-981-99-8949-2

MEDICAL DEVICE ADVERSE EVENT REPORTING FORM

Materiovigilance Programme of India (MvPI)

This form is intended to collect information on Medical Devices Adverse Event in India. The form is designed to be used voluntarily by Manufacturer/Importer/Distributor of Medical Devices, Healthcare Professionals and anyone with direct/indirect knowledge of Medical Devices Adverse Event.

General Information

1. Date of Report :
2. Type of Report : Initial ☐ Follow up ☐ Final ☐ Trend ☐
3. Reporter Reference for MDMC only: • Centre • Location • Month-Year • Case No.

Reporter Details

1. Type of Reporter : (a) Manufacturer ☐ (b) Importer ☐ (c) Distributor ☐ (d) Healthcare Professional ☐
   (e) Patient ☐ (f) Others ☐ specify ....
2. In case, where the reporter is not manufacturer, fill the following details:-
   (a) Has the reporter informed the incident to the manufacturer?
   Yes ☐ No ☐
   (b) Is the reporter also submitting the report on behalf of the manufacturer?
   Yes ☐ No ☐
3. Reporter contact information:
   a) Name :
   b) Address :
   c) Tel. /Mobile :
   d) Email :

Device Category

Medical Device	In Vitro Diagnostics (IVD)	Medical Equipments / Machines
I. Therapeutic ☐ Diagnostic ☐	I. Kits ☐	I. Therapeutic ☐ Diagnostic ☐
Both ☐ Preventive ☐	II. Reagents ☐	II. Therapeutic & Diagnostic ☐
Assistive ☐	III. Calibrator ☐	III. Preventive ☐
II. Implantable device ☐	IV. Control Material ☐	IV. Assistive ☐
Non-Implantable device ☐	V. Others ☐	V. Imaging ☐
III. Invasive ☐ Non-Invasive ☐	VI. IVD electronic reader/ Analyzer ☐	VI. Invasive ☐ Non-Invasive ☐
IV. Single use device ☐		VII. Others ☐
Reusable device ☐		
Reuse of manufacture marked Single use device ☐		
V. Sterile ☐ Non Sterile ☐		
VI. Personal use / Homecare use ☐		

Instruction for use Section A-F

- ***If Medical Devices/Equipments/Machines : Please fill all the sections i.e. A, B, C, D, E & F***
- ***If in Vitro Diagnostics (IVD) : Please fill sections i.e. A (except 6, 7, 8, 13, 14 & 16), B (except 1, 2, 6 & 8), D, E, & F***

(A) Device Details

Device Name / Trade Name / Brand Name: ....

Details	Name	Address
Manufacturer		
Importer		
Distributor		

1. a) Is the device notified/regulated in India : Yes ☐ No ☐

   b) Device Risk Classification as per India MDR 2017 : A ☐ B ☐ C ☐ D ☐
2. License No. (Manufacture/Import) :
3. Catalogue No. :
4. Model No. :
5. Lot / Batch No. :
6. Serial No. :
7. Software Version :
8. Associated Devices / Accessories :
9. Nomenclature Code if applicable; GMDN/UMDNS :
10. UDI No. (If applicable) :
11. Installation Date :
12. Expiration Date :
13. Last preventive maintenance date (dd/mm/yyyy) :
14. Last calibration date (dd/mm/yyyy) :
15. Year of manufacturing :
16. How long was device/Equipment/Machine in use :
17. Availability of device for evaluation : Yes ☐ No ☐

    If no, was the device destroyed ☐ Still in use ☐ return to manufacturer or importer/distributor ☐
18. Is the usage of device as per manufacturer claim /Instruction for use/user manual: Yes ☐ No ☐

    If no specify usage ....

    ....
19. For devices not regulated / notified in India : Regulator / Regulatory status in country of origin

    ....

(B) Event Description

1. Date of Event / Near miss incident:
2. Date of Implant/Explant (If applicable):
3. Location of Event:

   Hospital Premise ☐ Manufacture/Distributor premise ☐

   Home ☐ Others ☐
4. Device Operator:-

   Healthcare Professional ☐ Patient ☐ Others ☐

   Problem noted prior to use/near miss event ☐
5. Device disposition / Current location:
   a) Returned to company ☐ If yes, date ....../....... /.......
   b) Remains implanted in patient ☐
   c) Within the healthcare facility ☐
   d) At patient home ☐
   e) Destroyed ☐
   f) Others (specify) ☐
6. Is device in use after incidence : Yes ☐ No ☐
7. Serious event: ☐

   If serious, Tick the appropriate reason
   a) Death (DD/MM/YY) ☐ ..../............/............
   b) Life Threatening ☐
   c) Disability or permanent damage ☐
   d) Hospitalization ☐
   e) Congenital anomaly /birth defect ☐
   f) Any other serious (Imp. medical event) ☐
   g) Required intervention to prevent / permanent Impairment / damage device ☐
8. Non serious event ☐
9. Whether other medical devices were used at same time with above device if yes, please specify name(s)/use(s)

   ....

   ....

   ....

10. Detail description of Event:-

For manufacturer/authorized representative use only

	Year	No. of Similar Adverse Events	Total No. Supplied	Frequency of Occurrence (%)
11. Frequency of occurrence of similar Adverse Event in India in past 3 years				
12. Frequency of occurrence of similar Adverse Event in globally in past 3 years	Year	No. of Similar Adverse Events	Total No. Supplied	Frequency of Occurrence (%)

(C) Patient Information, History & Outcome

1. Patient Hospital ID :
2. Patient Initial :
3. Age :
4. Gender : Male ☐ Female ☐ Others ☐
5. Weight :
6. Other relevant history, including pre-existing medical conditions..

   ....

   ....

   ....

   ....
7. Patient Outcomes:
   a) Recovered Date (DD/MM/YY) ☐ ....../......./.......
   b) Not yet recovered ☐
   c) Death ☐ (DD/MM/YY) ☐ ....../......./.......
   d) Others ☐

      Please specify..

   ....

   ....

   ....

   ....

   ....

(D) Healthcare Facility Information (if available)

1. Name :
2. Address :
3. Contact Person Name at the site of event :
4. Tel. No. :

(E) Causality Assessment

1. Investigation action taken:

2. Root cause of problem (Applicable for follow up / final reports):

(F) Manufacturer/Authorized Representative Investigation & Action taken

1. Manufacturer/Authorized Representative device risk analysis report:

2. Corrective / preventive action taken:

3. Device history review:

Where to report?

Duly filled Medical Device Adverse Event Reporting Form can be sent to Indian Pharmacopoeia Commission, Ministry of Health and Family Welfare, Government of India, Sector-23, Rajnagar, Ghaziabad-20002, Tel-0120-2783400, 2783401 and 2783392, FAX:0120-2783311 or email to mvpi.ipcindia@gmail.com Or Call on Helpline no. 1800 180 3024 to report Adverse event.

Partnering Organizations

Disclaimer

Confidentiality: The patient's identity is held in strict confidence and protected to the fullest extent. Programme staff is not expected to and will not disclose the reporter's identity in response to a request from the public. Submission of a report does not constitute an admission that medical personnel or manufacturer or the product caused or contributed to the adverse event.

Annexure 9(b): Medical Device Adverse Event Reporting Form for HCPS (Version 1.1)

M. Nandave, A. Kumar (eds.), *Pharmacovigilance Essentials*,
https://doi.org/10.1007/978-981-99-8949-2

Version-1.1

IPC

MEDICAL DEVICE ADVERSE EVENT REPORTING FORM

Materiovigilance Programme of India (MvPI)

This form is intended to collect information on Medical Devices Adverse Event in India. The form is designed to be used voluntarily by Manufacturer/Importer/Distributor of Medical Devices, Healthcare Professionals and anyone with direct/indirect knowledge of Medical Devices Adverse Event.

General Information

1. Date of Report :
2. Type of Report : Initial ☐ Follow up ☐ Final ☐ Trend ☐
3. Reporter Reference for MDMC only: • Centre • Location • Month-Year • Case No.

Reporter Details

1. Type of Reporter : (a) Manufacturer ☐ (b) Importer ☐ (c) Distributor ☐ (d) Healthcare Professional ☐
   (e) Patient ☐ (f) Others ☐ specify
2. In case, where the reporter is not manufacturer, fill the following details:-
   (a) Has the reporter informed the incident to the manufacturer?
   Yes ☐ No ☐
   (b) Is the reporter also submitting the report on behalf of the manufacturer?
   Yes ☐ No ☐
3. Reporter contact information:
   a) Name :
   b) Address :
   c) Tel. /Mobile :
   d) Email :

Device Category

Medical Device	In Vitro Diagnostics (IVD)	Medical Equipments / Machines
I. Therapeutic ☐ Diagnostic ☐ Both ☐ Preventive ☐ Assistive ☐	I. Kits ☐	I. Therapeutic ☐ Diagnostic ☐
	II. Reagents ☐	II. Therapeutic & Diagnostic ☐
	III. Calibrator ☐	III. Preventive ☐
II. Implantable device ☐ Non-Implantable device ☐	IV. Control Material ☐	IV. Assistive ☐
	V. Others ☐	V. Imaging ☐
III. Invasive ☐ Non-Invasive ☐	VI. IVD electronic reader/ Analyzer ☐	VI. Invasive ☐ Non-Invasive ☐
IV. Single use device ☐ Reusable device ☐ Reuse of manufacture marked Single use device ☐		VII. Others ☐
V. Sterile ☐ Non Sterile ☐		
VI. Personal use / Homecare use ☐		

Instruction for use Section A-F

- ***If Medical Devices/Equipments/Machines : Please fill all the sections i.e. A, B, C, D, E & F***
- ***If in Vitro Diagnostics (IVD) : Please fill sections i.e. A (except 6, 7, 8, 13, 14 & 16), B (except 1, 2, 6 & 8), D, E, & F***

(A) Device Details

Device Name / Trade Name / Brand Name:

Details	Name	Address
Manufacturer		
Importer		
Distributor		

1. a) Is the device notified/regulated in India : Yes ☐ No ☐
   b) Device Risk Classification as per India MDR 2017 : A ☐ B ☐ C ☐ D ☐
2. License No. (Manufacture/Import) :
3. Catalogue No. :
4. Model No. :
5. Lot / Batch No. :
6. Serial No. :
7. Software Version :
8. Associated Devices / Accessories :
9. Nomenclature Code if applicable; GMDN/UMDNS :
10. UDI No. (If applicable) :
11. Installation Date :
12. Expiration Date :
13. Last preventive maintenance date (dd/mm/yyyy) :
14. Last calibration date (dd/mm/yyyy) :
15. Year of manufacturing :
16. How long was device/Equipment/Machine in use :
17. Availability of device for evaluation : Yes ☐ No ☐
    If no, was the device destroyed ☐ Still in use ☐ return to manufacturer or importer/distributor ☐
18. Is the usage of device as per manufacturer claim /Instruction for use/user manual: Yes ☐ No ☐
    If no specify usage
19. For devices not regulated / notified in India : Regulator / Regulatory status in country of origin

(B) Event Description

1. Date of Event / Near miss incident:
2. Date of Implant/Explant (If applicable):
3. Location of Event:

   Hospital Premise ☐ Manufacture/Distributor premise ☐

   Home ☐ Others ☐
4. Device Operator:-

   Healthcare Professional ☐ Patient ☐ Others ☐

   Problem noted prior to use/near miss event ☐
5. Device disposition / Current location:
   - a) Returned to company ☐ If yes, date ....../......./.........
   - b) Remains implanted in patient ☐
   - c) Within the healthcare facility ☐
   - d) At patient home ☐
   - e) Destroyed ☐
   - f) Others (specify) ☐
6. Is device in use after incidence : Yes ☐ No ☐
7. Serious event: ☐

   If serious, Tick the appropriate reason
   - a) Death (DD/MM/YY) ☐ ..../............/...........
   - b) Life Threatening ☐
   - c) Disability or permanent damage ☐
   - d) Hospitalization ☐
   - e) Congenital anomaly /birth defect ☐
   - f) Any other serious (Imp. medical event) ☐
   - g) Required intervention to prevent / permanent Impairment / damage device ☐
8. Non serious event ☐
9. Whether other medical devices were used at same time with above device if yes, please specify name(s)/use(s)

10. Detail description of Event:-

For manufacturer/authorized representative use only

	Year	No. of Similar Adverse Events	Total No. Supplied	Frequency of Occurrence (%)
11. Frequency of occurrence of similar Adverse Event in India in past 3 years				
12. Frequency of occurrence of similar Adverse Event in globally in past 3 years	Year	No. of Similar Adverse Events	Total No. Supplied	Frequency of Occurrence (%)

(C) Patient Information, History & Outcome

1. Patient Hospital ID :
2. Patient Initial :
3. Age :
4. Gender : Male ☐ Female ☐ Others ☐
5. Weight :
6. Other relevant history, including pre-existing medical conditions
7. Patient Outcomes:
   - a) Recovered Date (DD/MM/YY) ☐ ....../......./.......
   - b) Not yet recovered ☐
   - c) Death (DD/MM/YY) ☐ ....../......./.......
   - d) Others ☐

     Please specify

(D) Healthcare Facility Information (if available)

1. Name :
2. Address :
3. Contact Person Name at the site of event :
4. Tel. No. :

(E) Causality Assessment

1. Investigation action taken:

2. Root cause of problem (Applicable for follow up / final reports):

(F) Manufacturer/Authorized Representative Investigation & Action taken

1. Manufacturer/Authorized Representative device risk analysis report:

2. Corrective / preventive action taken:

3. Device history review:

(B) Event Description (Continued)

10. Detail description of Event:-

(E) Causality Assessment (Continued)

1. Investigation action taken:

2. Root cause of problem (Applicable for follow up / final reports):

(F) Manufacturer/Authorized Representative Investigation & Action taken (Continued)

1. Manufacturer/Authorized Representative device risk analysis report:

2. Corrective / preventive action taken:

3. Device history review:

Where to report?

Duly filled Medical Device Adverse Event Reporting Form can be sent to Indian Pharmacopoeia Commission, Ministry of Health and Family Welfare, Government of India, Sector-23, Rajnagar, Ghaziabad-20002, Tel-0120-2783400, 2783401 and 2783392, FAX:0120-2783311 or email to shatrunjay.ipc@gov.in Or Call on Helpline no. 1800 180 3024 to report Adverse event.

Partnering Organizations

Disclaimer

Confidentiality: The patient's identity is held in strict confidence and protected to the fullest extent. Programme staff is not expected to and will not disclose the reporter's identity in response to a request from the public. Submission of a report does not constitute an admission that medical personnel or manufacturer or the product caused or contributed to the adverse event.

Annexure 9(c): Medical Device Adverse Event Reporting Form for Consumers or Users

M. Nandave, A. Kumar (eds.), *Pharmacovigilance Essentials*,
https://doi.org/10.1007/978-981-99-8949-2

Version-1.0

IPC

MEDICAL DEVICE ADVERSE EVENT REPORTING FORM
Materiovigilance Programme of India (MvPI)
(For Consumers/Users)

Date of report (dd/mm/yyyy) **:......../......./..........**

(A) PATIENT INFORMATION, HISTORY & OUTCOME

1. Patient Hospital ID:
2. Patient Initial:
3. Age or (Date of Birth): (dd/mm/yyyy)
4. Gender: Male ☐ Female ☐ Others ☐
5. Weight (in kgs):

6. Other relevant medical history, including pre-existing medical conditions:

(B) SUSPECTED MEDICAL DEVICE DETAILS

Medical Device Name / Trade Name / Brand Name:

Details	Name	Address
Manufacturer		
Importer/ Distributor		

Model No.	
Lot / Batch No	
Serial No.	

(C) EVENT DESCRIPTION/ PRODUCT PROBLEM

1. **Date of Adverse Event / Near miss incident:** (dd/mm/yyyy)
2. **Type of report**
   Adverse Event ☐
   Product Problem ☐
   (e.g. defect/fault/error/malfunctioning)
3. **Date of Implant / Date of device used:** (dd/mm/yyyy)
4. **Date of Explant/ Device used up to date:** (dd/mm/yyyy)
5. **Location of Event:**
   Hospital Premise ☐
   Home ☐
   Others: .... ☐
6. **Is the device in use after the incidence**
   Yes ☐ No ☐

7. **Whether adverse event is**
   Serious event ☐ / **Non serious event** ☐
   If serious, Tick the appropriate reason
   a) Death (dd/mm/yyyy) ☐ ..../............/..........
   b) Life Threatening ☐
   c) Disability or permanent damage ☐
   d) Hospitalization ☐
   e) Congenital anomaly /birth defect ☐
   f) Any other serious events ☐
   g) Required intervention to prevent / permanent impairment / damage ☐
8. Whether other medical devices were used at the same time with the above device if yes, please specify the name(s)/use(s):

9. Detail Description of Event:

(D) Reporter contact information:

a) Name :
b) Occupation (optional):
c) Tel./Mobile:
d) Address :
e) Email.:

Version-1.0
हिन्दी संस्करण

IPC

चिकित्सीय उपकरण प्रतिकूल घटना सूचना फार्म
मैटीरिओविजिलैंस प्रोग्राम ऑफ़ इंडिया
(उपभोक्ताओं/ उपयोगकर्ताओं के लिए)

सुचना की दिनांक: (dd/mm/yyyy)

(A) रोगी के विषय में आवश्यक जानकारी

1. रोगी की अस्पताल पहचान संख्या :
2. रोगी का संछिप्त नाम :
3. आयु / जन्म तिथि): (dd/mm/yyyy)
4. लिंग: पुरुष ☐ स्त्री ☐ अन्य ☐
5. वज़न :

6. रोगी के पूर्व की अन्य चिकित्सा सम्बंधित स्थिति:

(B) संदिग्ध चिकित्सीय उपकरण का विवरण

चिकित्सा उपकरण का नाम/ व्यापरिक नाम/ बाजार में प्रचलित नाम:

विवरण	नाम	पता
निर्माता		
आयातकर्ता/ वितरणकर्ता		

प्रतिरूप क्रमांक	
लौट/ बैच क्रमांक	
श्रृंखला क्रमांक	

(C) प्रतिकूल घटना या उत्पाद की समस्या का विवरण

1. प्रतिकूल/ संभावित प्रतिकूल घटना की दिनांक: (dd/mm/yyyy)
2. सुचना का प्रकार
   प्रतिकूल घटना ☐
   उपकरण की समस्या ☐
   (e.g. कमी या खराबी)
3. चिकित्सा उपकरण प्रत्यारोपण या उपयोग की दिनांक:
4. चिकित्सा उपकरण को शरीर से निकालने या उपयोग बंद करने की दिनांक:
5. घटना किस स्थान पर घटित हुई:
   अस्पताल परिसर में ☐ / घर पर ☐
   अन्य किसी स्थान पर: .... ☐
6. क्या घटना के बाद उपकरण उपयोग में है:
   हाँ ☐ नहीं ☐

7. **प्रतिकूल घटना का प्रकार:**
   गंभीर प्रतिकूल घटना ☐ / गैर गंभीर घटना ☐
   यदि घटना गंभीर है, तो उचित कारण पर निशान लगाएँ
   a) मृत्यु (dd/mm/yyyy) ☐ ..../.........../...........
   b) जीवन के लिए खतरनाक ☐
   c) विकलांगता या स्थायी क्षति ☐
   d) अस्पताल में भर्ती ☐
   e) जन्मजात विसंगति/ जन्म दोष ☐
   f) कोई अन्य गंभीर कारण ☐
   g) घटना रोकने के लिए आवश्यक हस्तक्षेप/ स्थाई हानि होना या शारीरिक छतिग्रस्त होना) ☐
8. क्या उपरोक्त उपकरण के साथ एक ही समय में अन्य चिकित्सा उपकरणों का उपयोग किया गया था यदि हां, तो कृपया नाम/उपयोग निर्दिष्ट करें:

9. प्रतिकूल घटना का विस्तृत विवरण:-

(D) सूचना देने वाले का विवरण:-

a) नाम :
b) व्यवसाय (वैकल्पिक):
c) दूरभाष क्रमांक.
d) पता :
e) ई. मेल. :

WHERE TO REPORT?

Indian Pharmacopoeia Commission:

Duly filled Medical Device Adverse Event Reporting Form can be sent to Indian Pharmacopoeia Commission, Ministry of Health and Family Welfare, Government of India, Sector-23, Rajnagar, Ghaziabad-20002.

Helpline Number:

Adverse event associated with medical device can be reported via helpline No. i.e. **1800 180 3024**

[Available from: Monday to Friday (9:00 AM to 5:30 PM)]

Email Contact:

Scan copy of this form can be sent via email to mvpi-ipc@gov.in or shatrunjay.ipc@gov.in

DISCLAIMER:

Confidentiality: The patient's identity is held in strict confidence and protected to the fullest extent. A duly filled reporting form will be verified by the nearest monitoring centre of that report than only verified report will be submitted in the MvPI database. Submission of this report does not mean, the reporter /consumer will get compensation. Submission of a report does not constitute an admission that medical personnel or manufacturer or the product caused or contributed to the adverse event.

कहां रिपोर्ट करें?

भारतीय भेषज संहिता आयोग:

विधिवत भरे हुए चिकित्सा उपकरण सम्बंधित प्रतिकूल घटना सुचना फॉर्म को भारतीय भेषज संहिता आयोग, स्वास्थ्य एवं परिवार कल्याण मन्त्रालय, भारत सरकार, सेक्टर -23, राजनगर, गाजियाबाद -201002 पर भेज सकते है।

सहायता संपर्क :

चिकित्सा उपकरण सम्बंधित प्रतिकूल घटना को टोल फ्री नंबर **18001803024** पर कॉल कर प्रतिकूल घटना को दर्ज करा सकते है।

[उपलब्धः सोमवार से शुक्रवार (सुबह 9:00 बजे से शाम 5:30 बजे तक)]

ईमेल संपर्क:

चिकित्सा उपकरण सम्बंधित प्रतिकूल घटना सूचना फॉर्म की स्कैन कॉपी को ईमेल आई॰ डी॰ mvpi-ipc@gov.in or shatrunjay.ipc@gov.in पर भेज कर दर्ज करा सकते है।

उद्घोषणा:

गोपनीयता: रोगी की पहचान को पूरी तरह से गोपनीय और संरक्षित रखा जाता है। दर्ज कराई गयी सुचना को, सुचना के निकटतम स्थित निगरानी केंद्र से सत्यापित होने के उपरांत ही मैटीरिओविजिलैंस प्रोग्राम ऑफ़ इंडिया के डाटा बेस में शामिल किया जाएगा। इस रिपोर्ट को जमा करने का मतलब यह नहीं है कि रिपोर्टर/उपभोक्ता को किसी तरह का मुआवजा मिलेगा। किसी प्रतिकूल घटना कि सूचना को दर्ज कराने का अर्थ बिलकुल भी यह नहीं है कि प्रतिकूल घटना का कारण, चिकित्सा कर्मी या उपकरण के निर्माता या उपयुक्त उपकरण है।

Annexure 10: Blood and Blood Products

M. Nandave, A. Kumar (eds.), *Pharmacovigilance Essentials*,
https://doi.org/10.1007/978-981-99-8949-2

Annexure 10 Transfusion Reaction Reporting Form

National Institute of Biologicals
Ministry of Health & Family Welfare, Govt. of India
(National Coordinating Center)
HAEMOVIGILANCE PROGRAMME OF INDIA

Transfusion Reaction Reporting Form (TRRF) For Blood & Blood Components & Plasma Products (Version-2)

* Mandatory Field

(A) Patient Information

Hospital Code No.:						
Patient Initials*:	Gender*:	Blood Group*:				
Hospital Admission No.*:	Age/Date of Birth*:	......Yrs	......Month	......Days	......Hrs	......Mins
Primary Diagnosis*:						
Medical History:						

(B) Transfusion Reaction Details*

Was the patient under anaesthesia during transfusion: Yes/No if Yes type : GA/Spinal/LA

Pre-transfusion Vitals:	Temp:	Pulse:	BP:	RR:	SPO2:
Vitals at the time of reaction:	Temp:	Pulse:	BP:	RR:	SPO2:

Please tick mark the relevant signs and symptoms listed below

Generalised		Pain	Respiratory	Renal	Circulatory
☐ Fever	☐ Anxiety	☐ Chest Pain	☐ Dyspnoea	☐ Haematuria	☐ Tachycardia
☐ Chills	☐ Itching (Pruitus)	☐ Abdominal	☐ Wheeze	☐ Haemoglobinuria	☐ Hypertension
☐ Rigors	☐ Edema (Site)____	☐ Back/Flank Pain	☐ Cough	☐ Oliguria	☐ Hypotension
☐ Nausea	☐ Juandice	☐ Infusion Site Pain	☐ Hypoxemia	☐ Other______	☐ Raised JVP
☐ Urticaria	☐ Other______	☐ Other______	☐ Bilateral Infiltrates on Chest X-ray		☐ Arrhythmias
☐ Flushing					☐ Other______
☐ Restlessness					
☐ Vomiting			☐ Other______		

Any Other(Specify) : ....

(C) Transfusion Product(s) Details*

Select*	Select Component	Select Indication	Date & Time of Issue of Blood Component	Date & Time of onset Transfusion	Unit Id (Transfused)	Blood Group	Volume Transfused (ml)	Expiry date of Blood Component	Manufacturer of Blood Bag	Batch / Lot No. of the Blood Bag	1st time/ repeat Transfusion
☐	Whole blood										☐ 1st Time
☐	Packed Red blood cells (PRBC)										
☐	Buffy coat depleted PRBC										
☐	Leucofiltered PRBC										
☐	Random Donor platelets/ pooled										☐ Repeat 1 to 10
☐	Apheresis Platelets										
☐	Fresh Frozen Plasma										☐ Repeat > 10
☐	Cryoprecipitate										
☐	Any Other ____										

Add New Plasma Product

Select	Plasma Product	Indication	Date of Administration	Manufacturer	Expiry Date of the Plasma Product	Batch No. / Lot No.	1st Time / Repeat
							☐ 1st Time ☐ Repeat 1 to 10 ☐ Repeat > 10

(D) Investigations			
☐ Clerical Checks	Specify Error Found if any:		
Investigation	Pre-transfusion sample	Post-transfusion sample	
☐ Visual Check			
* ☐ Repeat Blood Grouping	O+ /A+ /B+ /AB+ /O- /A- /B- /AB-	O+ /A+ /B+ /AB+ /O- /A- /B- /AB-	
* ☐ Repeat Crossmatch	☐ Compatible ☐ InCompatible ☐ Not Done	☐ Compatible ☐ InCompatible ☐ Not Done	
* ☐ Repeat Antibody screen	☐ Negative ☐ Positive ☐ Not Done	☐ Negative ☐ Positive ☐ Not Done	
☐ Antibody Identification			
* ☐ Direct antiglobulin test	☐ Negative ☐ Positive ☐ Not Done	☐ Negative ☐ Positive ☐ Not Done	
☐ Hemoglobin			
☐ Plasma Hemoglobin			
☐ Urine hemoglobin			
☐ Bilirubin (Total/conjugated)			
☐ Platelet count			
☐ PT/INR			
* ☐ Blood culture of Blood Bag	☐ Negative ☐ Positive ☐ Not Done	Specify Organism if positive	
* ☐ Blood culture of Patient	☐ Negative ☐ Positive ☐ Not Done Specify Organism if positive	☐ Negative ☐ Positive ☐ Not Done Specify Organism if positive	
☐ Chest X-ray of the patient in case of suspected TRALI			
In case of Non-immune hemolysis (which of the following was the case?)			
☐ Hemolysis due to freezing of PRBC Units			
☐ Hemolysis due to inappropriate warming of PRBC Units			
☐ Hemolysis due to infusion of any other fluid through same BT set.	Specify Fluid:		
☐ Mechanical damage			
In Case of ABO Mismatch (which of the following was the case?)			
☐ Wrong Blood in tube			
☐ Grouping error			
☐ Labelling error			
☐ Wrong unit transfused			

(E) Nature of Adverse Reaction(s)*

Select	Reaction	Date & Time of Onset of Reaction	Date & Time of Recovery	Outcome
☐	Febrile Non Haemolytic Reactions (FNHTR) 1° C rise in temperature ☐ 2° C rise in temperature ☐ Only Chills & Rigors ☐			☐ 1. Death following the Adverse Reaction(s)
☐	Allergic reaction			
☐	Anaphylaxis			
☐	Immunological Haemolysis due to ABO Incompatibility			
☐	Immunological Haemolysis due to other Allo-Antibodies			
☐	Non Immunological Haemolysis			☐ 2. Recovered
☐	Hypotensive Transfusion Reaction			
☐	Transfusion Related Acute Lung Injury (TRALI) Definite ☐ Possible ☐			
☐	Transfusion Associated Dyspnoea (TAD)			
☐	Transfusion Associated Circulatory Overload (TACO)			☐ 3. Recovered with Sequelae
☐	Transfusion Transmitted Bacterial Infection			
☐	Transfusion Transmitted Parasitic Infection (Malaria)			
☐	Post Transfusion Purpura			☐ 4. Unknown
☐	Transfusion Associated Graft versus Host Disease (TAGvHD)			
☐	Other Reaction (s) Add New			

IMPUTABITLITY ASSESSMENT

(F) Imputability Assessment*

S. No.	Reaction Term	Transfusion Product/ Component	*Imputability Assessment (Please mention from the below list)

*Imputability: 1. Definite (Certain), 2. Probable (Likely), 3. Possible, 4. Unlikely (Doubtful), 5. Excluded, 6. Not Assessed

Monthly Denominator Reporting Form *

Hospital Code :	Month/Year:
Blood Component	**No.of Units Issued**
1) Fresh Frozen Plasma	
2) Whole Blood	
3) Packed Red Blood Cells (PRBC)	
4) Buffy Coat Depleted PRBC	
5) Leucofiltered PRBC	
6) Random Donor Platelets/ Pooled	
7) Apheresis Platelets	
8) Cryoprecipitate	
9) Any Other________	

National Institute of Biologicals
Ministry of Health & Family Welfare, Govt. of India

NATIONAL BLOOD DONOR VIGILANCE PROGRAMME

(Haemovigilance Programme of India)

Adverse Blood Donor Reaction Reporting Form

Version 2

A) Donor Information

Donor Id *: ________________

Type of Donation* (a) Whole Blood (b) Apheresis_______(Platelets/Plasma/Plasma + Platelets/RBC/Granulocyte/Peripheral Blood StemCells/ COVID-19 Convalescent Plasma)

Sex *__________ (Male/Female/Other)

Weight of Donor (kg) * ___________Height of Donor(cm)*________

Donor Type* (a) Voluntary (b) Replacement (c) Family Donor (d)Autologous (First Time/Repeat)

Age/ Date of Birth * Yrs: _____ Month:_____ Days:_____ OR ______

Site of Donation*__________ (Blood Centre/Camp)

Pre-Donation Vitals*Pulse: _____ per min BP (Systolic):_____ mmHg BP (Diastolic):____ mmHg

Date of Donation * ___________

Time of Donation Hr____ Min____

B) Whole blood Details of Blood Collected/Apheresis Details of Blood Collected

(a) Whole Blood

Lot No. of Blood Bag* _______________

Volume Collected (ml)* ______________

Manufacturer of Blood Bag* ________(Terumo Penpol Limited/Mitra Industries Pvt. Ltd/HLL Lifecare Ltd/Fresenius Kabi AG/Fenwal Inc/Polymed/Other)

Expiry Date of Blood Bag* ___________

(b) Apheresis

Lot No. Kit* ____________ Volume Collected (ml)* ________________ Expiry Date of Kit* ______________

C) Adverse Reaction Details

Date and Time of reaction* _________________ Hr________Min________

Type of Reaction* ____________(Localised/Generalized/Both/Other Reactions)

Vitals at the time of Reaction Pulse: ________ per min BP (Systolic): ____mmHg BP (Diastolic): ____mmHg

Data Captured* ______________ (Onsite/Call back by donor/Call back by Blood Centre)

Reaction Time* ______________ (Pre-Donation/During Donation/After Donation)

Venipuncture Site* ____________(Left/Right/Both)

Injury* ____________ (Yes/No)

Venipuncture* _____________(1/2/>2)

Site of Reaction* ______________ (At Donation Site/Outside Donation Site)

Donation Completed* ____________ (Yes/No)

D) Type of Complications:*

Localised Complications

☐ **A1-Complications mainly characterized by the occurrence of blood outside the vessels**

- (a) ☐ Haematoma (bruise)
- (b) ☐ Arterial puncture
- (c) ☐ Delayed(bleeding/Re-bleeding) ☐ (Within 30 minutes of Donation/After 30 minutes of Donation)

☐ **A2-Complications mainly characterized by pain**

- (a) ☐ Nerve injury/irritation
- (b) ☐ Other Painful arm

☐ **A3-Localised infection/inflammation along the course of a vein**

- (a) ☐ Thrombophlebitis
- (b) ☐ Cellulitis

☐ **A4- Allergy (local): Itching and redness at the ☐ (Venipuncture Site/Medical Adhesive Medicated Tape/Skin Disinfection Area)**

☐ **A5-Other major blood vessel injury -Serious conditions needing specialist medical diagnosis and attention**

- (a) ☐ Deep venous thrombosis (DVT)
- (b) ☐ Arteriovenous fistula
- (c) ☐ Compartment syndrome
- (d) ☐ Brachial artery pseudoaneurysm

Annexure : 11 ADR Reporting forms for Blood and Blood Products

सत्यमेव जयते

National Institute of Biologicals
Ministry of Health & Family Welfare, Govt. of India

NATIONAL BLOOD DONOR VIGILANCE PROGRAMME

(Haemovigilance Programme of India)
Adverse Blood Donor Reaction Reporting Form
Version 2

Generalized Complications

□ **B1-Vasovagal reactions**

(a) □ Generalized Weakness (b) □ Anxiety (c) □ Dizziness (d) □ Nausea
(e) □ Vomiting (f) □ Pallor(skin and lips) (g) □ Rapid Pulse (h) □ Convulsions
(i) □ Cold extremities (j) □ Hyperventilation (k) □ Hypotension (l) □ Low Vol Pulse
(m) □ Feeling of warmth (n) □ Tetany (o) □ Loss of bowel or bladder control (p)□ Cyanosis
(q) □ Sweating (r) □ Loss of Consciousness(LOC) __________(<60 Sec/>60 Sec)

□ **B2-Allergic reactions (Generalized)**

(a) □ Cyanosis (b) □ Wheezing (c) □ Flushing,swelling of eyes,lips or tongue
(d) □ Chest tightness (e) □ Cardiac a rrest

□ **B3-Other serious complications related to blood donation**

(a) □ Acute cardiac symptoms(other than myocardial infarction or cardiac arrest) (b) □ Myocardial infarction(MI)
(c) □ Cardiac arrest (d) □ Transient Ischemic attack (TIA) (e) □ Death

Apheresis Complication Yes/No

□ **C-Complications related to apheresis**

(a) □ Citrate reaction
□ tingling/vibrations-lips,fingers □ light-headedness □ Metallic taste □ Muscle twitching
□ Carpopedal spasm □ Shock □ Cardiac arrest □ Tetany
□ Prophylactic Calcium given before reaction □ (Yes/No)
(b) □ Haemolysis during procedure
(c) □ Air embolism
(d) □ Unable to return red cell(>200ml)

Other Complication

□ D-Other Reactions Please Specify ______________________________

Outcome* □ Resolved on donation site □ Resolved on follow up □ Recovered with Sequelae
□ Permanently disabled □ Death following the adverse reactions □ Unknown

Imputability* □ Definite (Certain) □ Probable (Likely) □ Possible
□ Unlikely (Doubtful) □ Excluded

Any Other Information or Predisposing Factors for Submitted Reactions : ______________

Reporter......................... **Date of Report............................**

Denominator Data about All Donor

Total Donation in the month (of reporting)

□ **Whole blood** [ ]

Volume of donation (Total)* No. of 350 ml bags [ ] No. of 450 ml bags [ ]

□ **Apheresis if apheresis** [ ] RBC [ ] Platelets [ ] Plasma [ ]
Plasma+Platelets [ ] Granulocyte [ ] Peripheral Blood Stem Cells [ ]
COVID-19 Convalescent Plasma [ ]

Gender of Donor(Total)* Male [ ] Female [ ] Other [ ]
Type of Donation(Total)* Voluntary [ ] Replacement [ ] Family Donor [ ] Autologous [ ]
Donor Types(Total)* First-Time Donors [ ] Repeat Donors [ ]
Site of Donation(Total)* Blood Centre [ ] Camp [ ]

Annexure 11(a): Who-UMC Causality Assessment

M. Nandave, A. Kumar (eds.), *Pharmacovigilance Essentials*,
https://doi.org/10.1007/978-981-99-8949-2

Uppsala Monitoring Centre

The use of the WHO-UMC system for standardised case causality assessment

Why causality assessment?

An inherent problem in pharmacovigilance is that most case reports concern *suspected* adverse drug reactions. Adverse reactions are rarely specific for the drug, diagnostic tests are usually absent and a rechallenge is rarely ethically justified. In practice few adverse reactions are 'certain' or 'unlikely'; most are somewhere in between these extremes, i.e. 'possible' or 'probable'. In an attempt to solve this problem many systems have been developed for a structured and harmonised assessment of causality (1). None of these systems, however, have been shown to produce a precise and reliable quantitative estimation of relationship likelihood. Nevertheless, causality assessment has become a common routine procedure in pharmacovigilance. The advances and limitations of causality assessment are reviewed in *Table 1*[(2)].

Table 1. Advances and limitations of standardised case causality assessment

What causality assessment can do	What causality assessment cannot do
Decrease disagreement between assessors	Give accurate quantitative measurement of relationship likelihood
Classify relationship likelihood	Distinguish valid from invalid cases
Mark individual case reports	Prove the connection between drug and event
Improvement of scientific evaluation; educational	Quantify the contribution of a drug to the development of an adverse event
	Change uncertainty into certainty

The WHO-UMC causality assessment system

The WHO-UMC system has been developed in consultation with the National Centres participating in the Programme for International Drug Monitoring and is meant as a practical tool for the assessment of case reports. It is basically a combined assessment taking into account the clinical-pharmacological aspects of the case history and the quality of the documentation of the observation. Since pharmacovigilance is particularly concerned with the detection of unknown and unexpected adverse reactions, other criteria such as previous knowledge and statistical chance play a less prominent role in the system. It is recognised that the semantics of the definitions are critical and that individual judgements may therefore differ. There are other algorithms that are either very complex or too specific for general use. This method gives guidance to the general arguments which should be used to select one category over another.

The various causality categories are listed in Table 2. The assessment criteria of the various categories are shown in a point-wise way, as has been developed for practical training during the UMC Training courses.

Uppsala Monitoring Centre

Table 2. WHO-UMC Causality Categories

Causality term	Assessment criteria*
Certain	• Event or laboratory test abnormality, with plausible time relationship to drug intake • Cannot be explained by disease or other drugs • Response to withdrawal plausible (pharmacologically, pathologically) • Event definitive pharmacologically or phenomenologically (i.e. an objective and specific medical disorder or a recognised pharmacological phenomenon) • Rechallenge satisfactory, if necessary
Probable/ Likely	• Event or laboratory test abnormality, with reasonable time relationship to drug intake • Unlikely to be attributed to disease or other drugs • Response to withdrawal clinically reasonable • Rechallenge not required
Possible	• Event or laboratory test abnormality, with reasonable time relationship to drug intake • Could also be explained by disease or other drugs • Information on drug withdrawal may be lacking or unclear
Unlikely	• Event or laboratory test abnormality, with a time to drug intake that makes a relationship improbable (but not impossible) • Disease or other drugs provide plausible explanations
Conditional/ Unclassified	• Event or laboratory test abnormality • More data for proper assessment needed, or • Additional data under examination
Unassessable/ Unclassifiable	• Report suggesting an adverse reaction • Cannot be judged because information is insufficient or contradictory • Data cannot be supplemented or verified

*All points should be reasonably complied with

The use of the WHO-UMC system

To illustrate how the system works, we suggest to first making a comparison of the criteria and wording of 'Probable' and Certain'. First of all there is one more criterion in the category 'Certain', the fourth: 'Event definitive pharmacologically or phenomenologically', i.e. an objective and specific medical disorder or a recognised pharmacological phenomenon (for instance 'grey baby syndrome' and chloramphenicol, or anaphylaxis immediately after the administration of a drug that had been given previously). This means that any other event is automatically excluded and can never qualify for 'Certain' (even in the case of a positive rechallenge observation). For 'Certain', rechallenge information with a satisfactory outcome is requested (i.e. what has happened when the drug was first stopped and later on resumed), unless the evidence in the report is already convincing without a re-exposure.

For 'Probable', on the other hand, a rechallenge is not required. To qualify as 'Certain' the interval between the start of the drug and the onset of the event must be 'plausible'; this means that there is in sufficient detail a positive argument in support of the view that the drug is causally involved, pharmacologically or pathologically. For 'Probable' the time relationship should be 'reasonable'; this is a more neutral term covering everything that is not unreasonable. Also, with regard to the second criterion, 'alternative causes', the wording is different in 'Probable'. For 'Certain' the occurrence of the event cannot be explained by any disease the patient is known to have or any other drug taken. For 'Probable', on the other hand, the event is 'unlikely' to be attributable to another cause. Also the dechallenge situations (i.e. what happened after stopping) are different. In a 'Certain' case report, the course of events constitutes a positive argument in favour of holding the suspected drug responsible, in pharmacological or pathological respects, whereas in a 'Probable' case it is sufficient if it is 'clinically reasonable' (i.e. not unreasonable).

The essential distinctions between 'Probable' and 'Possible' are that in the latter case there may be another equally likely explanation for the event and/or there is no information or uncertainty with regard to what has happened after stopping.

The criteria that may render the connection 'Unlikely' are firstly the time relationship is improbable (with the knowledge at the time), and/or another explanation is more likely. The term 'Unclassified/Conditional' is of a preliminary nature and is appropriate when, for a proper assessment, there is more data needed and such data are being sought, or are already under examination. Finally, when the information in a report is incomplete or contradictory and cannot be complemented or verified, the verdict is 'Unclassifiable'.

Since by far the most frequent categories in case reports are 'Possible' and 'Probable', the usual approach to using the system is to choose one of these categories (depending on the impression of the assessor) and to test if the various criteria fit with the content of the case report. If the report seems stronger one can go one step 'higher' (e.g. from 'Possible' to 'Probable'), if the evidence seems weaker one should try a 'lower' category. To see if that category is the right one or if it does again not seem to fit, the next adjacent term is tried.

For drug-drug interactions the WHO-UMC system can be used by assessing the actor drug, which influences the kinetics or dynamics of the other drug (which has usually been taken over a longer period), in the medical context of the patient.

Uppsala Monitoring Centre

How does it work?

How the WHO-UMC causality assessment system can be used will be illustrated with the aid of a few real-life case reports. These will be made available on the UMC website in the near future.

1. Meyboom RHB, Royer RJ. Causality Classification in Pharmacovigilance Centres in the European Community. Pharmacoepidemiology and Drug Safety 1992; 1:87-97.
2. Meyboom RHB. Causal or Casual? The Role of Causality Assessment in Pharmacovigilance. Drug Safety 17(6): 374-389, 1997.
3. Edwards IR, Biriell C. Harmonisation in Pharmacovigilance. Drug Safety 10(2): 93-102, 1994.

Uppsala Monitoring Centre

Summary description of Causality Assessment

Term	Description	Comment
Certain	A clinical event, including laboratory test abnormality, occurring in a plausible time relationship to drug administration, and which cannot be explained by concurrent disease or other drugs or chemicals. The response to withdrawal of the drug (dechallenge) should be clinically plausible. The event must be definitive pharmacologically or phenomenologically, using a satisfactory rechallenge procedure if necessary.	It is recognized that this stringent definition will lead to very few reports meeting the criteria, but this is useful because of the special value of such reports. It is considered that time relationships between drug administration and the onset and course of the adverse event are important in causality analysis. So also is the consideration of confounding features, but due weight must be placed on the known pharmacological and other characteristics of the drug product being considered. Sometimes the clinical phenomena described will also be sufficiently specific to allow a confident causality assessment in the absence of confounding features and with appropriate time relationships, e.g. penicillin anaphylaxis.
Probable/ Likely	A clinical event, including laboratory test abnormality, with a reasonable time sequence to administration of the drug, unlikely to be attributed to concurrent disease or other drugs or chemicals, and which follows a clinically reasonable response on withdrawal (dechallenge). Rechallenge information is not required to fulfil this definition.	This definition has less stringent wording than for "certain" and does not necessitate prior knowledge of drug characteristics or clinical adverse reaction phenomena. As stated no rechallenge information is needed, but confounding drug administration underlying disease must be absent.
Possible	A clinical event, including laboratory test abnormality, with a reasonable time sequence to administration of the drug, but which could also be explained by concurrent disease or other drugs or chemicals. Information on drug withdrawal may be lacking or unclear.	This is the definition to be used when drug causality is one of other possible causes for the described clinical event.

Uppsala Monitoring Centre

Unlikely	A clinical event, including laboratory test abnormality, with a temporal relationship to drug administration which makes a causal relationship improbable, and in which other drugs, chemicals or underlying disease provide plausible explanations.	This definition is intended to be used when the exclusion of drug causality of a clinical event seems most plausible.
Conditional/ Unclassified	A clinical event, including laboratory test abnormality, reported as an adverse reaction, about which more data is essential for a proper assessment or the additional data are under examination.	
Unassessable / Unclassifiable	A report suggesting an adverse reaction which cannot be judged because information is insufficient or contradictory, and which cannot be supplemented or verified.	

Annexure 11(b): Naranjo ADR Assessment Scale

Naranjo Adverse Drug Reaction Probability Scale				
Question	Yes	No	Do Not Know	Score
1. Are there previous *conclusive* reports on this reaction?	+1	0	0	
2. Did the adverse event appear after the suspected drug was administered?	+2	-1	0	
3. Did the adverse reaction improve when the drug was discontinued or a *specific* antagonist was administered?	+1	0	0	
4. Did the adverse event reappear when the drug was re-administered?	+2	-1	0	
5. Are there alternative causes (other than the drug) that could on their own have caused the reaction?	-1	+2	0	
6. Did the reaction reappear when a placebo was given?	-1	+1	0	
7. Was the drug detected in blood (or other fluids) in concentrations known to be toxic?	+1	0	0	
8. Was the reaction more severe when the dose was increased or less severe when the dose was decreased?	+1	0	0	
9. Did the patient have a similar reaction to the same or similar drugs in *any* previous exposure?	+1	0	0	
10. Was the adverse event confirmed by any objective evidence?	+1	0	0	
TOTAL SCORE:				

Modified from: Naranjo CA et al. A method for estimating the probability of adverse drug reactions. Clin Pharmacol Ther 1981; 30: 239-245.

M. Nandave, A. Kumar (eds.), *Pharmacovigilance Essentials*,
https://doi.org/10.1007/978-981-99-8949-2

Annexure 12: Causality Assessment for Vaccine

M. Nandave, A. Kumar (eds.), *Pharmacovigilance Essentials*, https://doi.org/10.1007/978-981-99-8949-2

	Y	N	UK	NA	Remarks
Immunization anxiety (Immunization stress related responses - ISRR)					
11. In this patient, could this event be a stress response triggered by immunization (e.g. acute stress response, vasovagal reaction, hyperventilation, dissociative neurological symptom reaction etc)?	☐	☐	☐	☐	
II (time): Was the event in section II within the time window of increased risk (i.e. "Yes" response to questions from II 1 to II 11 above)					
12. In this patient, did the event occur within a plausible time window after vaccine administration?	☐	☐	☐	☐	
III. Is there strong evidence against a causal association?					
1. Is there a body of published evidence (systematic reviews, GACVS reviews, Cochrane reviews etc.) **against** a causal association between the vaccine and the event?	☐	☐	☐	☐	
IV. Other qualifying factors for classification					
1. In this patient, did such an event occur in the past after administration of a similar vaccine?	☐	☐	☐	☐	
2. In this patient, did such an event occur in the past independent of vaccination?	☐	☐	☐	☐	
3. Could the current event have occurred in this patient without vaccination (background rate)?	☐	☐	☐	☐	
4. Did this patient have an illness, pre-existing condition or risk factor that could have contributed to the event?	☐	☐	☐	☐	
5. Was this patient taking any medication prior to the vaccination?	☐	☐	☐	☐	
6. Was this patient exposed to a potential factor (other than vaccine) prior to the event (e.g. allergen, drug, herbal product etc.)?	☐	☐	☐	☐	

Note: Y: Yes; N: No; UK: Unknown; NA: Not applicable.

The checklist is designed to assemble information on the patient-immunization-AEFI relationship in the following key areas:

- evidence for other causes;
- association of the event and the vaccine/vaccination with the vaccine product(s), immunization error or immunization anxiety (if there is an association, it is also important to find out if the event occurred within an plausible time window);
- evidence against a causal association;
- other qualifying factors for classification such as previous history of a similar event, the background rate of the event, pre-existing, present and past health conditions, potential risk factors, other medications, exposure to triggering factors etc.

The checklist and the questions are described in Table 1 with some suggestive examples. It is essential that all questions in the checklist be answered with any one of the options, "Yes", "No", "Unknown" or "Not applicable". When there is a positive response to any question, ("Yes" response), it is essential to provide an explanation for the positive response in the corresponding row under remarks. It will be observed that sometimes explanations for other responses ("No", "Unknown" or "Not applicable") are also important

Annexure 13: Reporting Form for Adverse Events for Immunization (AEFI)

M. Nandave, A. Kumar (eds.), *Pharmacovigilance Essentials*,
https://doi.org/10.1007/978-981-99-8949-2

Dec 2020

AEFI reporting id number:

STANDARD REPORTING FORM FOR ADVERSE EVENTS FOLLOWING IMMUNIZATION (AEFI)

***Patient name or initials:** ***Patient's full Address:** Telephone: Sex: ☐ M ☐ F (Pregnant - Trimester I☐ II☐ III☐ /Lactating ☐) ***Date of birth (DD/MM/YYYY):** _ _/_ _/_ _ _ _ *OR Age at onset:* ☐☐ *Years* ☐☐ *Months* ☐☐☐ *Days* *OR Age Group:* ☐ 0 < 1 year ☐ 1-5 years ☐ > 5 years - 18 years ☐ > 18 years – 60 years ☐ > 60 years	***Reporter's Name:** Institution: Designation & Department: Address: Telephone & e-mail: Date patient notified event to health system (DD/MM/YYYY): _ _/_ _/_ _ _ _ Today's date (DD/MM/YYYY): _ _/_ _/_ _ _ _

Health facility (or vaccination centre) name:

Vaccine							*Diluent*		
Name of vaccine (Generic)	***Brand Name incl. Name of Manufacturer**	***Date of vaccination**	***Time of vaccination**	Dose (1st, 2nd, etc.)	***Batch/ Lot number**	Expiry date	***Batch/ Lot number**	Expiry date	Time of reconstitution

***Adverse event (s):** ☐ Severe local reaction ☐ *>3 days* ☐ *beyond nearest joint* ☐ Seizures ☐ *febrile* ☐ *afebrile* ☐ Abscess ☐ Sepsis ☐ Encephalopathy ☐ Toxic shock syndrome ☐ Thrombocytopenia ☐ Anaphylaxis ☐ Fever≥38°C ☐ Other (specify).............................. Date & Time AEFI started (DD/MM/YYYY): ___ / ___ / _______ ☐☐ Hr ☐☐ Min	Describe AEFI (Signs and symptoms):

***Serious: Yes / No ;** ➔ If Yes ☐ Death ☐ Life threatening ☐ Disability ☐ Hospitalization ☐ Congenital anomaly ☐ Other important medical event (Specify_______________________________)

***Outcome:** ☐ Recovering ☐ Recovered ☐ Recovered with sequelae ☐ Not Recovered ☐ Unknown

☐ Died If died, date of death (DD/MM/YYYY): ___ / ___ / _______ Autopsy done: ☐ Yes ☐ No ☐ Unknown

Past medical history (including history of similar reaction or other allergies), concomitant medication and dates of administration (exclude those used to treat reaction) other relevant information (e.g. other cases). *Use additional sheet if needed:*

First Decision making level to complete:

Investigation needed: ☐ Yes ☐ No	If yes, date investigation planned (DD/MM/YYYY): ___ / ___ / _______

National level to complete:

Date report received at national level (DD/MM/YYYY): ___ / ___ / _______	AEFI worldwide unique ID:
Comments:	

**Compulsory field*

GPSR Compliance

The European Union's (EU) General Product Safety Regulation (GPSR) is a set of rules that requires consumer products to be safe and our obligations to ensure this.

If you have any concerns about our products, you can contact us on ProductSafety@springernature.com

In case Publisher is established outside the EU, the EU authorized representative is:

Springer Nature Customer Service Center GmbH
Europaplatz 3
69115 Heidelberg, Germany

Batch number: 10726133

Printed by Printforce, the Netherlands